Health in Child Care: A Manual for Health Professionals

4th Edition

American Academy of Pediatrics
141 Northwest Point Blvd
Elk Grove Village, IL 60007

CHOT

4th edition

3rd edition, 1987 (published as *Health in Day Care: A Manual for Health Professionals*)

2nd edition, revised, 1980 (published as *Recommendations for Day Care Centers for Infants and Children* and *Standards for Day Care Centers for Infants and Children*)

2nd edition, 1973 (published as *Recommendations for Day Care Centers for Infants and Children*)

1st edition, 1971 (published as *Standards for Day Care Centers for Infants and Children Under 3 Years of Age*)

Library of Congress Control Number: 2002107234
ISBN-1-58110-093-0
MA0213

Quantity prices available on request. Address all inquiries to:
American Academy of Pediatrics
141 Northwest Point Boulevard
Elk Grove Village, IL 60007

EDITORS
Jody R. Murph, MD
S. Donald Palmer, MD
Danette Glassy, MD

COMMITTEE ON EARLY CHILDHOOD, ADOPTION, AND DEPENDENT CARE 2001–2004
Chet D. Johnson, MD, Chairperson
Peter A. Gorski, MD, MPA, Past Chairperson
Deborah Ann Borchers, MD
Kerry L. English, MD
Danette Glassy, MD
Pamela High, MD
Susan E. Levitzky, MD
S. Donald Palmer, MD
Judith T. Romano, MD
Moira Szilagyi, MD, PhD
Dennis L. Vickers, MD, MPH

LIAISONS
Lorraine Brown, RN, BS
Maternal and Child Health Bureau

Claire Lerner, LCSW-C
Zero to Three

Pat Spahr
National Association for the Education of Young Children

Phyllis Stubbs-Wynn, MD, MPH
Maternal and Child Health Bureau

Ada K. White, LCSW, ACSW
Child Welfare League of America Inc

STAFF
Mary Crane, PhD, MA

TABLE OF CONTENTS

CONTRIBUTORS

Randall C. Alexander, MD, PhD
Morehouse School of Medicine, Atlanta, GA

Susan S. Aronson, MD
Pennsylvania Chapter, American Academy of Pediatrics, Narberth, PA

Sophie J. Balk, MD
Children's Hospital at Montefiore, Bronx, NY

Leanne C. Barrett
United Way of Southeastern New England, Providence, RI

Jay Belsky, PhD
Institute for the Study of Children, Families and Social Issues, Birkbeck College, University of London, London, England

Susan P. Berger, PhD
Children's Memorial Hospital, Chicago, IL

Robert W. Block, MD
University of Oklahoma-Tulsa, Tulsa, OK

V. Susan Bredekamp, PhD
Council for Professional Recognition, Washington, DC

Alice Bussiere, JD
Youth Law Center, San Francisco, CA

Judith A. Calder, BSN, MS
Alameda County Public Health—MCH, Oakland, CA

Carol Cohen Weitzman, MD
Yale University School of Medicine, New Haven, CT

Sarah Cohn
Yale-New Haven Hospital, New Haven, CT

Julie Cowan Novak, DNSc, RN, CPNP
Purdue University School of Nursing, West Lafayette, IN

Catherine Cowell, PhD
Mailman School of Public Health, Columbia University, New York, NY

Angela A. Crowley, PhD, APRN, CS, PNP
Yale University School of Nursing, New Haven, CT

Mary Dooling, RN, MSN
PediHealth Works, St Louis, MO

Kathryn M. Edwards, MD
Vanderbilt University School of Medicine, Nashville, TN

Margaret C. Fisher, MD
Monmouth Medical Center, Long Branch, NJ

Lilliam Gonzalez de Pijem, MD
University of Puerto Rico School of Medicine, San Juan, Puerto Rico

Peter A. Gorski, MD, MPA
Harvard Medical School, Boston, MA

Rene R. Gratz, PhD
University of Wisconsin—Milwaukee, Milwaukee, WI

Joseph F. Hagan, Jr, MD
University of Vermont College of Medicine, Burlington, VT

Bruce Hershfield, MS
Child Welfare League of America, Washington, DC

Barbara J. Howard, MD
The Johns Hopkins University School of Medicine, Baltimore, MD

Moniquin Huggins, MD
Child Care Bureau, Administration on Children, Youth, and Families,
US Department of Health and Human Services, Washington, DC

Jerri Ann Jenista, MD
St Joseph Mercy Hospital, Ann Arbor, MI

Chet D. Johnson, MD
Kansas University Medical Center, Kansas City, KS

Chris P. Johnson, MEd, MD
University of Texas Health Science Center at San Antonio, San Antonio, TX

Desmond P. Kelly, MD
AAP Section on Developmental and Behavioral Pediatrics, University of North
Carolina School of Medicine, Chapel Hill, NC

Pauline D. Koch
Koch Consulting, Newark, DE

Marjorie J. Kostelnik, PhD
College of Human Resources and Family Sciences, University of Nebraska,
Lincoln, NE

Nancy F. Krebs, MD, MS
Department of Pediatrics, University of Colorado, Denver, CO

Carole Logan Kuhns, RN, PhD
Virginia Polytechnic Institute and State University, Fairfax Station, VA

Claire Lerner, LCSW-C
Zero to Three, Washington, DC

Michael A. Lindstrom, AIA
Bright Horizons Family Solutions, Watertown, MA

Peter Michael Miller, MD, MPH
University of California San Francisco, San Anselmo, CA

Jody R. Murph, MD
Children's Hospital of Iowa, University of Iowa Hospitals and Clinics,
Iowa City, IA

Trudy V. Murphy, MD
National Immunization Program, Centers for Disease Control and Prevention,
Atlanta, GA

Linda Nathanson Lippitt, MD
Children's Healthcare of Atlanta, Smyrna, GA

Sheryl S. Nelson, MS
American Academy of Pediatrics, Elk Grove Village, IL

Leslie Nield-Anderson, PhD, APRN-BC
Florida International University, North Miami, FL

S. Donald Palmer, MD
Alabama Chapter, American Academy of Pediatrics, Sylacauga, AL

Mark D. Pavey, AIA
Children's Design Group, Montgomery, AL

Larry K. Pickering, MD
National Immunization Program, Centers for Disease Control and Prevention,
Atlanta, GA

James M. Poole, MD
Poole Pediatrics, Raleigh, NC

Douglas R. Powell, PhD
Purdue University, West Lafayette, IN

Jefferson B. Prince, MD
Massachusetts General Hospital/Harvard Medical School, Boston, MA

Patricia O. Quinn, MD
Washington, DC

Barbara Reisman, MBA, CPA
Schumann Fund for New Jersey, Montclair, NJ

Judith T. Romano, MD
Wheeling, WV

Ellen S. Rome, MD, MPH
Cleveland Clinic Foundation, Cleveland, OH

Lois S. Sadler, PhD, RNCS, PNP
Yale University School of Nursing, New Haven, CT

Edward L. Schor, MD
AAP Task Force on the Family, DesMoines, IA

Abby Shapiro, MEd
WFD Consulting, Watertown, MA

Mark D. Simms, MD, MPH
Medical College of Wisconsin, Milwaukee, WI

Gary A. Smith, MD, DrPH
Center for Injury Research and Policy, Children's Hospital, Columbus, OH

Karen Sokal-Gutierrez, MD, MPH
California Child Care Health Program, Piedmont, CA

Howard Spivak, MD
AAP Task Force on Violence
New England Medical Center, Boston, MA

Sarah H. Springer, MD
The Mercy Center for International Adoption, Mercy Hospital of Pittsburgh,
Pittsburgh, PA

Phyllis Stubbs-Wynn, MD, MPH
Maternal and Child Health Bureau, Rockville, MD

Moira Szilagyi, MD, PhD
Foster Care Pediatrics, Rochester, NY

Howard L. Taras, MD
University of California, San Diego, Division of Community Pediatrics,
La Jolla, CA

Donna J. Thompson, PhD
National Program for Playground Safety, Cedar Falls, IA

Susan B. Tully, MD
UCLA Medical Center, Pasadena, CA

J. M. Whitworth, MD
University of Florida, Jacksonville, FL

Flaura Koplin Winston, MD, PhD
University of Pennsylvania, Philadelphia, PA

Jean A. Wright, MD, MBA
Memorial Health, Savannah, GA

Wayne A. Yankus, MD
AAP Committee on School Health

PREFACE AND ACKNOWLEDGEMENTS

This manual has been written to serve as a resource for pediatricians, family practitioners, public health professionals, child care health consultants, and child care providers. It was also written with the express intent of serving as a text for pediatric residents or other professionals whose training includes issues relevant to child care. The actual process of writing, editing, and publishing this book has taken many years and has involved a legion of child advocates working tirelessly for something they believed in. I would like to thank, in particular the Committee on Early Childhood, Adoption, and Dependent Care, chaired successively by Ed Schor, Peter M. Miller, Peter Gorski, and Chet Johnson, who oversaw and lent support for this work. I wish to acknowledge all of the AAP staff members who shepherded this book from inception to completion. This long list includes (but is in no way limited to) Eileen Casey, Mary Crane, Rebecca Marshall, Rachael Hagan, Becky Marco, Jennifer Pane, Peg Mulcahy, Sheryl Nelson, Laura Aird, Scott Allen, and Alicia Siston, among many others. I would particularly like to express my appreciation and gratitude to the members of the Committee on Early Childhood, Adoption, and Dependent Care who were my support, my mentors, and my friends during this time. I would especially like to thank Ed Schor, Peter M. Miller, Peter Gorski, Neal Kaufman, Jim Poole, Jeri Ann Jenista, Mark Simms, Chet Johnson, Susan Levitzky, and Donald Palmer, who taught me more about children, about life, and about friendship than I could have ever imagined. My deepest respect and appreciation goes to all of the authors and the reviewers who contributed their time and expertise to this work. I also wish to thank my coeditors, Don Palmer and Danette Glassy, for their hard work, diplomacy, sense of humor, and unfailing support. Finally, I wish to thank all of the pediatricians, child care providers, child care health consultants, and others who work every day to make child care a better, safer experience for our children.

Jody R. Murph, MD, MS, FAAP, *Editor*

CHAPTER 1

Child Care in the United States

Abby Shapiro, MEd, and Leanne C. Barrett

LEARNING OBJECTIVES

From this introductory chapter, the reader will gain an understanding of the following child care-related issues:

- Prevalence of child care.
- Different types of care arrangements.
- Key national concerns.

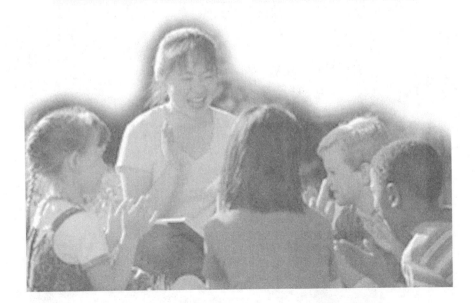

INTRODUCTION

A report from the Urban Institute stated that nearly three quarters (73%) of children younger than 5 years in the United States were in some form of regular child care, other than with a parent, during a typical week. This number represents 8.7 million preschool children in child care. More than three quarters (80%) of children 5 years of age with an employed primary caregiver were in some form of child care other than school. As children get older, fewer are in child care arrangements outside of school hours. Forty-nine percent of children 6 to 12 years of age were in some type of arrangement after school hours. Nearly two thirds of all children younger than 13 years currently have both parents or their only custodial parent in the workforce. Many 2-parent families in which 1 parent is not employed outside the home also use child care for early education and socialization. Still others use nonparental care while the parent is involved in activities in which the child's participation or presence is inappropriate. Such activities might require parents' attention to care for themselves or for another member of the family or to participate in a religious or community function not suitable for a young child. Nonparental child care has become a fact of life.

Child care has become increasingly significant in the lives of American families to the point that it has become an integral part of American childhood. In 2002, the US Census Bureau reported that close to 55% of mothers are returning to the workforce within a year of a child's birth and 72% of mothers with children older than 1 year are in the workforce. In all likelihood, these figures will continue to increase, particularly with the current welfare reform legislation requiring young mothers with dependent children to join the workforce.

In 2002, the US Census Bureau reported that close to 55% of mothers are returning to the workforce within a year of a child's birth and 72% of mothers with children older than 1 year are in the workforce.

Today, parents rely on a variety of arrangements to ensure their children are cared for and educated. The complexity and diversity of these child care arrangements has led some experts to characterize child care services in the United States as a "patchwork system." Care settings used by parents change repeatedly throughout childhood but also may vary considerably even within a given day or week. An infant may be home with his or her mother for the first few months of life and then receive care in a family child care home program with 2 to 5 other children younger than 6 years or in an infant classroom in a child care center. A toddler might be home with his or her mother on certain days of the week and stay at the grandparents' house or in a child care center on the remaining days. A preschool-aged child may attend a center 3 to 5 days a week, but when he or she is ill, the mother must call in sick to work or make hasty arrangements to drop the child off at a neighbor's. For parents who work evenings or weekends, a family child care provider, relative, or neighbor is most likely to be the child care provider if the parents can't share care between them. During the school year, an 8-year-old might be home alone before school most mornings, might attend an after-school program run by his or her church, school, or community center most afternoons, and might participate in special interest programs at the town recreation center during school vacations. During the summer, a child might attend day camp for 1 month, then go to residential camp for 2 weeks, and then visit a grandparent for the final 2 weeks before school starts.

By taking extended maternity and paternity leaves, arranging to work opposing shifts, working part-time, or finding work situations that do not require separation from their children, some working parents arrange their schedules so that their children are always in the care of either parent. For all families, child care arrangements are subject to disruption at any time, whether these arrangements are parental, relative, or more formal child care.

TYPES OF CHILD CARE

Informal or Relative Care

Care for an individual child or small group of children provided by relatives, close friends, or neighbors on a regular basis is referred to as informal or relative care. In most states this type of care, called by Gwen Morgan[1] "kith and kin," is exempt from licensing laws. The primary advantages to this type of care are that children are in the care of a familiar adult who may have an ongoing relationship with the parents and who may share similar values and child-rearing methods. Informal care may offer greater flexibility and affordability. Often, this type of care is the only option available to lower-paid workers and those working odd hours. A disadvantage of informal care is the fact that parents may worry about the educational quality of the care setting or disagree with their caregiver's discipline practices, but they may not be able to address these concerns effectively without jeopardizing their tenuous child care arrangement as well as their own relationship with the caregiver.

Child Care Center

A child care center offers care and educational activities to groups of children during the hours that their parents work, usually in a specifically equipped, dedicated facility. Centers are usually open all day (8 to 12 hours) and all year to meet the needs of working parents; some only operate half-days to provide early childhood education for children who do not need full-day care. Most centers serve children 3 to 5 years of age, but many also care for infants, toddlers, and school-aged children. They offer children a place to play and learn away from home, often with staff who have some training in child development and early childhood education. Developmentally appropriate learning experiences include fine motor and gross motor skill building, life experience, outdoor play, language stimulation with story reading and circle time, and social skill building play. These activities are integrated with meals, diaper changes, toilet learning, and time for naps. The activities usually include structured and unstructured times and teacher-directed and child-initiated experiences. Quality facilities have a written curriculum that defines their plans on a day-to-day basis. Many have family involvement activities as well.

Centers may offer part-time or flexible enrollment options for families who don't need full-time care for their children and may provide special enrichments, such as computers or dance and gymnastics, as well as a range of "convenience services" such as take-home meals, dry cleaning delivery, and occasional evening care for parents' night out. Some centers are even open 24 hours a day to accommodate children of shift workers.

The popularity of center-based care has soared over the last 3 decades. In 1965, only 1 of 20 preschool-aged children of working mothers was enrolled in a child care center, whereas recent Census reports show that nearly 40% of 3- to 5-year-olds are enrolled in this type of care. Center-based care is much more common for preschoolers than for infants and toddlers; in fact, when nonemployed mothers are considered, half of all children 3 to 5 years of age are enrolled in a center at least part-time. Many families with 1 parent who is not employed outside the home send their children to part-day child care centers for the enrichment and learning benefits. This trend has a long-standing historic basis and has been enhanced by public awareness that early childhood programs can provide a strong foundation for later school success.

Parents seem to recognize the advantages of exposing their children to the enriched environment a center can provide with specialized toys, trained teachers or caregivers, and other children. The chief disadvantage to center-based care is the relatively high cost for parents, who find that tuition expenses cost a significant portion of their earnings—at least $4000 to $10 000 per year for full-day, full-year quality care. These costs are comparable to tuition for private school for older children and are low compared with fees for higher education. Government subsidy of early childhood education costs helps some low-income families with child care expenses but is insufficient to meet the need. For babies and toddlers, quality center-based care is harder to find and usually more expensive than quality care for children in the 3- to 5-year age group.

About half of child care centers are operated on a not-for-profit basis. Common nonprofit auspices include government agencies, educational institutions, churches, synagogues, YMCAs/YWCAs, community centers, employer-linked centers, and parent cooperative nursery school programs. Some public schools provide early care and education during the preschool years. Since 1989 when Mitchell, Seligson, and Marx[2] reported that 1 in 5 public school districts offered programs for preschool children, many more schools have implemented full-day kindergartens and preschools. Any given community may offer a wide variety of early childhood services, including Head Start, early intervention services for children with special needs, part-day preschool, and full-day child care.

For-profit centers may be small "mom and pop" operations or may be affiliated with local or national chains. In recent years, for-profit child care has grown faster than not-for-profit private programs, with the most rapid growth occurring among large chains.[1] In fact, the provision of child care services now represents a $27 billion industry despite the reality that most for-profit centers operate on extremely slim margins.

An increasingly important type of child care center is an employer-sponsored center located at or near the work site. Recent counts by Work and Family Connection (http://www.workfamily.com), an organization that tracks workplace child care centers, reveals that there are now nearly 8000 employer-supported child care centers in the United States, including office parks, colleges, and hospitals. The most common supporter of workplace care for employees' children are hospitals, in which hundreds of on-site child care centers were developed during the 1980s to recruit and retain skilled nurses and other medical personnel. The federal government and the military operate more child care centers than any other system in the world. With support from Congress, higher standards have been set and met by child care centers run for military families and for civilian federal workers than for most other community programs. Many universities, colleges, and state and municipal governments have centers for employees and students. In addition, support for dependent care programs has grown among private industry.

There are now nearly 8000 employer-supported child care centers in the United States

A number of our nation's leading corporations, including Johnson & Johnson, Nations Bank, and Allstate Insurance Company, as well as smaller companies like BE&K Construction in Birmingham, Alabama, have built child care centers near major work sites. Many more have invested in community programs to expand the supply and enhance the quality of available care. In 1992, the American Business Collaboration (ABC) for Quality Dependent Care was launched to support this goal of ensuring adequate supply and quality of child care for employees. Currently, the collaboration comprises more than 18 member companies and has invested more than $36 million in more than 65 communities across the country. The ABC has created and funded more than 1500 innovative programs for dependent care.

Family Child Care Homes

Typical family child care homes provide care for up to 6 children, including the caregiver's own young children, usually in the residence of the caregiver. The care can include formal early childhood education curriculum in addition to household-type activities such as doing laundry, running errands, and cooking. Family child care is usually managed as an independent small business by each provider, although some providers are employed by or linked for support services with a sponsoring agency in a family child care system or network for support services. Large family child care homes (also called group child care homes) usually have 1 caregiver and at least 1 assistant providing care for 6 to 12 children in the caregiver's home. In most states, large family child care homes are considered a separate type of care; in some states they are regulated as small child care centers.

Family child care is generally less expensive than center-based care and may provide a more casual and flexible program for children. Unfortunately, studies of family child care indicate that, as with center-based care, only a small portion are of good quality. Unlike center-based care, of which most is of mediocre quality, much of family child care is unregulated and of poor quality. Annual turnover in family child care homes is high. Family child care providers earn little income, must relinquish some of their privacy at home, and usually work long hours. Family child care providers commonly go into business while their own children are young. Thus, discontinuity in child care arrangements may be more likely as caregivers go out of business or need to take a day off.

In-Home Care

In-home care is given in the parent's own home by someone the parent has hired and involves individuals who call themselves by any of a variety of names—eg, au pair (a live-in student who provides child care), sitter, housekeeper, mother's helper, student, relative, nanny. None of these terms ensure that the caregiver has any specific level of competence or training. In-home care may be provided by someone who lives elsewhere and comes to the home only for part of the day or by someone who lives in the home. Many au pairs are young adults seeking away-from-home experiences as foreign nationals or are from another part of the United States. They live with the family and are responsible for child care and light housework. Usually, these caregivers do not have extensive training or experience, and do not perceive child care as a permanent career choice. They use the opportunity to live with a family as an interesting way to achieve some level of independence, enroll in some classes to continue their education, and learn about a new culture while maintaining a subsistence-level income. Some nannies have formal training, and some have years of experience as child care professionals. Many are as young and inexperienced as au pairs.

Although in-home care is sometimes seen as the most convenient kind of child care for parents, especially those with long or erratic work hours, it is the most isolated type of care with the greatest demand on the parent to provide supervision with little opportunity to have an accurate view of the quality of care. For 1 or 2 children, it is more expensive than care from a center or family child care home. For more than 2 children, it may cost less than out-of-home options. It can take months to find an appropriate caregiver, and incompatibility or incompetence often surfaces later, causing sudden disruptions in arrangements. Salaries for in-home providers generally average $200 to $350 per week ($10 000 to $18 000 per year). Live-in caregivers usually receive a smaller salary, between $150 and $300 per week, because they receive room and board as part of their compensation. Some other disadvantages to this arrangement are the invasion of family privacy by someone who has needs of his or her own and the high rate of turnover. Because many in-home care providers don't consider their child care careers to be long-term, they may leave their jobs more frequently than other types of caregivers. Moreover, because there are no state regulations or standards for in-home care, careful recruiting, interviewing, and reference checks by parents and unannounced drop-in supervision are essential to ensure safe and appropriate care.

School-Aged Care

In addition to care in family child care homes, a wide variety of center-based school-aged programs provide supervised activities for children between 5 and 12 years of age at schools, community youth centers, or child care centers during the hours and days when schools are closed—before school, after school, and during summer vacation, holidays, teacher training days, etc. Before- and after-school programs are more commonly available for elementary school-aged children than for those attending middle school. For convenience, these programs may be located at the child's school or at other locations to which the child is taken with transportation services. Although full-day kindergarten is becoming more common, "wrap around" programming is used by many children in part-day kindergarten programs. Day camps are a common source of school-aged care during summer vacations, although some families use traditional overnight or residential programs. Day and overnight camps combine fun and learning experiences, and some focus on special interests, such as computers, sports, drama, and art. These programs are generally for children between 5 and 12 years of age, although some camps are open just to preschoolers and others include teenagers.

Care for school-aged children is among the most difficult to arrange, because most communities in the United States do not have a coordinated system for this age group. In some communities, after-school programs may be available only at certain elementary schools or community centers. Parents who cannot avail themselves of these programs must fend for themselves in arranging care. Because licensing regulations are often lax for school-aged child care, the quality of school-aged programs can vary tremendously. Standards of quality for this type of care are not as well known as are those for early childhood programs. One of the chief difficulties with after-school programs is the fact that most do not operate in dedicated space with full-time, professionally trained staff. Many are set up in the gymnasium or all-purpose room of a school and serve large numbers of children in the same space. Sports and games are more frequently offered than the long-term, more involved projects school-aged children enjoy, such as woodworking, cooking, and science experiments that may require special equipment and supplies that cannot be easily packed away at the end of the day.

As Michelle Seligson[3] notes, school-aged children have the propensity to "vote with their feet," and as they grow older, many refuse to attend programs they perceive as geared for younger children. Parents often face a difficult situation when their 9-year-old absolutely refuses to attend his or her after school-program anymore. To combat this problem, some families make elaborate arrangements for their school-aged children, combining after school lessons, activities, sports, and trips to friends' homes to ensure the child has little time home alone. But many school-aged children do spend at least some time home alone.

Backup or Drop-in Care

This type of care helps families when their regular care arrangements fail—their family child care provider is on vacation, their child care center closes for Christmas week, school is canceled because of a teachers' strike, etc. Some child care centers and family child care homes allow children who are not regularly enrolled to attend as long as space is available. Other centers solely provide backup child care and do not offer regular enrollment options. Boys and Girls Clubs often accept school-aged children on a drop-in basis. Sometimes emergency in-home care can be arranged on a same-day basis, although the cost of such arrangements is prohibitive for all but the most affluent if employers do not provide a subsidy. Traditional drop-in care programs continue to thrive so parents can work out at a health club, attend religious services, complete holiday shopping, or even go out for the evening.

Backup and drop-in care programs are attractive to today's busy and stressed families. Nevertheless, their main advantage—that they are available when regular arrangements fall through or are not feasible—is directly connected to their most significant disadvantage—their inability to build a stable caregiving relationship with a child. Some children adapt easily to care by unfamiliar adults in an unfamiliar environment, but others do not. Parents need to use their own best judgment when deciding whether this type of program is appropriate for their child. Sometimes parents who must work have no other alternative.

Care For Mildly Ill Children

Working parents of mildly ill children face a dilemma. Most parents would rather stay home with their ill children, but many employers do not provide leave for this purpose. Several types of programs have been developed to address this problem: hospital-based programs, stand-alone sick child care centers, "get-well rooms" at regular child care centers, and emergency in-home care programs. Keeping ill children at their regular programs seems to be the most desirable for parents who must work, because they will be cared for in a familiar setting by familiar people. For this reason, some centers and family child care homes offer arrangements to keep mildly ill children in the regular program or at least with familiar caregivers at the regular facility. Some centers are establishing "get-well rooms" for this purpose. Another service valued by parents is an emergency in-home care program in which trained caregivers or home health aids care for the child in the parent's home. Even though the child will be cared for by an unfamiliar person, the child will be in a familiar setting, allaying some of the parents' fears and feelings of guilt. More specialized programs, whether based in hospitals or dedicated sick child care facilities, have proven to be less popular with most working parents who have difficulty taking their ill child to an unfamiliar facility to be cared for by strangers among other unfamiliar ill children. There are a few of these programs in existence that have developed sufficient community support, but many specialized programs have closed in recent years, and few new ones have opened.

In most communities, very few options exist for parents with an ill child. Most must rely on a hastily made, informal arrangement with relatives, friends, or neighbors or stay home themselves. Care for a mildly ill child is usually more expensive than care for a well child. Plus, parents usually must continue to pay tuition for their child's regular program to maintain a reserved spot. Very few centers give parents rebates for care not used because of a child's illness.

Head Start

This early childhood enrichment program was established in 1965 at the peak of the federal government's War on Poverty campaign. Originally a federally funded and managed program for 3- and 4-year-olds in low-income families, the program has been extended to provide services to some infants and toddlers. Head Start combines an emphasis on children's education and health with social services for their families and a focus on parent involvement. Because Head Start originated as an educational intervention program for children regardless of whether their parents worked, many programs still only operate on a part-day and part-year basis. As low-income families have experienced the pressures of welfare-to-work requirements and other trends that encourage or require mothers to enter the workforce, child care for the full day and full year has become essential. Federal legislation in recent years has provided some additional funding to extend hours and days.

Care For Children With Special Needs

A variety of specialized programs exist to serve children with developmental delays, those who are "at risk" of developmental delay, or those with chronic illness. With the passage of Americans With Disabilities Act, federal law requires inclusion of such children in facilities that serve typically developing children. The special services available must be brought to the child now. Specialized services include early intervention programs, respite care programs, and protective care services.

Beginning with passage of the Education of the Handicapped Amendments of 1986 and subsequent amendments to the federal Act for the Education of All Handicapped Children, states have been required to provide educational services to disabled children younger than 6 years and provide early intervention programs to children and families at risk of developmental delay. This legislation resulted in the creation of a variety of services for children and families with special needs, including full- and part-day center-based programs as well as home visiting services that are now being reorganized to provide services in more inclusive settings. For children with chronic illnesses, such as allergies, asthma, seizure disorders, and diabetes, accommodation in settings for typically developing children requires planning and training of staff by the child's source of health care. No federal programs provide supplemental services for these children, but under the Americans With Disabilities Act, caregivers cannot refuse to serve them unless doing so would put the child care facility out of business.

Respite care programs have a longer history, originating with informal arrangements made between relatives and friends to watch a child with special needs so parents could attend to other duties, rest at home, or go on vacation. More recently, formal respite care programs for children and adults have emerged in many communities, providing a valuable service to highly stressed families. "Protective" care services also exist in many communities to provide an intermediary level of protective care for children at risk of abuse or neglect before foster care services are necessary. Usually funded by the state's child protection office, protective care services are often integrated into a community child care center or family child care home.

AVAILABILITY, AFFORDABILITY, AND QUALITY

According to a recent poll, 85% of registered voters believe it is difficult for parents to find after-school programs in their communities.[4,5] The demand for child care continues to grow at an estimated rate of approximately 4% to 5% per year.

The cost of child care can vary greatly, depending on the community, the age of the child, and the type of care. Most families spend between 10% to 20% of their gross income on child care, but some families living below the poverty line can spend more than one quarter of their income on child care. Full-day child care for infants can cost between $4000 and $15 000 per year, with costs generally higher in centers than in family child care homes. Care for preschoolers ranges from $3500 to $8000 per year, and part-day school-aged care ranges from $2000 to $5000 per year. Some federal and state funding subsidizes the cost of care for poor families waiting for subsidized care.

For many years, experts discouraged the use of full-day child care. It wasn't until researchers began to study children enrolled in *quality* programs that the benefits of child care became clear. Since the quality of care has been considered, researchers have found that quality child care does not harm children. In many cases, it enhances their development. Quality child care prepares children for academic success by fostering reasoning abilities, creativity, and communication skills and enhancing self-esteem and self-control. It also promotes positive social development by teaching children to share, empathize, and respect others. Furthermore, several studies of low-income children in quality early childhood programs documented significant improvement in cognitive outcomes compared with similar children at home.[6-7] Results from a longitudinal study of children enrolled in the Perry Preschool/High Scope Early Intervention Project indicate that quality education and care for young children can decrease the incidence of school failure, grade retention, special education placement, adolescent pregnancy, and delinquency; it is even associated with higher earning power and a greater commitment to marriage in adulthood.[8]

In recent years, researchers have begun to paint a picture of quality child care. Quality programs are those with warm, well-trained, well-compensated, and stable staff; low child-to-caregiver ratios; small group sizes; and developmentally appropriate activities and environments. All families and children deserve access to such child care. However, quality care is harder to find and more expensive than mediocre or poor care. The quality, availability, and affordability of child care are linked, and unfortunately, the higher the quality of care, the less affordable and less available it generally is.

Currently, the quality of child care in the United States is not good. The *Study of Children in Family Child Care*[9] reported that only 9% of the family child care homes studied were providing quality care (enhancing child development), 56% were providing adequate or custodial care (neither promoting nor harming child development), and 35% were providing inadequate care (impairing child development). Similarly, the final report of the *Cost, Quality, and Child Outcomes in Child Care Centers*[10] study revealed that of 398 child care centers in California, Colorado, Connecticut, and North Carolina studied, only 14% provided developmentally appropriate care. Nearly three quarters of the centers were rated as mediocre, and another 12% were poor. Not surprisingly, centers in states with less stringent regulations were more likely to be providing low-quality care.

Because no federally mandated standards for child care exist, the quality of child care available across the country varies significantly. Chapter 2 will detail the impact of state regulations on the supply of quality child care. The chart in Appendix A provides an overview of the range of state regulation and illustrates the disparate levels of quality (see also Table 1.1).

INTERNATIONAL PERSPECTIVE

Experts and commentators often point to other industrialized nations, particularly those in western Europe, as models for offering more accessible, quality, affordable care for working parents.[11] France and Denmark both provide heavy subsidies to support the care and education of young children, enabling most children to participate. In Denmark, about half of all children younger than 3 years are enrolled

TABLE 1.1. Caregiver-Child Ratios for Child Care Centers

Age Group	National Quality Standards for Accrediting Bodies*	California	Connecticut	Georgia	Indiana	Idaho
Infants (6 wk–1 y)	NAEYC[†] 1:3–1:4	1:4	1:4	1:6	1:4	1:6
Toddlers (1–3 y)	NAEYC 1:4–1:7	1:6	1:4	1:8–1:10	1:5–1:10	1:6–1:12
Preschoolers (3–5 y)	NAEYC 1:7–1:10	1:12	1:10	1:15–1:18	1:10–1:12	1:12
Kindergarten (5 y)	NAEYC 1:8–1:10	1:12	1:10	1:20	1:15	1:18
Elementary School (6–9 y)	NAEYC 1:10–1:12 NSACA[‡] 1:10–1:15	1:14	1:10	1:25	1:20	1:18
Middle School (10–14 y)	NAEYC 1:12–1:15 NSACA 1:10–1:15	1:14	1:10	1:25	1:20	1:18

* The National Association for Family Child Care does not publish ratios but advises child care centers to follow state regulations. See also National Association for Family Child Care. *Quality Standards for NAFCC Accreditation.* Salt Lake City, UT: National Association for Family Child Care; 2002.

† National Association for the Education of Young Children. *Accreditation Criteria and Procedures of the National Academy of Early Childhood Programs.* Washington, DC: National Association for the Education of Young Children; 1998.

‡ National School-Age Care Alliance. *The NSACA Standards for Quality School-Age Care.* Boston, MA: National School-Age Care Alliance; 1998.

in public child care programs, and nearly three quarters attend public preschool. Parents pay no more than 30% of the cost. In France, nearly all children 3 to 5 years of age attend preschool, and it is free of charge. Free after-school care is also widely available. French infants and toddlers are served by center-based programs called *crèches* or by home-based child care for which parents pay based on income. Other countries providing accessible, affordable care for preschoolers include Belgium, Finland, Germany, Italy, and Sweden. Arrangements for infant and toddler care vary. Many western European countries guarantee a generous maternity leave, so it is not uncommon to find mothers and fathers sharing care at home while their children are very young.[12,13]

Quality programs for preschool and school-aged children are traditional and abundant in many Scandinavian and eastern European countries, including the former Soviet Union. Those in Scandinavia are called *friditshem,* which translated means "free time homes." These programs are staffed by professionals who have completed a specialized 3-year training program with courses in recreation, arts and crafts, music, and dramatics.[2] Programs generally serve up to 20 children and keep the staff-child ratio at approximately 1:8. School-aged children attending these neighborhood-based programs can participate in such activities as woodworking, cooking, pottery, and sports in a home-based environment.

The former Soviet Union had preschool and school-aged programs, with educational, nutritional, and health services as integral parts of the programs. The preschool center was called a *detsky sad* and was easily recognized because it generally had a better-than-averagely maintained building where the equipment and furnishings were often enriched through parent involvement. The after-school programs were called children's palaces, in which recreational, educational, and social programs were arranged for out-of-school hours. With the breakup of the Soviet Union and economic hard times, these facilities have suffered from insufficient public resources but continue to be supported by parents.

PUBLIC POLICY AND PRIVATE ATTITUDES

American public opinion remains ambivalent about nonmaternal care, particularly for young children. Many remain convinced that stay-at-home mothers have the greatest potential to raise healthy, successful children. Others are concerned that the quality of child care currently available in most areas of the country may harm children, stating that the search for appropriate care amounts to a "cosmic crap shoot."[13]

However, most parents need child care to work and meet other personal and family responsibilities. Many have witnessed the positive relationships their children can form with warm caregivers and other children. Parents and others can see that young children can benefit from being exposed to a more enriched environment complete with diverse personalities, abilities, and appearances.

Many experts blame our lack of a national child care system on American ambivalence toward supporting families to meet their child care needs. We often pit adults against children by arguing whether child care should be a service for working parents or an educational program for children when, in reality, children and parents benefit greatly from quality, supportive programs.

Although child care legislation exists in the United States, including the Child Care and Development Block Grant of 1990, America's system of child care still does not approach those that exist in many parts of Europe. As federal investment has increased in child care over the past decade, new systems have been developed for training caregivers, for making subsidized care available to low- and low-to-middle-income parents, and for resource and referral services to help parents find good quality care. Although these developments are encouraging, much remains to be done to bring the full benefits of quality child care for children in the United States to the level achieved in other developed countries.

CONCLUSIONS AND RECOMMENDATIONS
- Give parents clear information about what constitutes quality child care.
- Support efforts to strengthen and improve state child care regulations.
- Support community resource, referral, and caregiver training services.
- Advocate for adequate public and private funding to support the development and provision of quality care.

NATIONAL ORGANIZATIONS WITH CHILD CARE EXPERTISE
American Academy of Pediatrics
Healthy Child Care America Campaign
141 Northwest Point Boulevard
Elk Grove Village, IL 60007
800/433-9016
Web site: http://www.healthychildcare.org

Child Care Aware
1319 F Street NW, Suite 500
Washington, DC 20004
800/424-2246
Web site: http://www.childcareaware.org

Children's Defense Fund
25 E Street NW
Washington, DC 20001
Web site: http://www.childrensdefense.org

Families and Work Institute (FWI)
267 Fifth Avenue, Floor 2
New York, NY 10016
Web site: http://www.familiesandwork.org

National Association for Family Child Care (NAFCC)
5202 Pinemont Drive
Salt Lake City, UT 84123
Web site: http://www.nafcc.org

National Association for the Education of Young Children (NAEYC)
1509 16th Street NW
Washington, DC 20009
Web site: http://www.naeyc.org

National Association of Child Care Resource and Referral Agencies (NACCRRA)
1391 F Street NW, Suite 500
Washington, DC 20004
Web site: http://www.naccra.org

National Child Care Information Center (NCCIC)
243 Church Street NW, 2nd Floor
Vienna, Virginia 22180
Web site: http://www.nccic.org

National Institute on Out-of-School Time
Wellesley Centers for Women
106 Central Street
Wellesley, MA 02481
Web site: http://www.niost.org

National School-Age Care Alliance (NSACA)
1137 Washington Street
Dorchester, MA 02124
Web site: http://www.nsaca.org

Zero to Three
National Center for Infants, Toddlers, and Families
2000 M Street NW, Suite 200
Washington, DC 20036
202/638-1144
Web site: http://www.zerotothree.org

REFERENCES

1. Morgan G. *A Hitchhiker's Guide to the Child Care Universe.* Washington, DC: National Association of Child Care Resource and Referral Agencies; 1998
2. Mitchell A, Seligson M, Marx F. *Early Childhood Programs and the Public Schools: Between Promise and Practice.* Dover, MA: Auburn House; 1989
3. Seligson M, Fink DB. *No Time to Waste: An Action Agenda for School-Age Child Care.* Wellesley, MA: Wellesley College; 1989
4. Charles Stewart Mott Foundation. *Special Report: 21st Century Schools.* Flint, MI: Charles Stewart Mott Foundation; 1999
5. The Urban Institute. *What Happens When the School Year Is Over? The Use and Costs of School-Age Children During the Summer Months.* Washington, DC: The Urban Institute; 2002. Available at: http://www.urban.org/UploadedPDF/310497_OP58.pdf. Accessed March 19, 2004
6. American Orthopsychiatric Association. *Day Care: Scientific and Social Policy Issues.* Zigler EF, Gordon EW, eds. Boston, MA: Auburn House Publishing Co; 1982
7. Peth-Pierce R. *The NICHD Study of Early Child Care.* Rockville, MD: National Institutes of Health; 1998. NIH Publication No. 98-4318

8. Schweinhart LJ, Barnes HV, Weikar DP. *Significant Benefits: The High/Scope Perry Preschool Study Through Age 27.* Ypsilanti, MI: High/Scope Press; 1993

9. Galinsky E, Howes C, Kontos S, Shinn M. *The Study of Children in Family Child Care and Relative Care: Highlights of Findings.* New York, NY: Families & Work Institute; 1994

10. Helburn S, Culkin M, Howes C, et al. *Cost, Quality and Child Outcomes in Child Care Centers.* Denver, CO: University of Colorado at Denver; 1995

11. Lubeck S. *Nation as Context: Comparing Child-Care Systems Across Nations.* New York, NY: Teachers College Record; 1995

12. Cochran M. *International Handbook of Child Care Policies and Programs.* Westport, CT: Greenwood Publishing Group; 1993

13. Zigler EF, Lang ME. *Child Care Choices: Balancing the Needs of Children, Families, and Society.* New York, NY: Free Press; 1991

ADDITIONAL RESOURCES

Kisker EE, Hofferth SL, Phillips DA, Farquar E. *A Profile of Child Care Settings: Early Education and Care in 1990.* Washington, DC: US Government Printing Office; 1990

The Urban Institute. *Child Care Arrangements for Children Under Five: Variation Across States.* Washington, DC: The Urban Institute; 2000

The Urban Institute. *Child Care Patterns for School-Age Children With Employed Mothers.* Washington, DC: The Urban Institute; 2000

The Urban Institute. *Primary Child Care Arrangements of Employed Parents: Findings From the 1999 National Survey of America's Families.* Washington, DC: The Urban Institute; 2002

The Urban Institute. *Who's Caring for Our Youngest Children? Child Care Patterns of Infants and Toddlers.* Washington, DC: The Urban Institute; 2001

US Census Bureau. *Who's Minding the Kids? Child Care Arrangements: Spring 1999.* Washington, DC: US Census Bureau; 2003. Available at: http://www.census.gov/population/www/socdemo/child/ppl-168.html. Accessed March 19, 2004

US Census Bureau. Fertility of American Women: June 2002. Washington, DC: US Census Bureau; 2003. Available at: http://www.census.gov/prod/2003pubs/p20-548.pdf. Accessed March 19, 2004

CHAPTER 2

Regulation, Licensing, and Accreditation

Pauline D. Koch and V. Susan Bredekamp, PhD

LEARNING OBJECTIVES

From this chapter, the reader should gain an understanding of the following:

- The definition, basic principles, and components of regulation and child care licensing.
- Research on quality child care related to regulation.
- The role of other agencies in the regulatory process.
- Criteria for effective licensing and review of current state practices.
- Issues, challenges, and recommendations for regulatory reform facing state child care licensing agencies.
- Coordinated roles of child care licensing and accreditation.

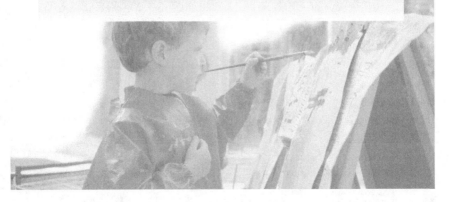

INTRODUCTION

The research is compelling at this point on the importance of the early years and education in shaping the lives of young children. Everyone has a role to play in ensuring that children receive the care and education they need to grow into healthy, successful, and productive adults. The protection of children is a partnership among parents, child care providers, regulatory agencies, funding agencies, resource and referral agencies, and the community at large.

With the increased demand for child care by the labor force and as a result of welfare reform, greater attention must be given to the role of governmental regulation of child care as a means to achieve and maintain quality child care in the United States. Parents, as consumers of child care at all income levels, seek the security of knowing that their children are receiving care that is safe, trustworthy, and of good quality.

● Mandatory regulatory systems for licensing and monitoring child care programs and voluntary accreditation systems for recognizing programs that meet high professional standards play a fundamental role in creating a safe, healthy, nurturing, and developmentally sound setting for children provided early care and education.

REGULATION AND LICENSING

A major function of government is the protection of its citizens through regulation in areas in which the average citizen is not able to determine the safety of a service or whether the service provider is qualified to deliver that service. Thus, human care regulation achieves consumer protection by establishing and enforcing standards designed to decrease the risk of harm to consumers of the services.[1] The term "standards" will be used in this chapter in a broad, generic manner, and "rules" or "requirements" will refer to standards required for state licensing.

Although regulation is found at national, state, and local levels, child care is primarily regulated at state and local levels. There are a number of baseline permissions a child care provider must seek and receive before being granted the right to operate—licensing, registration, and zoning, construction, fire code, and health and sanitation approvals. Often, these permissions come from different agencies, each with its own statutory authority and requirements. Regulatory coordination is critical to an efficient and responsive licensing process, which facilitates rather than impedes the growth of much-needed child care services. In the current climate of regulatory reform, there is an increased effort in many states to simplify and improve these often unconnected processes by removing rule inconsistencies (Hawaii), creating local inspection teams (Oregon and Ohio)[2] and improving coordination and communication among all regulatory agencies (Delaware).

WHAT IS CHILD CARE LICENSING?

Child care licensing is consumer protection through prevention. The fundamental purpose of licensing is to protect the health, safety, and well-being of children receiving care away from their homes and families. The state grants permission to operate to child care facilities that meet certain minimum requirements or rules designed to protect children from the following:

- unsafe buildings;
- fire hazards;
- infectious diseases;
- poisoning;
- injury;
- harm from developmental impairment; and
- harm from lack of supervision.

All of these forms of harm are equally devastating to children and must be prevented to ensure the basic health, safety, and appropriate care of children.[2]

Equal protection is at the core of a sound licensing system. Licensing must apply equally to all private, public, for-profit, and not-for-profit facilities. All children are entitled to a basic level of protection, regardless of child care provider. Thus, all programs providing out-of-home child care should be regulated, without exception, to ensure that all children, regardless of race, ethnicity, religion, geographic location, age, or length of time in care, are afforded the protection and safeguarding that comes from an effective regulatory program.

As a preventive program, licensing is heavily dependent on the education of child care providers to teach and reinforce the rules. Each rule can be considered a right that children and parents have in child care programs and, as such, is a legal requirement that must be met for licensure. Failure to comply with licensing rules results in penalties, including removal of the license, and failure to be licensed is considered a criminal offense. Although the purpose of licensing is not to close programs but to assist child care providers to achieve compliance with the rules, licensing agencies must have the power to eliminate harmful care when programs demonstrate willful violation of rules or inability to provide safe care.

Licensing rules are formulated through a democratic process of consensus building, using citizen task forces that represent diverse interests, including child care providers, advocates, parents, child development and other experts, and licensing staff with the licensing agency coordinating the process. Rules must be clear and easily understood, measurable, shown by research findings to decrease the risk of harm, and economically feasible. Rules cannot be successfully implemented without support from the community and agreement on the part of those being regulated.

Licensing rules are, in reality, the community's consensus on the acceptable minimum standards of care critical to the protection of children. Rules vary across states, and standards of care can be set as high as the public will tolerate. Research finds that outcomes for children are better in states with higher licensing standards. Research has clearly established that only a small percentage of care in this country can be rated as good—14% of center-based care, 8% of infant care,[3] and 9% of family child care homes.[4] Further, the studies found an alarming proportion of inadequate (below minimal quality) care.

As the professional practice of early child care and education improves through the influence of research, increased child care provider training and education, and wider use of accreditation, the community's expectations of quality increase as well as, usually, licensing rules. Informed citizens and advocates for quality child care can play a strong role in raising the level of licensing standards or rules. Strong advocacy is critical to ensure that there is a safety net in place for all children. Regulation then is the essential means of ensuring that the lower limit of quality established by the state as critical to decrease the risk of harm is maintained.

Strong advocacy is critical to the adoption of licensing rules, which decrease the risk of harm across all areas of risk. For example, over the years, states have responded to the pressure for strong licensing rules relating to health concerns, particularly in the areas of immunization, hand washing, standard precautions, caring for mildly ill children, health training of staff, and criminal record and child abuse registry checks. In the same way, states are making great strides in improving requirements for child care provider training and staff qualifications in response to the results of new research and the movement to create comprehensive career systems for early childhood teachers and child care providers.

States are making great strides in improving requirements for child care provider training and staff qualifications

Similar improvements are not evident in other areas of health and safety. In the 1995 status update of state licensing efforts in the 1990 report "Who Knows How Safe," the Children's Defense Fund found that many states still do not require basic health and safety protections, such as first aid training in family child care, resilient surfaces beneath climbing equipment in centers, and smoke detectors and fire drills in family child care homes.[5,6] In the 1998 report, "Child Care: Use of Standards to Ensure High Quality Care," the US General Accounting Office reviewed state licensing rules against health and safety standards of the 1992 *National Health and Safety Performance Standards: Guidelines for Out-of-Home Child Care Programs*. This study found that states licensing rules more often parallel the National Health and Safety Performance Standards for indoor and outdoor square footage than for other standards for pinch and crush points and surface coverings of playground equipment, hand washing, sanitation of surfaces, and toys for infants and toddlers[6] (see also Appendix B).

Advocacy to improve standards will be critical to ensure that the safety net of necessary quality is in place for all children. The field of practice continuously improves as influenced by ongoing research, increased child care provider training, and wider use of accreditation. As the field of practice improves, so does the community standard of quality. These factors, along with the influence of licensing rule comparisons across states, all help to continuously raise licensing standards, which are the lower limits of quality that are considered safe and acceptable. Strong advocacy to retain what is essential to protect children from the risk of harm will be especially important in light of the current challenges facing the reform of regulation of human service programs to eliminate unnecessary rules and streamline regulatory procedures. It is also important to note that as critical as strong licensing standards are for the protection of children, they are only one component of the regulatory function.

Licensing rules are just one method to achieve quality, although they are critical as they serve as the floor below which no program may fall. Other regulatory and nonregulatory mechanisms are also used by various segments of the community to improve the health, safety, and quality of child care. As delineated in Table 2.1, beyond the basic floor or lower limit of quality, other regulatory approaches specify higher levels of standards, in ascending order:

- Standards for approving publicly operated programs, which should be equal to the quality required of privately operated programs.
  - ~ Many states make exempt from the licensing law programs operated by public and private schools, but few have standards for approving and monitoring such programs.
- Standards for government-funded programs (eg, Head Start performance standards, higher standards set for child care services purchased by the state).
- Standards for credentialing of individuals (eg, state certification of public school teachers).
- Accreditation standards established as model standards to recognize higher quality.
- Goal standards in the field that represent best practices or the "ceiling" of quality.

Credentialing and accreditation are usually administered by the private sector and are voluntary, although there is a beginning movement for state-required credentialing of child care providers, combined with or separate from facility licensing. With this movement, there is much discussion about whether staff-child ratio requirements could or should be set in relation to the level of staff qualifications, permitting higher-qualified staff to care for more children.

There are, in addition, a large number of nonregulatory methods used by various segments of the community to promote and achieve quality. Studies by the Children's Defense Fund, Wheelock College (The Center for Career Development in Early Care and Education), and the US General Accounting Office indicate that states are placing greater emphasis and funding on a variety of nonregulatory methods

TABLE 2.1. Achieving Quality Child Care					
QUALITY					
Nonregulatory Approaches					
Training	Technical assistance	Consultation	Consumer education	Resource and referral	Peer support associations
Regulatory Approaches					
Goals and best practices		Accreditation standards		Funding standards	Credentialing of individuals
Licensing/Minimal Standards—Reducing the Risk of Harm					
Zoning	Building safety	Fire safety		Health and sanitation	Facility licensing standards

Exemptions

Some programs are not regulated in many states. These exemptions may include:
- few children in family child care home
- half-day nursery school/preschool
- church/synagogue-operated centers
- school-based programs

Criminal sanctions may be issued against programs that operate illegally.

to promote compliance with rules and improve quality, such as accreditation, child care provider training and education, peer support, and consumer education about quality. A large part of the impetus and funding for these activities has been the federal funds for quality improvements in child care available since 1992. In some states, there seems to be more emphasis on funding these quality initiatives without equal emphasis on maintaining an effective licensing system, which provides the foundation of quality.

One prime example of an effective nonregulatory method has been the strong movement for states to develop comprehensive professional development systems for child care providers. This movement began with an initiative titled "Delaware First...Again: The First Statewide Training System for Child Care Staff," developed in consultation with Gwen Morgan and Joan Costley of Wheelock College and Nancy Brown (then of North Carolina State University).[6] This program, resulting in a large increase in progressive, role-related, and appropriate training opportunities in states with improved articulation to institutions of higher learning, requires coordination and collaboration among all segments of the community for success. Because training is linked to all levels of quality but has a clear link to licensing rules, which decrease the risk of harm to children, the licensing agency must be involved and is a logical agency to administer the system, as is the case in Delaware. All of these methods, regulatory and nonregulatory, improve health, safety, and quality in child care settings and are most effective when implemented within a coordinated child care system.

An effective regulatory program is critical to adequately decrease the risk of harm to the millions of children in early care and education. Effectiveness is determined by the ability of the agency to carry out its licensing functions, which include the following:

1. The formulation of clear, reasonable, and valid requirements, updated in response to new research findings and experience, sensitive to diversity, and developed by a democratic citizen-based process.
2. The fair and uniform implementation and strong enforcement of the requirements with a solid licensing law, legally sound enforcement procedures that include a wide range of enforcement options and tools, sufficient qualified and well-trained staff, adequate funding, and strong administrative and community support.
3. Strong technical assistance to applicants and licensees to achieve and maintain compliance and encouragement to exceed the lowest acceptable limit set by the standards.
4. Consumer education about "what licensing is" and the roles of the licensing agency, child care providers, parents, and community in that process.

HOW EFFECTIVE IS LICENSING?

A number of studies since the late 1980s have examined state licensing policies and provided examples of effectiveness as well as areas of weakness. In a study by the Office of the Inspector General of the US Department of Health and Human Services, caseloads for licensing staff were almost double the recommended limits, and fewer than half of all regulated family child care homes were inspected in 1988, despite the finding that licensing officials considered frequent on-site monitoring as the best way to maintain compliance.[7]

A US General Accounting Office study in 1992 found that 18 states reported a decrease in the frequency of visits since 1989, and 20 states failed to conduct one unannounced visit per year to child care facilities.[8] In the 1990 Children's Defense Fund report *Who Knows How Safe?* many states reported they lacked sufficient resources to monitor and enforce the rules. However, the report noted some encouraging efforts by states to strengthen their licensing systems by decreasing exemptions, improving licensing rules, and refining their monitoring and enforcement efforts.[9] In their 1995 update, the Children's Defense Fund reported that in 1993, 1 in 5 states still exempted family child care homes caring for 5 or fewer children from licensure and, therefore, all basic protection, and only 9 states required all family child care homes to be regulated. In addition, the study found that many states conduct extremely infrequent inspections of family child care homes or none at all. This study stated, "Furthermore, [underfunding] and inadequate numbers of staff to inspect programs are major causes of inadequate enforcement efforts to protect children."[5]

A study by the US General Accounting Office in January 2000 found that in 1999, 27 states reported child care licensing staff increases, with an average 44% increase from 1996. Only 3 states reported decreases in staff from 1996–1999.[10] In this study, child care licensing experts and the literature recommended several licensing and enforcement practices as critical to ensure that child care providers comply with state licensing rules. These activities included:

- Conducting background checks of all adults working alone with children before granting a license.
- At least 1 unannounced inspection per year for child care centers and large family child care homes; 1 unannounced inspection every 5 years for small family child care homes.
- Enforcement sanctions should be a part of the regulatory system, including an array of enforcement options, such as fines and revocation of license.
- Licensing staff should be required to have appropriate education and experience for their assigned category of child care with at least 24 hours of continuing education per year.
- Caseloads for licensing staff should consist of no more than 75 licensed programs.

When comparing data across states, the General Accounting Office study found that states were generally following the recommended practices regarding background checks, frequency of monitoring visits, use of unannounced visits, enforcement of sanctions, and training for licensing staff. Most states reported that they did not have caseloads at the recommended level, and they did not regulate all out-of-home child care providers, as recommended by experts. Eleven states reported caseloads at or below the recommended level of 75 facilities; one third of the states reported caseloads more than double the recommended levels.[11]

In many states, quality improvement federal funding has been used to help licensing agencies to improve their licensing and monitoring activities, to increase the number of licensing staff, to improve licensing rules, and to increase training opportunities for licensing staff. These funds continue to have a powerful positive effect on the protection of children with states using varying amounts to improve the licensing function. Strong advocacy is still needed in states and nationally to ensure that the necessary level of funding is maintained and increased.

Recent publications have clearly pointed out the problems with the current regulatory system. Criticizing the lax enforcement in many states, Gormley reported in *Everybody's Children* on the low number of license revocations across the country. He finds this data especially disturbing in light of the large percentage of inadequate care found by studies on child care quality. He attributes lax enforcement to the following causes: "inspectors have mixed feelings about punitive sanctions; they possess a limited range of tools to deal with code violations; and they are put off by a cumbersome legal process." Gormley makes a strong case for the use of an array of intermediate sanctions, "regulatory bargaining," and greater regulatory attention to facilities with "bad track records."[12] Howard, in *The Death of Common Sense: How Law Is Suffocating America*, eloquently describes the unintended consequences of too much regulation bogged down in detail, which restricts innovation. He strongly recommends giving more discretion to regulators to interpret a small number of general rules with flexibility as dictated by the regulated setting.[13]

Despite the problems with current regulation, recent research on child care quality has shown that state regulation and monitoring of child care do improve quality. In 1 study, states with stronger licensing standards had fewer poor-quality child care centers.[14] Another study found that in Florida, child-staff ratios and training requirements in their licensing rules improved the intellectual and emotional development of children in child care centers.[8] In a third study, regulated family child care homes provided better quality than unregulated child care—that is, 13% of regulated homes provided "inadequate" care, in contrast to 50% of the unregulated homes.[8] These are just a few of the many research studies on quality early care and education that have shown the importance of licensing for positive outcomes for children.

There are many continuing challenges facing human care regulation to remove unnecessary bureaucratic processes, improve efficiency, and be more responsive to consumers and the industry. As states respond to the current climate of deregulation and reinvention of government, it is important to keep in mind that, despite general criticism, public support has grown stronger for regulation that provides consumer protection through prevention. In addressing the challenges to reform the way they do business, it will be critical for states to satisfy the criteria for effective licensing to ensure out-of-home care that appropriately decreases the risk of harm.

RECOMMENDATIONS TO REFORM THE REGULATORY SYSTEM

To remain viable and to improve efficiency and effectiveness, sound child care regulatory programs have continually worked to refine their monitoring and enforcement efforts, taking advantage of the latest technology and information. Class, Morgan, and others have over the years provided much guidance to the field on regulatory refinement and reform. Without federal support of the licensing function, licensing agencies have operated at the whim of state legislatures and consequently reflect a very uneven pattern of consumer protection.

In the 1980s, states' commitment to strengthening licensing programs diminished with a trend toward decreasing staff and regulatory coverage as the mechanism to decrease licensing caseloads. At the same time that greater emphasis was placed on streamlining licensing functions to make use of available resources, most states experienced a period of tremendous growth in the numbers of facilities, resulting in increased demands on the licensing system. States were often faced with expanding caseloads and diminished fixed resources. In some states, there were efforts by the legislature to erode or eliminate child care licensing programs by legislative exemptions, severe reduction, or elimination of funding.

NATIONAL PERSPECTIVE

Since the 1970s, early care and education professionals have advocated for a strong national policy recognizing the rights and needs of children, their parents, and child care providers. Appropriate early care and education require a healthy environment with good working conditions and well-trained, adequately compensated child care providers. Such a national policy will provide the framework necessary to ensure the appropriate investment at national, state, and local levels in early care and education.

Strong leadership and sufficient financial commitment from the federal government are needed to stimulate the conditions necessary to permit state and local communities to provide the supports necessary to parents, government, and child care providers for appropriate, affordable, and accessible early care and education for all children. Some progress has been made, but more is needed. In the area of regulation, strong federal support is needed for state regulatory functions and for an effective mix of regulatory and nonregulatory methods, as described earlier, to improve the quality of care.[15] Federal financial assistance to states, earmarked for sound regulatory reform, is recommended.

It is essential that there be a strong commitment to research in child care licensing to provide the data needed to support the components of regulatory programs and to study the impact of enforcement efforts and licensing rules in preventing harm to children in out-of-home care. Strong support is needed for educational and training standards for child care licensing staff to ensure that they are knowledgeable in child development as well as in the principles of regulatory administration. Funding and support is necessary to assist the National Association for Regulatory Administration in the development of national credentialing for licensors.

STATE PERSPECTIVE

States must continue to make a strong commitment to licensing and provide needed resources, including sufficient, qualified, well-trained staff to ensure effective regulation. States must focus on strong enforcement of rules in their reform of the regulatory process. In a 1994 supplement to *Pediatrics,* Morgan discussed the regulatory issues being debated today and set forth clear, well-justified solutions and recommendations for reform in the areas of enforcement and improved compliance.[16]

Gormley recommends a "bargaining model" of regulation that emphasizes regulatory enforcement rather than standard setting and encompasses greater flexibility by regulators, encouraging them to negotiate, use a variety of enforcement methods and intermediate sanctions, and "improvise, strike bargains, make deals, reward good performers, and punish bad performers." His model focuses attention and resources toward problem facilities for the most efficient use of scarce resources.[17]

Among the methods for reform proposed by Morgan and Gormley are some that have been in place in many states for a number of years and others that are still under discussion. The methods stress coordinated licensing, streamlined monitoring, giving more attention to problem facilities, and empowering licensors. To improve the regulatory process, states can:

- Streamline the regulatory system through better coordination and communication among zoning, building, fire safety, health agencies, and licensing to eliminate or minimize barriers to licensing—the creation of local teams is one suggested approach.
- Streamline the monitoring process through the use of licensing indicator systems to predict level of compliance with the comprehensive rules, portable computers on-site to decrease paperwork and time on site, differing attention to licensees on the basis of performance, and elimination of license renewal.
- Place emphasis on strong enforcement of rules, removing licenses from child care providers who willfully, deliberately, or frequently violate rules, and using a variety of intermediate sanctions, such as consent agreements and fines, to achieve compliance.
- Empower well-qualified licensors trained in consumer protection, law enforcement, and rights of licensees with greater discretion in licensing decisions.
- Institute reward systems for good compliance; require posting by licensees of compliance record and notices of noncompliance and negative sanctions; publish names of licensees in good compliance and those with negative sanctions.
- Institute improved coordination among all agencies and organizations that monitor programs, with staggered visits where feasible, to ensure consistent reinforcement of basic health and safety rules and communication of noncompliance.
- Update licensing statutes and policies to eliminate or decrease exemptions and strengthen monitoring and enforcement options.
- Improve rule-making process to ensure a democratic process and regular review of all rules.
- Provide parents with licensing records of compliance and substantiated complaints through resource and referral agencies.
- Provide consumer education on licensing through state Web sites.
- Provide parents with quality ratings of facilities or agency responsible for quality beyond licensing, including information about accreditation of programs.
- Provide computerized training records for all child care providers, including training beyond that required for licensing, and certificate of training record or qualifications.
- Develop comprehensive, coordinated career development systems for early child care providers and educators with involvement of licensing agency. Where possible, the licensing agency may provide management for the system.

In summary, regulation and child care licensing play a strong role in creating a safe, healthy, and nurturing setting for children receiving early care and education. The goal of licensing, as a form of consumer protection, is to decrease the risk of harm to children in out-of-home care. Licensing sets a lower limit of standards below which a program may not legally operate. Effective licensing is critical to promote safe, healthy, and appropriate care for all children. Programs are encouraged, by a mix of regulatory and nonregulatory methods, to achieve a higher level of quality. Coordination among all agencies and organizations in a state is important for effective safeguarding of children and advocacy for the development and enforcement of strong licensing standards. In the current climate of deregulation and regulatory reform, a number of recommendations were set out to create a more effective and appropriate regulatory system.

NATIONAL ASSOCIATION FOR THE EDUCATION OF YOUNG CHILDREN ACCREDITATION

An important complement to state licensing of early childhood programs is national, voluntary accreditation. As in other fields, such as health care, the early childhood profession developed and implements an accreditation system that is designated to achieve 2 goals: to improve the quality of care and education provided for young children in group programs and to recognize those programs that achieve substantial compliance with high standards for quality. The system described here, the National Academy of Early Childhood Programs, is sponsored by the National Association for the Education of Young Children (NAEYC), the nation's largest professional organization of early childhood educators, with a membership of more than 100 000. Other accreditation systems also exist, including 1 sponsored by the National Child Care Association, the National Early Childhood Program Accreditation, and an agency accreditation that encompasses child care services sponsored by the Council on Accreditation of Services for Children and Families. Family child care homes can be accredited by the National Association for Family Child Care. Child care and youth programs for school-aged children can be accredited by the National School-Age Care Alliance.

The NAEYC's accreditation system has been in operation since 1985 and is currently the largest, with nearly 8000 accredited programs and more than 8000 in the process. The NAEYC's system addresses all types of center-based early childhood programs, including full- and part-day centers, public and private child care, preschool, kindergarten programs, and school-aged child care centers. The enormous diversity of types of programs for young children is represented in NAEYC's system, including Head Start, public school, for-profit and nonprofit, employer-sponsored, parent cooperative, church and synagogue housed or operated, military child care, and many others. Programs accredited by the NAEYC are in all 50 states and many countries overseas where US military personnel are served.

The accreditation system is based on a set of national standards and involves a 3-step process: self-study, on-site validation visit, and commission decision. Accreditation is valid for 3 years. The self-study process involves all the key players in a program—administrator, teachers, parents, and even children—in a process of self-evaluation and improvement. A major piece of the process is an observation instrument that is used by teachers and administrators to determine the actual quality of children's experiences in classrooms. The process also incorporates questionnaires of administrators, directors, and parents and various documents related to program policies. These same tools are used by validators who go on-site to verify the accuracy of the program's report of its compliance with the accreditation criteria. The accreditation decision is based on a professional judgment of the program's overall compliance with the criteria.

The criteria for accreditation[18] are professionally approved standards. They address all components of an early childhood program: interactions among teachers and children, curriculum, relationships among teachers and families, staffing, administration, staff qualifications and professional development, health and safety, nutrition and food service, physical environment, and evaluation. The system is designed to build on rather than replace licensing standards and monitoring. Licensing is a prerequisite to accreditation.

Licensing is a prerequisite to accreditation.

Accreditation is also designed to complement licensing in that it emphasizes areas of the program that define the actual quality of the child's experiences (interactions among teachers and children and curriculum). These areas are also highly subjective and, therefore, less open to regulation by governmental bodies. Licensing, by contrast, can and should emphasize the more objective, measurable determinants or predictors of quality (such as staff-child ratio, physical environment, and health and safety provisions). Validators for accreditation (the individuals who conduct on-site visits) are early childhood professionals, not experts in health and safety. They are more qualified to observe and interpret the appropriateness of the curriculum than the safety of the physical structure. Nevertheless, because numerous states exempt various types of early childhood programs from licensure and because there is a very real lack of funds for regular monitoring of licensed programs in many states, accreditation standards and procedures must also address the regulatable characteristics of programs as much as possible.

The relationship of accreditation and licensing is a complex one.[19] Ideally, national accreditation standards are set higher than every state's minimum licensing standards. However, the wide range of diversity of state licensing standards in the United States complicates this simple assumption. As a result, in some states such as

Massachusetts or Connecticut, where licensing standards are closer to accreditation standards, achieving accreditation is not as difficult. In other states, where, for example, the licensing regulation allows twice as many children per adult as accreditation recommends, achieving accreditation can be a daunting economic challenge. In short, licensing standards tend to establish a market value for child care in a state that even the best intentioned of child care providers cannot ignore. Operating a national accreditation system in such diverse regulatory contexts is among the greater challenges facing the NAEYC.[20]

Many important issues confront accreditation systems in the field of early childhood education. One is the great difficulty of educating parents about accreditation.[21] Parents need to understand that neither licensing nor accreditation is a guarantee of a quality experience for their children, but they also need to understand that both licensing and accreditation provide important consumer protection and education services that need to be safeguarded. Child advocates of all types, including pediatricians, can play an important role in helping educate parents to the reality that all early childhood programs are not equal, that licensing is designed to ensure adequate rather than potentially harmful quality, and that accreditation is a tool to improve and recognize better-quality programs. Parents can contact the NAEYC or visit their Web site (http://www.naeyc.org/) for information about which programs are accredited and should inquire about accreditation status of programs they are considering.

A second major challenge facing accreditation is the trend toward deregulation of all human services. A private, professionally operated accreditation system may be an excellent alternative to government regulation, especially for services close to the family, such as child care. Nevertheless, voluntary accreditation cannot and should not replace the important consumer protection responsibility of state licensing. Accreditation is designed to identify good programs, but licensing is designed to protect every child from harm; these are complementary but not interchangeable functions.[19]

CONCLUSIONS AND RECOMMENDATIONS

Research indicates the components of a program most likely to result in positive outcomes for children (enhanced language, social, and cognitive development).[22] The biggest concern is that a great deal is known about what constitutes a high-quality, developmentally appropriate early childhood program, yet most American children are not experiencing this type of program.[23] Accreditation, in conjunction with state licensing, is an important strategy for moving research and theory to practice and improving the child care experiences of America's most vulnerable citizens.

REFERENCES

1. Class NE. Safeguarding day care through regulatory programs: the need for a multiple approach. In: *Proceedings of the Annual Meeting of National Association for the Education of Young Children*. Seattle, WA: National Association for the Education of Young Children; 1969:4–5

2. Morgan G. *New Approaches to Regulation*. Boston, MA: Wheelock College Institute for Leadership and Career Initiatives; 1995:4

3. Helburn S, Culkin ML. *Cost, Quality, and Child Outcomes in Child Care Centers: Executive Summary*. Denver, CO: University of Colorado at Denver; 1995:2

4. Galinsky E, Howes C, Kontos S, Shinn M. *The Study of Children in Family Child Care and Relative Care: Highlights of Findings*. New York City, NY: Families and Work Institute; 1994:1–6

5. Adams GC. Summary and introduction. In: *How Safe? The Status of State Efforts to Protect Children in Child Care*. Washington, DC: Children's Defense Fund; 1995:1–13

6. Brown N, Costley JB, Morgan G. *Delaware First...Again: The First Comprehensive State Training Plan for Child Care Staff*. Boston, MA: The Center for Career Development in Early Care and Education; 1990

7. Kusserow RP. *Enforcing Child Care Regulations*. Washington, DC: US Department of Health and Human Services; 1990

8. Howes C, Smith E, Galinsky E. Brief summary of findings. In: *The Florida Child Care Quality Improvement Study: Interim Report*. New York, NY: Families and Work Institute; 1995:1–2

9. Adams GC. *Who Knows How Safe?* Washington, DC: Children's Defense Fund; 1990:41–53

10. US General Accounting Office. *Child Care: State Efforts to Enforce Safety and Health Requirements*. Washington, DC. US General Accounting Office, 2000

11. US General Accounting Office. *Child Care: States Face Difficulties Enforcing Standards and Promoting Quality*. Washington, DC: US General Accounting Office; 1992

12. Gormley WT Jr. *Everybody's Children: Child Care as a Public Problem*. Washington, DC: The Brookings Institution; 1995

13. Howard PK. *The Death of Common Sense: How Law Is Suffocating America*. New York, NY: Random House; 1994

14. Helburn S, Culkin ML. *Cost, Quality, and Child Outcomes in Child Care Centers: Executive Summary*. Denver, CO: University of Colorado at Denver; 1995:4

15. Galinsky E, Howes C, Kontos S, Shinn M. Predictors of quality: regulation. In: *The Study of Children in Family Child Care and Relative Care: Highlights of Findings*. New York City, NY: Families and Work Institute; 1994:47–51

16. Koch PD. Regulation and guidelines toward a healthy child-care setting. *Pediatrics*. 1994;94(6 Pt 2):1104–1107

17. Morgan G. New *Approaches to Regulation*. Boston, MA: Wheelock College Institute for Leadership and Career Initiatives; 1995:14–16

18. National Association for the Education of Young Children. *Accreditation Criteria and Procedures of the National Association for the Education of Young Children*. Washington, DC: National Association for the Education of Young Children; 1998

19. Morgan G. Licensing and accreditation: How much quality is *quality*? In: Bredekamp S, Willer BA, eds. *NAEYC Accreditation: A Decade of Learning and the Years Ahead.* Washington, DC: National Association for the Education of Young Children; 1996: 129-138

20. Bredekamp S, Glowacki S. *The First Decade of NAEYC Accreditation: Growth and Impact on the Field.* Washington, DC: National Association for the Education of Young Children; 1996:1-10

21. Reisman B. What do parents want? Can we create consumer demand for accredited child care programs? In: Bredekamp S, Willer BA, eds. *NAEYC Accreditation: A Decade of Learning and the Years Ahead.* Washington, DC: National Association for the Education of Young Children; 1996:139-148

22. Bredekamp S, Willer BA. *NAEYC Accreditation: A Decade of Learning and the Years Ahead.* Washington, DC: National Association for the Education of Young Children; 1996

23. Cost, Quality, and Child Outcomes Study Team. *Cost, Quality, and Child Outcomes in Child Care Centers.* Denver, CO: Economics Department, University of Colorado at Denver; 1995

ADDITIONAL RESOURCES

Child Care Aware
1319 F Street NW, Suite 500
Washington, DC 20004
Phone: 800/424-2246
Web site: http://www.childcareaware.org/en/licensing/

Healthy Child Care America (HCCA)
American Academy of Pediatrics
141 Northwest Point Boulevard
Elk Grove Village, IL 60007
Phone: 800/433-9016
Web site: http://www.healthychildcare.org

National Association for the Education of Young Children (NAEYC)
1509 16th Street NW
Washington, DC 20036
Phone: 800/424-2460
Web site: http://www.naeyc.org
Accredited program search: http://www.naeyc.org/accreditation/center_search.asp

National Association for Family Child Care (NAFCC)
5202 Pinemont Drive
Salt Lake City, UT 84123
Phone: 801/269-9338
Web site: http://www.nafcc.org

National Child Care Association (NCCA)
1016 Rosser Street
Conyers, GA 30012
Phone: 800/543-7161
Web site: http://www.nccanet.org

National Child Care Information Center (NCCIC)
Web site: http://www.nccic.org
243 Church Street NW, 2nd Floor
Vienna, VA 22180
Phone: 800/616-2242

National Early Childhood Program Accreditation (NECPA)
126C Suber Road
Columbia, SC 29210
Phone: 800/505-9878
Web site: http://www.necpa.net

National Resource Center for Health and Safety in Child Care
UCHSC at Fitzsimmons
Campus Mail Stop F541
PO Box 6508
Aurora, CO 80045
Phone: 800/598-KIDS
Web site: http://nrc.uchsc.edu

National School-Age Care Alliance (NSACA)
1137 Washington Street
Dorchester, MA 02124
Phone: 617/298-5012
Web site: http://www.nsaca.org

The Nation's Network of Child Care Resource and Referral (NACCRRA)
1319 F Street, NW, Suite 500
Washington, DC 20004-1106
Phone: 202-393-5501
Web site: http://www.naccrra.org

CHAPTER 3

Financing: Issues of Cost and Quality in Child Care

Barbara Reisman, MBA, CPA

LEARNING OBJECTIVES

- The reader will understand that good-quality child care (care that meets the developmental and educational needs of children and the workforce needs of their parents) costs more to provide than does poor-quality care.

- The reader will learn that child care is, by necessity, a labor-intensive service and that the compensation and training of staff have a direct relationship to the quality of early childhood education.

- The reader will understand why the price of care is high for parents, and yet quality in most programs is mediocre to poor.

- The reader will understand the current sources of funding for child care: primarily parent fees, with a significant but secondary investment from federal, state, and local governments and a very small level of participation from employers and private philanthropies. Comparisons are made to the dramatically different funding structure for public schools and higher education.

INTRODUCTION

Thirteen million children younger than 6 years and 17 million school-aged children are in child care for all or part of their day. Parents use child care for a variety of reasons: to give their children social and educational experiences that help them develop and be ready for school; to provide a safe haven and opportunities for enrichment before and after school; or to enable parents to work, confident that their children are well cared for. Parents select the type of child care that will meet the needs of their child and their work schedules. To understand the economic impact of child care on families, it is important to distinguish between paid and unpaid care, as well as among the types of care. Parents do not usually pay relatives who care for their children, although 17% of relative-care arrangements are reimbursed. According to data from the Urban Institute from 1999, parents or other relatives were the primary caregivers for 54% of preschool children with an employed parent. Fourteen percent of preschool children are cared for in family child care homes and 28% are in child care centers, Head Start programs, or nursery or prekindergarten programs. As children approach school age, parents tend to favor more formal types of child care arrangements, most of which they pay for, including child care centers, nursery schools, Head Start, and prekindergarten programs. For parents who pay for care, and especially for low-income working families, child care represents a significant cost. In 1993, families who paid for care for preschool children and had incomes less than $14 400 per year paid an average of 25% of their income for child care. Families with incomes more than $54 000 per year paid about 6% of their incomes for child care.

This chapter will outline the factors contributing to the cost of providing child care, describe the current sources of funding, and outline recommendations for increasing investment in child care to improve quality and ensure that all families have access to the type and quality of child care their children need.

THE RELATIONSHIP BETWEEN COST AND QUALITY

The quality of care children receive is dependent on the following 3 factors: the safety of the environment, the attentiveness and responsiveness of the adults who staff the program, and the opportunity the children have to engage in stimulating activities appropriate to their age and level of development. Each of these factors contributes to the cost of providing out-of-home care, but the most significant component of child care cost is the cost of labor. Labor costs represent 70% to 80% of the total cost of a good-quality child care program, whether it is a center-based program or a family child care home.

The quality of child care and its impact on the child and the family are directly correlated with the cost of providing it. High quality in child care programs requires high staff-child ratios, small groups, and well-trained and well-compensated staff. All of these factors make child care a labor-intensive service to provide. Child care is similar to public schooling and higher education in terms of the social benefits that accrue with improved educational outcomes. However, unlike public schooling or higher education, both of which are more generally viewed as public goods, child care is largely paid for by parent fees. As shown in Fig 3.1, parent fees account for 60% of all child care expenditures. Government at the federal, state, and local levels provides 39% of funding, primarily by subsiding low-income working families and by providing tax credits. The private sector, including employers and philanthropies, contributes about 1% of the total fees.

Good-quality child care contributes to family stability, children's health, and later school success. Longitudinal studies demonstrate that these gains are greatest for children from low-income families, that the gains persist throughout the child's life, and that the value of these gains far outweighs the cost. However, most children (74%) are in care that is mediocre, which neither harms the child nor provides the stimulation or stable relationships that maximize child development.

A significant proportion of children, approximately 12% overall but half of all infants, are in care that can only be described as poor and that may in fact be dangerous to the child. For infants and toddlers, this may mean that caregivers are not responsive to children's needs, that they fail to respond when children cry, that diapers are not changed, that children are not held when they are fed, or even that children are exposed to unsanitary conditions or dangerous substances. Similar results were found for centers and family child care homes.

AFFORDABILITY: THE GAP BETWEEN WHAT PARENTS CAN PAY AND WHAT QUALITY COSTS

Families who pay for child care spend, on average, about $3800 per year for 1 or more preschool children. By contrast, national experts peg the cost of providing good-quality care at $5000 to $8300 per child per year. These latter figures represent 26% to 44% of the gross income for a family of 4 earning the median income and paying for child care for 2 children. Clearly, most working families cannot afford to pay this high a proportion of their family income for child care. Some families decide to work fewer hours to decrease their need for child care. In about 25% of all 2-parent families, the parents work different shifts to decrease their need for care. Other parents choose a lower-priced alternative, sacrificing quality.

CHILD CARE SUBSIDIES: PRICE VERSUS COST

The price parents pay for child care is related to but not the equivalent of the cost of providing it. Some parents receive subsidies that help decrease their cost. These subsidies come in several forms: direct government subsidies, tax credits, and employer benefits. Government subsidies are available primarily to families leaving welfare to enter the workforce or to families whose low income makes them eligible for supplemental government support. Much of these subsidies come from the federal government in the form of block grants to the states. The states are then free to decide which families will get help paying for care. With the implementation

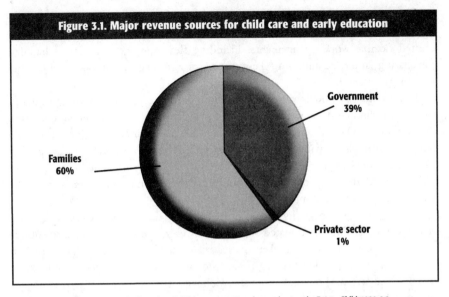

Figure 3.1. Major revenue sources for child care and early education

Government
39%

Families
60%

Private sector
1%

Source: Stoney L, Greenberg M. The financing of child care: current and emerging trends. *Future Child.* 1999;6:2.

of the Personal Responsibility Act (welfare reform), most states are directing the largest proportion of their subsidies to families moving from welfare to work. Low-income working families (the working poor) are increasingly relegated to waiting lists for child care assistance, despite the fact that their incomes are low enough to qualify them for child care support. Even mothers moving from welfare to work who are eligible for transitional child care often do not receive these benefits, usually because they are unaware that the benefits are available to them.

Single-parent families and 2-parent families in which both parents have earned income qualify for the Child and Dependent Care Tax Credit. The credit, which is nonrefundable, allows a credit equal to a percentage of the employment-related expenditures for any form of child care and entitles families to as much as a $720 credit for 1 child and $1440 for 2 or more children. In practice, virtually no families are able to claim the maximum credit, because it is available only to families whose incomes are below $10000. The maximum credit for families with incomes over $28000 is $480 for 1 child or $960 for 2 or more children. Thirty-one states also have child care tax credits, most of them calculated as a percentage of the federal Child and Dependent Care Tax Credit.

In the past 5 years, major corporations and some small employers have invested more than $350 million in child care initiatives. Although these investments have garnered significant public attention, they account for less than 1% of total spending on child care. The funds have been used primarily to help start new child care centers, to recruit and train family child care providers, and to improve the quality of child care services. Many employers have established dependent care assistance plans, which enable employees to pay for child care in pretax dollars. Others have created flexible work arrangements, including flex-time and part-time schedules, job sharing, and telecommuting. Few employers subsidize the ongoing cost of child care for their employees.

Many states are now investing public funds to create prekindergarten programs, usually for children deemed to be at risk of some form of developmental, cognitive, or social delay. These programs often operate on a part-year and part-day basis, making them difficult for parents who are working full-time to use them. Many parents use these programs by making multiple arrangements for their children, for example, a prekindergarten program in the morning, and a family child care home in the afternoon and for the summer.

Many child care programs also receive charitable donations, including rent-free space, volunteer time, or donated supplies. However, the biggest source of subsidy for child care is the below-market salaries that teachers and other child care staff receive. Child care providers struggle, too often unsuccessfully, to get by on fees that parents can afford. Low staff compensation and the resulting high rates of staff turnover have a deleterious impact on children; they disrupt the trusting relationships with parents and caregivers that form the foundation of cognitive and social development. Whether in a center or family child care home, revenue from parent fees alone does not allow most child care providers to offer children the trained staff, small group sizes, and low child-to-adult ratios that encourage frequent, responsive adult interactions with each child that are at the heart of good-quality child care.

Low staff compensation and the resulting high rates of staff turnover have a deleterious impact on children.

Staff, directors, teachers, aides, and other personnel are key to the quality of any early childhood program. Child care providers need to be well trained and adequately compensated if they are to provide children with the attention, stimulation, and continuity children need to thrive. Yet, child care teachers are among the lowest paid of any professional occupational category. Low pay and poor working conditions cause 31% of child care staff to leave their jobs each year.[1] For the director of a child care center, turnover is a constant disruption; children experience this turnover as loss. Repeated changes in caregivers may contribute to lower cognitive outcomes as well as difficulty in forming secure attachments to other adults and children. A recent study by the Center for the Child Care Workforce, a follow-up to its comprehensive 1988 *National Child Care Staffing Study*, found that staff in child care centers earn just slightly more than the minimum wage, and only 21% of centers provide paid health insurance. Child care teachers, most of whom have college degrees in early childhood education, earn about

$18 988 annually, less than the average salary of working women with a high school diploma.

RESEARCH RELATES COST TO QUALITY

Two recent studies have examined the operating costs of child care centers and of family child care homes. Both of these studies found that:

1. Parent fees are the single largest source of revenue for both types of care.
2. Salaries and other personnel costs are the single largest item in child care program budgets, comprising about 70% of total operating costs.
3. The cost structures in family child care homes and centers are different, but the fees charged to parents are similar for preschoolers and lower for infants in family child care homes.
4. Nonprofit and for-profit centers have different revenue sources and allocate costs differently, but there are no significant differences in variable costs per child hour between the 2 sectors.

The study of *Cost, Quality, and Child Outcomes in Child Care Centers*,[1] one of the few studies of the relationship between cost and quality of child care services, found "positive, significant, but modest relationships between cost and quality. Specifically, the results suggest that raising quality from mediocre to good would increase total variable costs by about 10%. This assumes that wages, hours of service provided, space, and volunteer hours remain about the same." The study also found that child care teachers and other staff provide what the researchers describe as a supply subsidy in the form of forgone wages. This assumption about forgone wages, its relationship to high staff turnover, and the resulting diminution in quality becomes a critically important factor in estimating the cost of increasing quality from mediocre to good. The researchers' estimate of those costs holds wages equal; were they to increase to a level that child care providers could earn in occupations requiring similar experience and education, the cost of increasing quality would be much greater.

CONCLUSIONS AND RECOMMENDATIONS

Despite the fact that child care provides educational, social, and developmental experiences for nearly 30 million children at a key point in their development, it is viewed primarily as a consumer good; a product that parents can choose to use. This view persists even though 80% of all children are in some form of out-of-home care or preschool setting before they reach kindergarten. Although policy makers tend to make a distinction between early childhood education and child care (one is designed to help children be ready for school and the other is primarily to provide a safe place for children while their parents work), young children are learning and developing from birth, and their earliest social and educational experiences help determine how well they will do in school and as adults.

The plain fact, now borne out of research that delves into the microeconomics of child care centers and family child care homes, is that child care cannot be of good quality and affordable to most working parents. Without additional investment from the public (local, state, and federal government) and private (employers and private philanthropies) sectors, child care for most families will remain mediocre at best and poor to even dangerous for some.

Most recent studies of child care have proposed greater public investment, stricter state licensing standards, and increased efforts to educate parents about the value of good-quality child care and its characteristics. These recommendations may also call for greater flexibility on the job and some form of paid parental leave. These proposals often face stiff opposition from those who claim that such investments would favor families with working mothers over those with mothers who stay at home. This opposition seems particularly disingenuous given the passage and implementation of the Personal Responsibility Act, which requires poor single mothers with children as young as 12 weeks to go to work or engage in some work-related activity to be eligible for any form of welfare, food stamps, or Medicaid.

The health care profession can play a key role in helping parents understand the importance of good-quality child care, make appropriate choices for their children, and get better information about resources that help parents pay for care. Resource and referral agencies are community-based agencies that provide information to parents about the child care available in their community. These agencies usually have printed materials for parents that can be made available for distribution in doctors' offices and clinics.

Medical professionals in many communities are volunteering to provide well-child examinations and immunizations for young children and to screen for developmental delays that can be reversed with early intervention. Child care programs are eager to collaborate with such efforts.

Finally, doctors and nurses can play an important role as advocates for better quality child care and for more public investment that will improve the quality of care and make it more accessible to working families. They are a trusted voice in their communities, with personal and profound knowledge of the challenges families with young children face. When they speak on behalf of the families they care for, health care professionals can be eloquent and persuasive.

REFERENCE

1. Helburn S, Culkin ML. *Cost, Quality, and Child Outcomes in Child Care Centers: Executive Summary.* Denver, CO: University of Colorado at Denver; 1995

ADDITIONAL RESOURCES

Children's Defense Fund. *The High Cost of Child Care Puts Quality Care Out of Reach for Many Families.* Washington, DC: Children's Defense Fund; 2000. Available at: http://www.childrensdefense.org/pdf/highcost.pdf

Council of Economic Advisers. *The Economics of Child Care.* Washington, DC: Council of Economic Advisers; 1997

David and Lucile Packard Foundation. Long-term outcomes of early childhood programs. *Future Child.* 1995;5:3

Mitchel A, Stoney L, Dichter H. *Financing Child Care in the United States.* Kansas City, MO: Ewing Marion Kauffman Foundation; 2001

The Urban Institute. *Child Care Expenses of America's Families.* Washington, DC: The Urban Institute; 2000

US Census Bureau. *Who's Minding the Kids? Child Care Arrangements.* Washington, DC: US Census Bureau; 1999

US Department of Agriculture. *Expenditures on Children by Families: 2001 Annual Report.* Washington, DC: US Department of Agriculture; 2002

CHAPTER 4

Designing a Safe and Healthy Child Care Environment

Mark D. Pavey, AIA, and Michael A. Lindstrom, AIA

LEARNING OBJECTIVES

After reading this chapter, the reader will:

- Be able to describe elements of playground design and layout necessary for safe use.

- Be familiar with construction elements that are important to prevent hazardous situations (eg, no dangling blind cords; correct water temperature, light, and ventilation; etc).

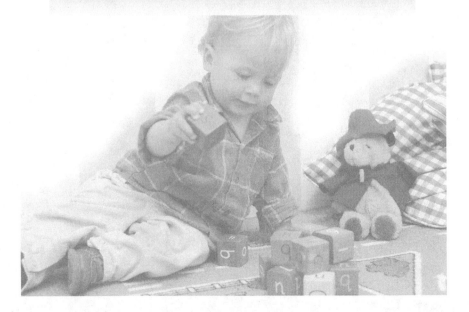

INTRODUCTION

As parents flock to child care centers in ever increasing numbers, their primary concern is for the safety of their children. Placing a child in a center with many other children raises concerns about injuries and disease control. Health care professionals must be prepared to counsel parents about how to compare and select a center. It is important that the center balances health and safety while providing an environment that promotes appropriate child development. There are many ways a center can help protect and nurture a child without creating a cold, sterile environment.[1,2]

At least as important as the physical environment is to a safe, nurturing learning environment are the quality, training, enthusiasm, and creativity of the child care providers. For example, a rich, challenging outdoor learning environment may be more or less safe depending on the training, involvement, and attentiveness of the staff.

SITE DESIGN

Initially, the location of a center should be considered with safety in mind. The neighborhood is an issue, as are ease of evacuation, noise levels, and traffic volume. A center should not be located too close to a railroad, airport, or major highway. It should not be situated within another building in a way that would impede evacuation of the center in an emergency. The location should be free of obvious hazards, including open pools, unprotected ledges or cliffs, dangerous equipment, drainage ditches, or open storm drainage structures. Although there is conflicting data on the effect of electromagnetic fields, it may be prudent not to locate a center near telecommunication towers.

Soil contamination is a serious problem in many parts of the country, particularly in urban areas where there is a high concentration of manufacturing or industrial facilities. An environmental audit should be completed on any new site or playground area to assess for lead, polychlorinated biphenyls, or other hazardous substances. In existing buildings, testing for lead paint and asbestos will probably be required and should be undertaken even if not required.[3,4] Radon is a lethal gas that occurs naturally in many areas of the country and in many common building materials, such as concrete block and drywall. Radon has been estimated by the US Environmental Protection Agency (EPA) to be the leading cause of lung cancer in nonsmokers. The local EPA office or state agency will provide inexpensive test kits and offer guidance on mitigation. Generally, radon can be controlled with ventilation (typically under a concrete slab) and sealing.[5]

The site should be laid out to permit access by emergency vehicles. The parking area and building entries should be well lit. Parking areas should be screened or fenced if they are adjacent to a hazardous area, such as a roadway with heavy traffic. Parking and drop-off areas should be designed to minimize pedestrians crossing vehicle lanes. Security phones or duress alarms may be desirable in high-security settings. Parking lot lighting is essential, because staff members and some parents leave the center after dark, particularly in the winter months, when most other employees have left the premises. Ideally, an unobstructed line of sight should be provided from the director's office to the parking lot.

PLAYGROUNDS

The layout and selection of equipment in playgrounds is critical to child safety. The US Public Interest Research Group and the Consumer Federation of America have said, "Too many children are getting hurt and killed on our playgrounds. Approximately 170 100 children are injured seriously enough on public playground equipment to require emergency room treatment each year. Tragically, an average of 17 children die each year playing on playgrounds. Many of these deaths and injuries could be prevented if playgrounds—from equipment to surfacing to layout—were designed with safety in mind."[6]

The prevailing philosophy in the past was to install a large play piece and a couple of swings in the yard and call it a playground. This created high densities of active children in relatively small areas. The new thinking about playground design provides many activities spread out over the entire yard. Children have more choices, are more dispersed, and are less prone to injury.

In the past 10 years, investigators have learned that fall zones and impact materials are the most critical safety factor on playgrounds. The Consumer Product Safety Commission (CPSC)[7] and American Society for Testing of Materials (ASTM) maintain guidelines covering many aspects of playground equipment safety. Some state child care licensing regulations reference 1 or both. The 2 sets of guidelines do not always contain the same recommendations. Wood mulch pits (often called engineered wood fiber) are 1 recommended option for fall zone material appropriate in most areas of the country. Mulch generally has a low first cost but must be replenished at least once a year. Rubber impact mats and resilient rubber surfacing are satisfactory fall zone materials, providing a low maintenance, wheeled toy-friendly, wheelchair accessible surface. There are limitations to the material; it does not have the inherent play value of sand and is somewhat monotonous when overused. Rubber also has a relatively high first cost and may be slippery when wet. Mats may lose their color or harden, leaving a hot black surface exposed. Sand is an excellent playground material; however, one cannot dismiss the maintenance problems it creates inside and outside the center or the potential health hazards created by open sandpits. Sand can pose challenges; however, all other things being equal, a playground without sand will not provide as rich an experience as a playground with sand. Round rock and pea gravel can provide an excellent impact material; however, they tend to be of the size that easily gets put into ears and noses as well as swallowed and thrown and have little inherent play value. Tire chips have good resiliency and a low cost; however, they stain clothing and shoes easily.

The playground equipment itself must be carefully evaluated. Slides more than 6 feet high, which is higher than necessary for play value, only increase the risk of injury. Improperly sized openings in play equipment pose a head entrapment hazard (3-9 inches) that may lead to strangulation. Swings can be very hazardous. If provided, they should be placed away from travel paths to avoid collisions. Swing seats that are made of wood, metal, or other rigid material increase the severity of injury if impact occurs. Small gaps, open s-hooks, and other protrusions pose clothing entanglement hazards, in particular for drawstrings on clothing. A play yard should not contain metal slides that may burn a child when hot. Traditional seesaws become very hazardous when a child jumps off. Spring riders are heavy moving objects that can easily collide with a passing child. Wooden playground structures might be treated with carcinogenic creosote, and splinters likely will be a major problem.[8]

A well-planned playground should have a high-quality fence 6 feet tall at the perimeter with locking gates. Fire codes may require that gates not be locked from the inside while playgrounds are occupied. Childproof latches are available for unlocked gates.[9] A 6-foot fence is generally the best height to provide security for children (preventing child snatching) as well as vandalism control. Gates should be self-closing and self-latching. Like interior doors, the gates must prevent finger pinching. Fence elements must be smooth, with no finials or sharp pickets on which children might be

A well-planned playground should have a high-quality fence 6 feet tall at the perimeter with locking gates.

injured. Fences must discourage climbing, with no horizontal rails except at the bottom and top. Fastening devices should project outward to prevent injury. Wood fences should be splinter free and nontoxic. Guardrails, bollards, or planters should be provided to protect playgrounds located next to roads or driveways.

The playground should be laid out so that staff can observe many activities from 1 location, with no hidden areas. Activities should be separated and swings should be located away from pedestrian circulation. All edges on equipment, benches, landscape edging, etc should be rounded, with no protruding bolts or rusty sharp edges. Any potentially poisonous plants should be removed. Table 4.1 contains a list of common plants considered to be poisonous.

Children require some play area that is protected from the sun as well as accessible to drinking fountains. The importance of shade in warmer climates cannot be overestimated. In general, one should not count on newly planted trees to provide shade for 4 or 5 years. Building overhangs and porches are very effective and are also useful on rainy days. Commercially available or custom-made shade structures can be used to supplement porches and mature trees and to create dramatic play and interest areas within larger play spaces.

TABLE 4.1. Poisonous Plants

Amaryllis	English ivy	Monkshood
Arrowhead/nephthytis	English yew	Morning glory
Asparagus	Euonymous	Mother-in-law
Autumn Crocus	Four-o'clock	Mountain laurel
Azalea	Foxglove	Mushrooms (certain ones)
Barberry	Fruit pits or seeds	Narcissus
Belladonna	Gladiola	Nightshade family
Birds of paradise	Green parts of tomato	Oak (acorns)
Bittersweet	Holly	Oleander
Black locust	Horse chestnut, buckeye	Peony
Bleeding heart	Hyacinth	Philodendron family
Boxwood	Hydrangea/snowball bush	Poinsettia
Buttercup	Indian hemp	Poison ivy, oak, sumac, and tobacco sumac
Caladium	Iris	Pokeweed
Castor-oil plant (bean)	Jack-in-the-pulpit	Privet
Chinaberry	Jequity bean (Rosary pea)	Rhododendron
Chinese evergreen	Jerusalem cherry	Rhubarb leaves
Chokecherry	Jimsonweed	Skunk cabbage
Chrysanthemum	Jonquil	Snow on the mountain
Crown of thorns	Juniper	Sprouts and green parts of potato
Daffodil	Larkspur	Water hemlock
Dumbcane/dieffenbachia	Lily of the valley	Wisteria
Elderberry	Mistletoe	Yew

Children will experiment with running, throwing, and climbing. At times, they seem to dare death and destruction by running up the slide, sliding or swinging on stomachs, climbing to scary heights, and standing on top of a "mountain." Equipment and materials should be continuously monitored for safety and repair as well as safe use. Swings are not unsafe in and of themselves, even swings where children can stand or swing on their stomachs. Platforms, ladders, or slides also are not inherently unsafe. However, if supervision is lax, if there are too many children and/or too few things to do, if the playground is too small, or if there are hard objects nearby that increase the potential for injury, the use of active playground equipment does present a threat.[10] Climbing equipment should be age appropriate, and equipment that is not challenging enough may encourage inappropriate use (eg, 5-year-olds climbing on the roof of a play piece intended for toddlers).

Hilly playgrounds are not necessarily unsafe; topography can add to the play experience if designed properly. Jack and Jill should run up the hill, and when they run down, there should not be a fence or other hard object to run into.

BUILDING DESIGN AND PHILOSOPHY

Along with industry growth, center design philosophy has changed dramatically as providers are moving from child care to child development. Centers are becoming more homelike in design, often in opposition to health and safety concerns. Providing a homelike setting has meant providing spaces that are more residential in scale and feeling than typical commercial construction. These centers may include finishes and materials such as wood cabinets, soft window treatments, area rugs, pillows, residential furniture, and the like. These elements, which act to warm the center and make it more appealing, need to be of appropriate materials to meet basic health and safety standards.

Home is where people feel familiar and secure; it is predictable. Children's settings require ordered space—space that furthers the program goals while creating a pleasant place to live and work for all those who inhabit the center. Hazards inside a center include falls, falling objects, burns, fires, poisoning, choking, cuts, punctures, etc. The goal should be to eliminate the chance of serious accidents that might lead to permanent injury and to minimize minor injuries. In a sterile, padded world with insufficient stimulation, children turn themselves off or turn to and on each other for stimulation. Too much concern for safety and containment prevents learning autonomy and responsibility.

VISUAL CONTROL

A controlled exit that allows teachers to observe as each child is dropped off and picked up is absolutely essential. Parents must be required to come into the building and sign their child in and out. A secured vestibule with a security keypad will keep unwanted visitors away. There should be limited access for children to areas that are dangerous. With rare exception, children should only have access to classrooms, playgrounds, and common areas. Kitchen areas should be designed so that unsupervised children do not have access. Exit doors (which cannot be locked from the inside) leading to unsupervised or dangerous areas (parking lot, dumpster, etc) should have alarms to alert teachers if the door is opened.

Staff must be able to supervise children's activities at all times, including times when they are changing diapers, children are in restrooms, or children are on the playground. The plan of the building should avoid blind spots or areas that are not easy to observe and give the teachers the ability to view their class as well as other classes. This can be accomplished by consciously designing view windows and the strategic use of mirrors with sight lines in mind (between classrooms, from corridor to classroom, as well as between the classroom and the playground).

Children's bathrooms should be designed to provide teachers with clear visible access. Children's bathroom doors should generally be low gates to facilitate supervision by sight and sound. Classroom and playground doors should have full glass vision panels to permit supervision, increase natural light, and avoid opening doors into small children.

CURRICULUM SUPPORT

The facility should be planned to allow maximum efficiency and organization for staff. Adequate storage within a workable plan is essential to a child's health and safety. When staff can easily keep areas orderly and clean, they can better supervise the children and provide them with a safer environment from a sanitary and practical standpoint.

Within the room, a barrier or distance must separate diapering and food preparation areas. Individual children's personal items must be kept separate with divided cubbies and well-spaced coat hooks (at least 12 inches apart). Storage closets should be lockable, and at least 1 lockable cabinet should be located in each classroom for the teacher's personal items.

FIRE SAFETY

Every child care center should have an emergency plan and highly visible evacuation plan posted in each room. At a minimum, smoke detectors should be provided in every classroom and the kitchen. A full fire alarm and smoke detection system that automatically notifies the fire department when activated is highly desirable. A fire extinguisher should be provided in every classroom and the kitchen. If the budget allows, a sprinkler system should be installed. Although not always required by building codes, sprinklers provide the highest level of fire safety to centers. There has been wide acceptance of residential sprinkler systems in child care centers. Typically, this type of sprinkler system can be installed at a third of the cost of a commercial system.

The center should be planned to allow for quick evacuation. Every classroom should have an alarmed exterior door leading directly to a fenced play area.

BUILDING MATERIALS

Toxic woods, lead paints, asbestos, and other hazardous materials have no place in a child care setting. Two-year-olds love to chew on whatever is available at their height. The use of pressure-treated lumber is discouraged in fences, fall zone borders, or as a part of any building element within 4 feet of the ground. Off-gassing of new building materials can be a far greater threat to children than to adults, because they have proportionally less internal tissue to absorb airborne pollutants.

Low-emitting volatile organic compound building products, especially carpet, should be used. If new carpet is installed, it should be allowed to freely ventilate for at least a week. Other possible contaminants are paints, polishes, pesticides, cleaning fluids, and particle board (formaldehyde). Every child care center should have a no-smoking policy on the premises.

All materials should be selected and specified without sharp corners or edges. Concrete sidewalks should have rounded edges. Brick rowlocks should be rounded. Sharp edges and abrasive surfaces should be avoided on millwork and other surfaces. Casework edges should be "eased," and countertops should be rounded. All interior wood trim should be rounded or smooth along its length and at corners.

All glass below 42 inches from the ground should be tempered or laminated safety glass. When screened windows are provided, guards should be provided to prevent children from falling through the screens.[11]

BUILDING FINISHES

All surfaces (especially in areas with diapering and toileting activities) should be made of durable and cleanable materials. Avoid seams and penetrations. Floors should be a seamless, resilient material, preferably with a turned up "hospital cove" base to facilitate cleaning and disinfecting. Area rugs, which can be removed and cleaned periodically, provide an additional soft surface for play. Vinyl pads and blocks are a better choice than fabric, because they are easily cleaned.

Wall hangings should be made from materials that meet class A flame spread requirements. Rugs should be finished so that the edges lay flat on the floor, preventing tripping. A closed cell carpet backing is preferable, because it doesn't absorb spills or promote the growth of microorganisms.

FURNISHINGS

Window treatments should be made of fire-rated fabrics and should have no dangling blind cords or loose parts that present a strangulation hazard. Some vinyl mini-blinds have high lead content and should be avoided.

In the infant room, 1 evacuation crib should be provided. In case of an emergency, all the babies are placed in this crib and wheeled outside. A direct exit route from this area to the outside should not require wheeling the crib up or down steps or other impediments.

The importance of commercial quality furnishings over residential quality is stressed for safety and durability. Furnishings and equipment in a child care center are exposed to much more use and abuse than in a home. They should be built to last.

Tacks and staples should not be used on bulletin boards in classrooms, because they pose a dangerous choking hazard. Magnetic boards or pliable adhesive are safer options for mounting paper.

All furniture and fixtures should be firmly secured to walls and floors. The tipping over of furniture is a leading cause of injury and death in child care centers. In earthquake-prone areas, it is more essential to secure as many pieces of the environment as possible.

DOORS AND HARDWARE

Doors are very dangerous in child care center settings. Fingers are commonly injured in child care center doors. The use of continuous nonpinch hinges is encouraged on all doors that are accessible and readily used by children. Lightweight, hollow-core doors also are encouraged in lieu of heavy solid doors with closers. The maintenance negative is far outweighed by the increased safety and lower first cost. Dutch doors should be avoided, again because of the increased risk of pinching. Devices are available that attach to the front and back of the hinge side of a door to prevent pinching. Closers, if properly adjusted, slow the speed at which the door closes and are essential on exterior doors that could be blown shut by the wind or slammed by a child. The Americans With Disabilities Act (ADA) now requires lever handle hardware on all doors. The lever design should be rounded and turn back toward to the door to help prevent eye injuries. All cabinet doors and drawers accessible to children should be provided with childproof latches mounted on the interior of the cabinet.

PLUMBING

Hand washing is the most important element in prevention of transmission of infectious diseases and food poisoning. Almost every area of a children's center should have access to water for washing hands, for drinking, for activities, and for cleanup. Sinks should be sized appropriately for the ages of the children using them. This encourages hand washing but also discourages the use of step stools at children's sinks, which can create a fall hazard. Every changing table should have an adjacent hand wash sink. The design of the table should consider the weight of the children being diapered. Many teachers have injured their backs lifting heavy 2-year-olds. There are changing tables available with pullout steps to eliminate lifting toddlers. However, the risk of back injury needs to be weighed against the less likely but potentially more serious possibility of head injury that might result from a child's fall from such a ladder or stair. Therefore, pullout steps should only be provided for tables in older children's rooms (those with 2- and 3-year-olds), and impact mats should be installed adjacent to the steps.

In infant and toddler rooms, toilets or flush rim sinks should be provided only if the center allows the use of cloth diapers and only if the center allows the caregiver to dump the feces instead of wrapping it up in the diaper. The most sanitary situation is the mandatory use of disposable diapers, with the baby changed in a manner that provides as little contact with the feces as possible (ie, wrap up the diaper and throw it in a plastic-lined can that is foot-pedal operated and closes tightly). Dumping of feces from either type diaper should be discouraged. For health reasons, the center should have a policy of not allowing cloth diapers.

Hot water should be readily accessible not because it kills germs, but rather because it makes hand washing a more pleasant task, encouraging more frequent washing. The need to restrict the temperature of hot water is sometimes overlooked. The center water heater should be set at 110°F for handwashing sinks. A tempering valve or a separate water heater should be included to provide 140°F water to the kitchen, laundry, and janitor's fixtures. A circulating pump is ideal for providing instant hot water. Water controls should be provided to minimize contamination; large "wrist blades" or electronic sensors are recommended at diapering stations. Storage for diapering supplies (diapers, wipes, lotion, etc) should be readily accessible and stored on open shelves or individual open cubbies to eliminate having to touch a cabinet door handle during the diapering process. Paper towel or changing table cover dispensers should not require hand contact. A dishwasher is useful and encourages teachers to frequently wash and disinfect toys.

Drinking fountains, if provided, should have angled mouthguards, because many children put the spout in their mouth before turning the water on. The safest method is to provide paper cups near a drinking fountain or sink.

Solder used to assemble copper piping should be lead free.

ELECTRICAL

Receptacles should be liberally provided to eliminate the use of extension cords. Outlets should be a safety type or have safety covers and should be mounted at least 18 inches above the floor and higher for shelf-mounted compact disc players and electronics. Adult-height counters should be provided with higher outlets. The ADA conflicts with child safety by requiring switches, fire alarm pulls, and other devices to be mounted at low heights. Fire alarm pulls can be provided with flip-up acrylic plastic covers to discourage children from playing with them. Switches, intercoms, etc may be mounted at 54 inches above the floor (the side reach for an adult in a wheelchair). Computer wiring, telephone wiring, and extension cords should be encased or attached to solid construction to prevent strangulation or electrocution.

Electrical meters (as well as all utility meters) should be located to allow reading without entering the playground. Light fixtures should have lenses, lamps with protective sleeves, or another mechanism to prevent a broken lamp from becoming a hazard to children. Light bulbs and fluorescent fixtures all should have lenses or protective sleeves to prevent shattering.

HEATING, VENTILATION, AND AIR CONDITIONING

Fresh air and natural light should be maximized in a child care center. Operable window area should be equal to a minimum of 5% of the floor area. The State of Georgia controls the capacity of the child care space on the basis of the amount of available window area. Windows should be sized to allow emergency evacuation if an exterior door is not provided. No room used for child care should be without windows. Exhaust vents should be provided above all diaper changing tables and in all toilet areas.

Gas-fired heating units must be properly vented and supplied with combustion air from outdoors. Heating units, grilles, and ductwork should be inaccessible to children. Carbon monoxide monitors should be provided if there is possibility of oxygen depletion of the interior air.

The temperature should be maintained from 68°F to 72°F 1 foot from the ground, although state requirements may vary. A high mixture of outside air in the heating, ventilating, and air conditioning system is desirable. Humidity of 50% to 55% is desirable to control the growth of mold and mildew. Controlling odors through ventilation is a real concern. If the budget allows, high volumes of outdoor air should be introduced to the center. A heat and cool air exchanger can recapture a high percentage of energy that would otherwise be exhausted. Quality and crispness of the air in centers with ventilation energy recovery units have been found to be far better than centers without them.

CODES AND THE ADA

Building codes and the ADA have been found not to address the concerns of children in child care settings adequately. Their concerns for fire egress and accessibility often ignore child safety concerns. Egress is important in case of a fire; however, children escaping and running out to the street is a far greater concern. The architect must educate many entities that govern the construction of a center to provide an acceptable balance of safety, accessibility, and age-appropriate learning spaces.[12]

CONCLUSIONS AND RECOMMENDATIONS

It is critically important to be able to evaluate a center during a quick tour from a standpoint of health and safety. Parents should have a basic awareness of the physical elements within a child care environment that would affect their children's well-being. Choosing a home away from home for their child can be intimidating. Hopefully, the information presented herein will provide some basic criteria for evaluating facilities.

REFERENCES

1. *ABCs of Safe and Healthy Child Care: An On-Line Handbook for Child Care Providers.* Atlanta, GA: Centers for Disease Control and Prevention, US Public Health Service, Department of Health and Human Services; 1997. Available at: http://www.cdc.gov/ncidod/hip/abc/abc.htm. Accessed March 19, 2004

2. American Academy of Pediatrics, Pennsylvania Chapter. Appendix Q. In: *Model Child Care Health Policies.* 4th ed. Rosemont, PA: American Academy of Pediatrics, Pennsylvania Chapter; 2002

3. *Lead Based Paint Interim Guidelines for Hazard Identification and Abatement in Public and Indian Housing.* Washington, DC: US Department of Housing and Urban Development; 1990

4. Environmental Protection Agency. *Lead in School Drinking Water.* Cincinatti, OH: National Service Center for Environmental Publications; 1989. Publication No. EPA 5709-89/001

5. US Environmental Protection Agency. *Radon in Water Sampling Program.* Washington, DC: Environmental Protection Agency, Office of Radiation and Indoor Air; 1978. Publication No. EPA/EERF-78-1

6. *Playing it Safe: A Fifth Nationwide Safety Survey of Public Playgrounds.* US Public Interest Research Group and The Consumer Federation of America; 2000. Available at: http://pirg.org/reports/consumer/playground2000. Accessed March 19, 2004

7. US Consumer Product Safety Commission. *Handbook for Public Playground Safety.* US Consumer Product Safety Commission; 2001. Available at: http://www.cpsc.gov/cpscpub/pubs/325.pdf. Accessed March 19, 2004

8. National Program for Playground Safety. *Selecting Playground Surface Materials: Guidelines for Selecting the Best Surface Material for Your Playground.* Cedar Falls, IA: National Program for Playground Safety, University of Northern Iowa. Available at: http://www.uni.edu/playground/products.html#surfacing_guide. Accessed March 19, 2004

9. Child safety latch. Hoover Fence Co. Available at: http://www.hooverfence.com/catalog/cpage32.htm. Accessed March 19, 2004

10. Olds AR. *Child Care Design Guide.* New York, NY: McGraw-Hill; 2001

11. Safety Standard for Architectural Glazing. US Consumer Product Safety Commission, 16 CFR §1201

12. *Child Care: State Efforts to Enforce Safety and Health Requirements.* Washington, DC: US General Accounting Office; 2000. Available at: http://www.gao.gov/new.items/he00028.pdf. Accessed March 19, 2004

ADDITIONAL RESOURCES

American Academy of Pediatrics, American Public Health Association, and Maternal and Child Health Bureau. *Caring for Our Children. National Health and Safety Performance Standards: Guidelines for Out-of-Home Child Care Programs.* 2nd ed. Elk Grove Village, IL: American Academy of Pediatrics; 2002

American Academy of Pediatrics, American Public Health Association, and Maternal and Child Health Bureau. *Stepping Stones to Using Caring for Our Children.* Elk Grove Village, IL: American Academy of Pediatrics; 2004

Bunnett R, Kroll D. Transforming spaces: rethinking the possibilities. Turning design challenges into opportunities. *Child Care Information Exchange.* Jan/Feb 2000;131

Child Care Bureau, Administration on Children, Youth, and Families. *Tribal Child Care Facilities: A Guide to Construction and Renovation.* Washington, DC: Child Care Bureau; 1999. Available at: http://www.nccic.org/pubs/tribguid.html. Accessed March 19, 2004

Child Care Law Center Web site. Available at: http://www.childcarelaw.com. Accessed March 19, 2004

Greenman J. *Places for Childhoods: Making Quality Happen in the Real World*. Redmond, WA: Exchange Press

Head Start Bureau, Administration on Children, Youth, and Families. *Head Start Center Design Guide for Head Start Facilities*. Arlington, VA: Head Start Bureau; 2000. Available at: http://www.headstartinfo.org/pdf/hscenterdesignguide.pdf. Accessed March 19, 2004

National Children's Facilities Network and Community Investment Collaborative for Kids Web site. Available at: http://www.liscnet.org. Accessed March 19, 2004

National Institute of Environmental Sciences. Electric and magnetic fields: basics. In: EMF Questions and Answers. Research Triangle Park, NC: National Institute of Environmental Sciences; 2002. Available at: http://www.niehs.nih.gov/emfrapid/booklet/basics.htm. Accessed March 19, 2004

National Resource Center for Health and Safety in Child Care Web site. Available at: http://nrc.uchsc.edu. Accessed March 19, 2004

Olds AR. *Child Care Design Guide*. New York, NY: McGraw-Hill; 2001

Ruth LC. *Design Standards for Children's Environments*. New York, NY: McGraw-Hill; 2000

Silverman FL, Driscoll D. Design collaborations—successes and failures in developing a child care center design. *Child Care Information Exchange*. Nov/Dec 2000;136

Spaces for Children. *Designing an Early Head Start Facility: Tips for Start Up*. Berkeley, CA: Spaces for Children; 2001. Available at: http://www.spacesforchildren.com/ehssetup.html. Accessed March 19, 2004

Spaces for Children. *Eight Steps in the Design Process for Child Care Centers*. Berkeley, CA: Spaces for Children; 2001. Available at: http://www.spacesforchildren.com/8steps.html. Accessed March 19, 2004

Spaces for Children. *Landscape for Learning: The Impact of Classroom Design on Infants and Toddlers*. Berkeley, CA: Spaces for Children; 2001. Available at: http://www.spacesfor children.com/landc1.pdf. Accessed March 19, 2004

Spaces for Children. *Landscapes for Learning Design Manual: Designing Group Care Environments for Infants and Toddlers*. Berkeley, CA: Spaces for Children; 1999

US Architectural and Transportation Barriers Compliance Board. *Guide to ADA Accessibility: Guidelines for Play Areas*. Washington, DC: US Access Board; 2001. Available at: http://www.access-board.gov/play/guide/guide.pdf. Accessed March 19, 2004

US General Services Administration. *Child Care Center Design Guide*. Washington, DC: US General Services Administration; 1998. Available at: http://www.gsa.gov/attachments/ GSA_PUBLICATIONS/pub/000000000041.pdf. Accessed March 19, 2004

Whole Building Design Guide Web site. Available at: http://www.wbdg.org. Accessed March 19, 2004

Developmentally Appropriate Programming: A Guide to Best Practices in Child Care Settings

Marjorie J. Kostelnik, PhD

LEARNING OBJECTIVES

This chapter will help the reader:

- Understand of the definition and importance of developmentally appropriate practices in child care.

- Learn how to support parents and caregivers in selecting and accessing high-quality child care.

- Recognize learning styles and appreciate differing preferences.

- Understand social and cultural considerations in the child care setting.

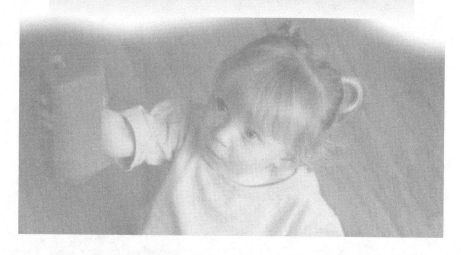

INTRODUCTION

Health care professionals are often asked for advice regarding the best way to approach particular health issues. What is the best remedy for a cold? What is the best way to handle an ear infection? What strategies work best for decreasing children's contact with infectious disease? In each case, they make a judgment about what advice to give a particular family on the basis of their knowledge of: 1) children's health and physical development; 2) the home and community environment in which the child is living; 3) the individual characteristics of the child in question; and 4) an understanding of current medical practices most favored by the profession.

This match between the health care professional's understanding of best medical practices and recommended actions is similar to judgments child care providers make to effectively meet the needs of the children in their care. Child care professionals who act on such judgments are said to be using "developmentally appropriate practices." In child care circles, developmentally appropriate practices represent standards of best practice on which many professionals agree. Such practices are used to differentiate high-quality child care programs from poor-quality programs.

QUALITY MAKES A DIFFERENCE IN CHILDREN'S LIVES

High-quality child care benefits children and their families; poor-quality care is detrimental to them. Children whose care is described as high quality enjoy a variety of benefits. Such children demonstrate higher levels of language development, greater social competence, a better ability to regulate their own behavior, and better academic performance than do their peers whose care is described as poor quality.[1] There also is evidence that children who have high-quality early childhood experiences outperform peers who have no such experiences before they enter formal school. These results hold true in the short and long term. On the other hand, poor-quality experiences yield negative outcomes, such as increased behavior problems and poorer academic progress in children.[2,3] Families may not be able to compensate for the negative impact of poor-quality care, at least for children who spend 20 or more hours per week in such settings.[1] This makes it essential for parents to have some sense of what differentiates high-quality from poor-quality child care.

CHARACTERISTICS OF HIGH-QUALITY CHILD CARE

Researchers have spent years identifying factors that contribute to high-quality child care. Two types of variables are most commonly identified; those that are structural and those that are process related. Structural variables are regulable factors, such as the adult-child ratio in a setting (optimal ratios vary with children's ages; ratios that allow for personal interaction among children and adults as well as among peers are best); group size (optimal size varies with children's ages); and education and training of child care providers (training specifically related to child development and early childhood education is optimal). Process variables center around activities offered to children and the kinds of relationships established between adults and children in the setting. In high-quality child care programs, these activities and relationships support and enhance children's physical, emotional, social, language, and intellectual development. They also support and complement the family in its child-rearing role.

High-Quality Child Care is Developmentally Appropriate

As the characteristics of high-quality child care have become more commonly understood in the field, efforts have been made to catalogue them into a single document for easy reference and comprehensive coverage. The most significant work in this regard has been carried out by the National Association for the Education of Young Children (NAEYC). A professional organization with more than 100 000 members, the NAEYC first put forward guidelines for best practices in 1987 and released an updated version in 1997.[4] Throughout the past decade, the principles and strategies it contains have been corroborated by other professional organizations, such as the National Association of State Boards of Education, the National Association of Elementary School Principles, and the National Education Association. Today, early childhood settings throughout the United States are attempting to match their programming with the NAEYC criteria. As a result, practices identified as developmentally appropriate (covering structural and process-oriented variables) have come to be viewed as synonymous with high-quality child care. Strategies at odds with these practices represent poor quality-care and are described as developmentally inappropriate.

The Essence of Developmentally Appropriate Practice

Developmentally appropriate practices provide a resource for thinking about, planning, and implementing high-quality programs for children from birth through 8 years of age. Early childhood professionals who use such practices make judgments about child care programs on the basis of their understanding of 3 important concepts[4]:

1. How children develop and learn.
2. The strengths, needs, and interests of individual children.
3. The social and cultural contexts in which children live.

In other words, child care providers who use developmentally appropriate practices think about what children are like and how they learn at a given age. They appreciate, for instance, that 2-year-olds are significantly different from 5-year-olds and that the interests and capabilities of the 2 age groups are distinct. This understanding of what is age appropriate helps them establish reasonable expectations for what might be interesting, safe, achievable, and challenging for children.[4] At the same time, such child care providers recognize that all children within a given age group are not identical. Consequently, they also evaluate to what extent the child care program is individually appropriate. This means that, in their daily programming, they accommodate variations in children's learning styles, temperament, interests, and developmental capacities. Developmentally appropriate early childhood programs also reflect social and cultural contexts experienced by children and families enrolled. In these settings, early childhood professionals make a deliberate effort to know about and demonstrate respect for beliefs, values, and customs children learn at home. This focus on socially and culturally appropriate practices yields programs that children find to be relevant and meaningful and that families view as supportive.

CONCEPT 1: IN DEVELOPMENTALLY APPROPRIATE PROGRAMS, EARLY CHILDHOOD PROFESSIONALS UNDERSTAND HOW CHILDREN DEVELOP AND LEARN

Child care providers who understand child development and learning are the most likely to engage in developmentally appropriate practices.[3] They recognize common developmental threads among all children and understand significant variations among cultures. Instead of treating their interactions with children as wholly intuitive, child care professionals who engage in developmentally appropriate practices use factual information to think about children and how to respond to them. This expands their notions of what constitutes normal child behavior. As a result, they are more likely to accept typical variations among children and accurately recognize potential problems that may require special intervention. Familiarity with child development also offers clues to child care providers about the sequence in which activities might be presented to children and the degree of developmental readiness necessary for children to achieve particular goals.[5]

There are similar benefits when early childhood professionals have a strong background in how children learn. Although there is a lack of unanimous agreement on the exact manner in which learning takes place, it is accepted that children from birth to 8 years of age think and acquire knowledge in ways that differ significantly from those demonstrated by older children and adults. Understanding how young children think and act is the key to creating appropriate physical environments for children and determining appropriate adult-child interactions, activities, and routines that support, rather than undermine, children's natural ways of learning.

Characteristics of Child Development

Children Develop Holistically
Aesthetic, cognitive, emotional, language, physical, and social development are interrelated. Although one facet of development may appear to be more dominant than others at times, in truth, children function in an integrated fashion. Consider the following example of children playing in the housekeeping area of a child care

center. As the youngsters "play house," their activity is influenced by many developmental processes, including:

1. Aesthetic (eg, appreciating the beauty of a hat or scarf donned by another child, enjoying arranging cups and saucers in certain ways, etc).
2. Cognitive (eg, determining how many children can fit in the space available; remembering who has had a chance to play and who has not; analyzing what behaviors fit the roles of mother, father, baby; etc).
3. Emotional (eg, coping with the disappointment of not playing the role of mother, accepting compliments, figuring out how to deal with criticism from other players, expressing anger about a disputed way to carry out the play, etc).
4. Language (eg, determining what scripts to use to enter or exit out of the play, using words to signal changes in roles, describing a sample scenario to another child, etc).
5. Physical (eg, writing a grocery list, setting out plates and cups, dressing the baby, climbing a climber while pretending to scale a hill on the way to work).
6. Social (eg, negotiating roles and actions, signaling others about one's desire to change the direction of the play, making way for a new player, working out disagreements about scenarios and props, etc).

This holistic picture is true for every task in which children engage. Cognitive processes shape social ones, social processes promote or restrict cognitive capabilities, and physical processes influence language and cognition.[6]

Child Development Follows a Normative Sequence

Development is sequential and progresses predictably. For instance, children's earliest attempts to write messages are to create scribbles. In cultures in which the alphabet is used, scribbles gradually turn into linear repetitive movements, then into letter-like forms, then into single consonants representing entire words, then into combinations of letters based on children's interpretation of phonetic spellings. This sequence proceeds in an uneven, rather than uniform, fashion. Individual children may spend more or less time involved in a certain behavior; they may move forward for a while, then back a little, then forward again. Regardless of the timing, such sequences tend to remain constant, with phases associated with each sequence appearing in the same order.

Child Development Proceeds at Varying Rates Within and Among Children

Every child develops according to his or her own genetic timeline. Differences in child development appear intrapersonally and interpersonally. Within every individual, various facets of development are dominant at different times throughout childhood. Such internal variations explain why the same child may cry easily, have difficulty cutting with scissors, climb nimbly to the highest rung on the slide, and recite numbers from 1 to 20 with ease. Such unevenness among developmental domains is to be expected.

Variations in rates also occur interpersonally. Even though normative sequences still apply, the pace at which youngsters move through them differs. Hence, children of approximately the same age often exhibit widely varying behaviors and understandings. For instance, one could expect some 4-year-olds to enter a child care program already adept at making conversation and establishing peer relationships. Other 4-year-olds in the same group might have little idea of how to enter a play group or how to engage in the give-and-take necessary to keep a play episode going. Such variations are normal, and similar differences could be found in every aspect of development.

Development is Epigenic

Development is based on a foundation; past, present, and future are related and build one on the other in succession. New capabilities and understandings arise out of, and elaborate on, what is already there.[6] The idea that children's writing evolves from scribbling illustrates the epigenic principle. So does the fact that children develop independence only after they have developed a sense of trust and that fluent, expressive language is founded on earlier babblings. In each of these instances, certain developmental processes are carried forward throughout time, providing continuity from one phase of development to the next.

Characteristics of Childhood Learning

Children Are Active Learners

Children are not passive beings waiting for something to happen; rather, they actively participate in shaping their own experiences. Recent studies of children's brain growth development underscore the active nature of the young brain and the connection between children's physical activity and subsequent cognitive development.[7] Motorically, children are people on the move. They are biologically programmed to reach out, pull up, stand upright, and move forward. Such physical activity stimulates children's senses, enhancing their intellectual functioning. Thus, young children are compelled to taste, touch, hear, look at, and smell objects and spaces to find out about them—what their properties are, how they function, and how they fit in with the rest of the world. It is in this way that children connect thought with action—exploring, discovering, and learning.[6]

Children's Learning Is Affected by Maturation

As human beings mature, new possibilities for learning are created that could not have been realized earlier. This is illustrated by the fact that children's ability to recognize other people's emotions increases with age.[5] Initially, children rely on facial expressions to tell them how someone else is feeling. A crying peer is sad, and a smiling peer is happy. As children progress from toddlerhood into the primary years, their cognitive capacities mature to the point that they are able to recognize that situational cues also contribute to an accurate interpretation of another person's emotional state. Thus, a crying peer may be sad because his dog died or sad because his toy was broken, not simply because tears are running down his face. Eventually, children reach a level of cognitive maturation that allows them to recognize the difference between tears of sadness and those that come about because of happiness, embarrassment, or fear.

Conversely, if suitable maturation has not taken place, it is futile to demand that children demonstrate mastery of particular knowledge or skills. For instance, to share, children must first develop the ability to recognize another person's point of view and techniques for interacting cooperatively. These cognitive milestones are generally beyond the capabilities of most toddlers. Thus, trying to make a 14-month-old share materials will likely result in failure, because a child that age lacks prerequisite skills necessary for success. In this way, biologic characteristics of each child place some limits on the sequence and speed at which particular competencies emerge. This timetable can be impeded by environmental insults and slightly accelerated by environmental stimulation. However, the rate of maturation is not completely elastic.[6]

Children's Learning is Influenced by the Environment

Children do not gain knowledge and skills from maturation alone. Environmental factors play an essential part in the learning process too. These can be described according to the following 3 environmental contexts[8]:

1. Biologic environment (eg, nutrition, medical care, physical exercise, and drugs).
2. Physical environment (eg, clothing, shelter, materials available, climate, and energy).
3. Social environment (eg, family, peers, child care programs, schools, community, media, and culture).

These environments combine to enhance or detract from children's ability to learn. We know, for instance, that children learn best when they feel psychologically safe and secure.[4] Kostelnik et al said, "For children ages birth to eight years, this translates into knowing that they are in a place where routines and expectations are suited to their capacities and are predictable. Security also comes from being in the company of adults who like them, who tolerate mistakes, and who support their efforts to explore and experiment. Children's learning is further enhanced when the child care environment is stimulating, but not overwhelming. If the latter conditions prevail, children tend to 'shut down' cognitively; becoming less sensitive to environmental cues, less likely to process information, and less able to transfer information from one situation to another."[5] Under the latter conditions, children are likely to act out in some way or withdraw. These circumstances are not conducive to effective learning.

Children's Preferred Learning Styles Differ

Although most children use all of their senses to learn, for many, one modality tends to overshadow the rest. That is, children come to prefer one sensory channel to others. These preferences are described as differences in learning style. For instance, if Michael is primarily a visual learner, he will respond best to what he sees and will envision something in his mind as a way to recall it. Sarah, an auditory learner, relies on hearing and talking as her primary means of learning. For her, sound is the message, and she may sometimes move her lips or talk herself through tasks to make them easier. Douglas, a kinesthetic or tactile learner, must move and constantly touch things in order to grasp concepts. It is also not unusual for him to have to touch himself in some way to remember or process information. These modalities, or patterns of learning, are not mutually exclusive. Some children might use a combination of modalities as their preferred learning style.

Harvard researchers Gardner and Hatch have taken the idea of preferred modalities a step beyond the 3 modalities described earlier in this chapter and have expanded the construct further than simple perceptual processing. They believe that everyone possesses at least 7 intelligences or frames of mind and that a person's blend of competencies in each area produces a unique learning profile. Gardner and Hatch suggest that "each of these (intelligence or competency) areas may develop independently (in the brain). Individuals may be 'at promise' in some areas while being average or below average in others."[9] The 7 intelligences are described in Table 5.1, along with ways children learn best in relation to each. They further postulate that people possess various degrees of know-how in all 7 categories, yet there are certain categories that eventually dominate, making those the methods by which an individual learns best.

Table 5.1. Seven Intelligences That Contribute to a Child's Learning Profile	
Intelligence	**Child Learns Best By**
Linguistic	Using words orally or in writing
Logical-mathematical	Looking for logical patterns and relationships
Musical	Experiencing rhythm, melody, pitch, timbre, or tone relative to a musical piece
Spatial	Visualizing, graphically representing visual or spatial ideas
Bodily-kinesthetic	Touching, moving, responding to bodily sensations
Intrapersonal	Working alone; being aware of inner moods, intentions, motivations, temperaments, and self-desires
Interpersonal	Sharing, comparing, relating to others, cooperating

Children Learn Through Play

Children play at home, at the child care center, and everywhere in between. They play with people, things, and ideas. Kostelnik et al said, "When more fundamental needs are met—when children are not sleeping, eating, or seeking emotional support from others—children choose to play and can remain occupied that way for hours at a time. Play is the province of children from the time they are born throughout the elementary school years."[6]

All facets of development are enhanced through children's play. Play is the primary means children use to gather and process information, learn new skills, and practice skills already acquired.[10] Within the context of their play, children come to understand, create, and manipulate symbols as they take on roles and transform objects into something else. Children explore social relationships too. They experiment with various roles, such as leader and follower or novice and expert. As children play with peers, they come to recognize points of view unlike their own, working out compromises and negotiating differences. Play enables children to expand their physical skills, language capabilities, and creative imaginations. Play also provides a safe means for children to release tensions, express emotions, and explore anxiety-producing situations, such as the arrival of a new baby at home, uncertainties of moving, or loss of a family member through divorce or death. In all of these ways, play is of considerable value to young children, and most scientists agree that it is central to children's learning.[4]

CONCEPT 2: IN DEVELOPMENTALLY APPROPRIATE PROGRAMS, EARLY CHILDHOOD PROFESSIONALS TREAT CHILDREN AS INDIVIDUALS

Child care providers are called on daily to make decisions that require them to see each child as distinct from all others. Adults must weigh such variables as a child's age, what a child's current level of comprehension might be, and what experiences a child has had. Although age is not an absolute measure of a child's capabilities and understanding, it does serve as a guide for establishing appropriate expectations. For instance, knowing that preschoolers do not yet have a mature grasp of sharing, child care providers would not consider a 4-year-old who wants all of the crayons for herself as being bad; rather, they would help her learn how to divide or take turns with the materials. Likewise, child care providers coach and support children who are learning to take turns in a game. They would not expect children to automatically know how to do this. Thus, child care providers are constantly teaching children the day-to-day knowledge and skills they must have to get along in the world.

The kinds of previous knowledge and skills a child brings to a situation should also be taken into account. Obviously, children with little or no exposure to a particular situation or skill would not be expected to perform at the same level of competence as children whose experience is greater. For instance, standards for eating independently would be different for a 3-year-old than for a 6-year-old, not only because of differences in maturity but also because the older child has had more practice. Furthermore, a child who has never seen or eaten with chopsticks would not be expected to demonstrate the same degree of proficiency in using them at a meal as would a child from a family in which such utensils are commonplace.

Circumstantial factors also contribute to determining the developmental appropriateness of certain decisions. Under normal circumstances, a home-based child care provider's goal is to foster independence among the children in her care. Ordinarily, children are given time to make their own decisions, to repeat a task to gain competence, and to do as much as possible for themselves. However, these goals and strategies have to be modified, for instance, when a child vomits at the table. Under such circumstances, children have no choice about going to the bathroom to get cleaned up, and they cannot choose to not take off their soiled clothes. In this case, children have fewer choices than the child care provider might ordinarily provide.

CONCEPT 3: IN DEVELOPMENTALLY APPROPRIATE PROGRAMS, EARLY CHILDHOOD PROFESSIONALS RESPECT THE SOCIAL AND CULTURAL CONTEXTS THAT SHAPE CHILDREN'S LIVES

Child development and learning occurs within the embedded contexts of family, community, and culture. These contexts influence all elements of child care and early education. Typical examples include the following[11]:

- Adult expectations for children of different ages
- Sleep patterns and rest time and bedtime routines in which children participate
- The role of children in the family, early childhood program, and neighborhood
- Toilet training
- Diet and mealtime behavior
- Discipline and child guidance techniques
- How adults talk to children
- How adults show affection for children and build relationships with them
- Gender roles children learn
- Dress and personal hygiene practices
- Acceptance of, and response to, children's crying
- Children's attachment to, and separation from, adults

As a result of variations among children's social and cultural experiences, individual children come to the child care setting with different needs, expectations, and response patterns. Child care providers who ignore these variations damage children by communicating to them that significant beliefs and practices in their lives are unacceptable or deficient in the eyes of the program.[12,13] This can have devastating effects on children's self-esteem, cognitive capacities, and ability to function effectively in society.[14] Conversely, when child care providers demonstrate respect for children's social and cultural heritage, children are affirmed and their learning is enhanced. This is most likely to occur when children perceive a connectedness between home and the child care setting. The more early childhood program strategies and content build on what is familiar to children, the more comfortable children feel. The more congruent expectations are between home and early childhood environments, the more productively children learn.

Practical Implications

The concepts described earlier in this chapter ultimately determine the ways adults interact with children, the kinds of environments they create for them, and the expectations they have for childrens' behavior. Some specific child care practices parents should look for in determining whether the program they are considering for their child is developmentally appropriate are presented in Table 5.2.

Practices that counter these are characterized as developmentally inappropriate. Some of these include:

- Neglecting children's basic needs for safety, nurturance, and stimulation.
- Emphasizing one aspect of child development and learning (such as cognition or social development) to the exclusion of all others.
- Expecting all children to learn the same thing, at the same time, in the same way.
- Treating play as trivial or unacceptable.
- Expecting children to learn mostly through listening and engaging in abstract activities that have little meaning or relevance to them.
- Ignoring or demeaning children's cultural backgrounds.
- Treating parents as inconsequential or as adversaries.

Developmentally Appropriate Practices Are Adaptable Across Program Settings

Strategies associated with developmentally appropriate practices can be carried out in an assortment of child care settings—part-time or full-day, home-based or center-based, private or public, or not-for-profit or for-profit. They are equally applicable to programs that serve infants, toddlers, preschoolers, school-aged children, and children with special needs. Developmentally appropriate practices can be observed in large and small programs and in urban, suburban, and rural locations. Practices regulated through licensing of child care programs represent a minimum but incomplete level of best practices mostly related to basic health and safety standards. Child care programs that have progressed to the level of accreditation (as described in Chapter 2) are most likely to demonstrate the broader array of developmentally appropriate practices listed here.

Developmentally Appropriate Practices Are Adaptable Across Program Models

Early childhood programs differ not only in physical characteristics and clients served but also in theoretical foundations. Most of these variations center on different beliefs about how much biology or environment influence child development and

Table 5.2. Developmentally Appropriate Child Care Practices

Child-Focused Assumptions	Developmentally Appropriate Practices
Children develop holistically.	Daily activities and routines in the child care setting address all aspects of children's development—aesthetic, emotional, intellectual, language, physical, and social
Child development follows a normative sequence.	Child care providers use their knowledge of developmental sequences to appropriately challenge children and to determine reasonable expectations for individual children.
	Child care providers avoid attempting to unduly accelerate children's progress through certain developmental sequences, such as those associated with handwriting, sharing, or playing games with rules.
Child development proceeds at varying rates within and among children.	The daily schedule gives children opportunities to pursue activities at their own pace. Children are not required to rotate from activity to activity on a predetermined schedule throughout the day.
	Activities are repeated throughout the year so that children benefit from their participation according to their changing needs and abilities throughout time.
Child development is epigenic.	Child care providers interact with children and observe them carefully to discover what they know and can do.
	Activities are planned on the basis of children's level of performance and understanding.
	Child care providers help children make connections between new and past experiences.
	The program is designed to support children's progress toward more elaborate concepts and skills as children exhibit interest and mastery.
Children are active learners.	Children are provided many opportunities to directly explore and handle objects every day.
	Large portions of the day are devoted to times when children can move about the room freely.
	Daily schedules allow for quiet times followed by longer, more active periods. Inactive segments of the day are kept short.
	Children have opportunities to engage in active, large-muscle play daily.
Children's learning is affected by maturation.	Child care providers demonstrate an understanding of how children mature and what might be reasonably expected of children throughout time.
	Activities are provided to children that are within their ability to master. Child care providers simplify, maintain, or extend activities in response to children's demonstrated levels of functioning and comprehension.
	Children have opportunities to interact with children whose abilities vary. This allows children chances to learn from other children and serve as models for peers with whom they come in contact.

Table 5.2. Developmentally Appropriate Child Care Practices, continued

Child-Focused Assumptions	Developmentally Appropriate Practices
Children's learning is influenced by environmental variables.	The child care environment is safe and secure and complies with legal requirements of the appropriate licensing or accrediting agency.
	Children's biologic and physical needs are met. For instance, children may use the toilet whenever they need to, they may rest when they are tired, and they are provided with snacks and meals as appropriate. Classrooms and outdoor areas offer ample space for safe, unencumbered movement. Adequate ventilation is provided, and temperatures are maintained at a comfortable level. Children's wet or soiled clothing is changed promptly.
	A daily routine is established that is relatively stable and predictable to children. Changes in routine are explained in advance so children can anticipate what will happen next.
	Activities, transitions, and routines are designed keeping in mind children's attention span; physical development; and need for activity, social interaction, and attention from caring adults.
	Staff schedules are designed to provide children with consistent adult supervision. Children can readily identify a specific adult from whom to seek help, comfort, attention, and guidance.
	Positive discipline techniques are used to enhance children's self-esteem and self-control.
	Two-way communication between program and home is established. Home events are considered in planning children's educational experiences, and those experiences are communicated to families.
Children's learning styles differ.	Activities address a variety of modalities—seeing, hearing, tasting, touching.
	Children may choose from an array of different activities every day.
	The same information and skills are presented through different modalities.
	Children have opportunities to work and play on their own and with others.
Children learn through play.	Play is integrated throughout the entire day and within all aspects of the early childhood program.
	There are a variety of props and other manipulative objects with which children may play.
	Child care providers are joyful and playful as they interact with children.
	Child care providers enhance children's play sometimes as observers and sometimes as participants.

Table 5.2. Developmentally Appropriate Child Care Practices, continued	
Child-Focused Assumptions	**Developmentally Appropriate Practices**
Children are individuals.	Child care providers take time to observe children carefully in order to recognize individual patterns of behavior.
	Child care providers accommodate the needs and interests of individual children throughout the day rather than requiring all children to do the same thing, at the same time, in the same way all day long.
Children are shaped by the social and cultural environments in which they live.	Children are treated with warmth, consideration, and caring (regardless of socioeconomic, cultural, ethnic, or family background; appearance; behavior; or any disability).
	Early childhood professionals make a special effort to know what objects, practices, and beliefs are relevant to individual children and their families.
	Children have access to images, objects, and activities in the early childhood program that reflect their home experiences.
	Child care providers work collaboratively with children's family members and others in the community to develop shared goals for children.
	Each child and his or her family is treated as a valued member of the early childhood program.
	Family traditions are honored.
	Child care providers establish 2-way communication between the early childhood program and families. This communication takes a variety of forms, including verbal and written methods. Various modes of family involvement are offered, including at-home, on-site, and extracurricular opportunities.

learning. These differences in theoretical orientation lead to variations in program models and in the curricula children experience. A brief overview of 4 theoretical perspectives prevalent among today's early child care providers is described here.

The Maturationist Perspective

Some child care providers carry out programs designed primarily to support the natural unfolding of children's developmental capacities. They believe that the proper program for each child can best be determined by referring to norms for that age range. Activities and materials are then provided to support children's current levels of functioning. Self-discovery by children, rather than adult-initiated activities, dominates the program. Attempts to train children before they are ready for certain kinds of learning are believed to be ineffective or even harmful. If children do not seem ready to engage in certain tasks, they are left to grow into them without adult intervention. This practice is known as giving children "the gift of time."

The Mental Health Perspective

The work of Sigmund Freud and Erik Erikson underscores the significance of early personality development, giving rise to the view that early childhood programs can help prevent mental illness. Child care programs espousing a Freudian-Eriksonian mental health perspective use play-based activities to enhance children's sense of well-being. Children are free to choose activities in which they will participate, all of which emphasize play as a primary vehicle for involvement. Child care staff provide materials, such as sand, water, clay, and blocks, to help children gain personal satisfaction as they act on their emotions and internal drives. They assume that children will become emotionally functional human beings with support, but little direct intervention, from adults.

The Behavioral Approach

Child care providers who focus on children achieving specific behavioral outcomes (eg, reciting the alphabet, tying a bow, counting to 10) rather than internal affective processes are described as having a behavioral orientation. The programs they create are often associated with teaching children academics and basic self-help skills. To achieve their goals, these child care providers rely on direct instruction and external rewards to shape children's behavior in certain directions. Such shaping involves the following steps: 1) targeting a desired behavior; 2) establishing a baseline; 3) selecting relevant reinforcers; 4) sequencing instruction; and 5) systematically applying reinforcers until the goal is achieved.

The Interactionist Perspective

The models described thus far represent polar views of child development and learning. Whereas the maturationist and mental health philosophies emphasize the dominant role of biology, the behavioral approach focuses on environmental factors almost exclusively. The interactionist point of view represents a combination of the 2. On the basis of the work of Jean Piaget and Lev Vygotsky, child care providers espousing an interactionist philosophy believe that children are holistic beings who pass through a series of cognitive stages throughout childhood and adolescence. These stages are influenced by biology and children's interactions with the physical world and other people. This philosophical orientation suggests that children benefit from a balance between opportunities for self-discovery and direct instruction—from chances to play freely and to participate in teacher-directed activities. The interactionist point of view maintains that children's self-esteem should be enhanced along with their physical, language, and cognitive skills. Currently, this philosophy dominates the early childhood scene in terms of research and program implementation.

Developmentally Appropriate Practices Are Most Closely Associated With the Interactionist Approach to Early Childhood Intervention

The assumptions about child development and learning described earlier in this chapter are fundamental to an interactionist philosophy. However, because the interactionist approach combines many suppositions characteristic of the other perspectives discussed, developmentally appropriate practices can also be observed in well-executed programs more closely aligned with maturational, mental health, and behavioral orientations. In addition to these theoretical origins, early childhood programs may be designed around certain life perspectives, such as a particular religious or cultural orientation. These variations have led to a proliferation of program models and claims, which parents sometimes find confusing. When faced with questions regarding which programs might be best or how one program model compares with another, it is better to come back to the notion of developmental appropriateness than to advocate for one particular model as opposed to another. Regardless of the name given to any early childhood program (eg, Montessori, developmental, High/Scope, play-based, academic readiness, Reggio Emilia, back-to-basics), the most important criteria for selecting an early childhood program is the extent to which program personnel demonstrate developmentally appropriate practices.

Programs That Use Developmentally Appropriate Practices May Be Hard for Parents to Find

Identification of best practices has not ensured that every setting in which children receive care uses such strategies. In fact, there is evidence that many children in the United States receive care that is inadequate at best and detrimental at worst. Recent findings suggest that we have a lack of high-quality care in this country. Zigler and Stevenson estimate that one third of children in America have child care experiences that will compromise their development.[15] Many children are ignored for long periods of time, lost in a crowd of other children, made to sit for hours unoccupied or in front of a television, forced to engage in activities far below or beyond their years, and deprived of nurturance from adults who are consistently in their lives. There are several reasons for this dilemma, including lack of trained professionals in early childhood education, low wages in the child care industry, lack of public understanding of what constitutes high-quality care, and lack of political will to ensure that high-quality care is generally available to families at a price they can afford.

Public Confusion About Developmentally Appropriate Practices

Another dilemma faced by proponents of developmentally appropriate practices is widespread public confusion as to what such practices entail. In the absence of true understanding, myths have surfaced about what it all means. These myths are often based on false assumptions (eg, child care providers in developmentally appropriate programs never teach children anything, children just play all day long, children never learn to read, write, or spell correctly). Other myths result from people's superficial understanding of child development and learning (eg, if children aren't reciting the alphabet, they are not learning anything about reading). Still more myths have been created as a way for groups to advance their political agendas (eg, opponents proclaim that by advocating respect for children whose family configurations vary widely, developmentally appropriate programs undermine family values). All of these myths make the erroneous assumption that developmentally appropriate practices consist of a rigid set of strategies that child care providers adopt unthinkingly and universally. In reality, the concept of developmentally appropriate practice is evolving, and its application is contextually based, as discussed earlier in this chapter. Developmentally appropriate practices help child care providers make informed decisions; they are not a substitute for decision making. Every day, child care providers find themselves in situations in which they must figure out how to apply the guidelines in ways best suited to meet the individual needs of children in their care. Consequently, early childhood professionals continually make judgments about whether or not their actions and programs enhance or detract from the quality of children's lives. Such decision making is one characteristic associated with high-quality child care. Finally, public confusion and concern is most often associated with tangential details (such as what holidays to celebrate with children or the role of phonics in reading instruction) that are not directly tied to guidelines published by the NAEYC. These arguments miss the essence of developmentally appropriate practices represented by the concepts featured in this chapter. It is these tenets that provide the foundation for defining high-quality early childhood programs. The bottom line is that developmentally appropriate programs are those in which children of all abilities, ages, races, cultures, creeds, and socioeconomic and family lifestyle backgrounds feel loveable, valuable, and competent.

The Role of the Health Care Professional in Helping Parents Recognize and Consider Developmentally Appropriate Practices in Their Child Care Decisions

It is natural for parents to turn to health care professionals for advice about which child care program to select for their child. When faced with such queries, health care professionals should acquaint parents with the 3 concepts of developmentally appropriate practices described in this chapter and some practices associated with those concepts. Parents should be advised to consider these concepts as part of their decision making. The following strategies can help parents evaluate child care settings in which they are interested:

1. Take the time to choose a child care situation carefully.
2. Prepare questions in advance aimed at determining the quality of care provided in the setting.

3. Visit the early childhood program in person. Do not rely on phone calls or advertisements alone. Ask to see the actual room, group of children, and adults with whom your child will be interacting.
4. Talk to other families whose children are enrolled in the program to determine their degree of satisfaction and the extent to which they feel respected by program personnel.
5. Ask program staff to what extent they know about and practice developmentally appropriate strategies in the program.
6. Make sure you are allowed to make unannounced visits at any time to visit your child and see the program in operation.
7. Select a licensed program, and whenever possible, an accredited one.

CONCLUSIONS AND RECOMMENDATIONS

Information provided by health care professionals to parents about what constitutes high-quality child care can make a significant contribution to children's well-being. Evidence suggests that, whether from desperation or lack of knowledge or money, many parents accept the unacceptable in terms of child care. Advice from health care professionals about how to make more informed choices could ultimately enhance the quality of children's lives. Focusing on developmentally appropriate practices is the best way to ensure that this happens.

REFERENCES

1. Doherty-Derkowski G. *Quality Matters: Excellence in Early Childhood Programs.* Don Mills, Ontario: Addison-Wesley Publishers; 1995
2. Dunn L, Kontos S. What have we learned about developmentally appropriate practice? *Young Child.* 1997;52:4-13
3. Hart CH, Burts DC, Charlesworth R. Integrated developmentally appropriate curriculum: from theory to research to practice. In: Hart CH, Burts DC, Charlesworth R, eds. *Integrated Curriculum and Developmentally Appropriate Practice: Birth to Age Eight.* Albany, NY: State University of New York Press; 1997:1-27
4. Bredekamp S, Copple C, eds. *Developmentally Appropriate Practice in Early Childhood Programs.* 3rd ed. Albany, NY: Delmar Publishers; 1998
5. Kostelnik MJ, Stein LC, Whiren AP, Soderman AK. *Guiding Children's Social Development.* 3rd ed. Albany, NY: Delmar Publishers; 1998
6. Kostelnik MJ, Soderman AK, Whiren AP. *Developmentally Appropriate Curriculum: Best Practices in Early Childhood Education.* 2nd ed. Upper Saddle River, NJ: Merrill; 1999
7. Begley S. Your child's brain. *Newsweek.* 1996;Feb 19:54
8. Santrock JW. *Children.* 6th ed. Boston, MA: McGraw-Hill; 2000
9. Hatch T, Gardner H. New research on intelligence sheds light on how children use their brains to make sense of the world. *Learning.* 1988;17:36-39
10. Sroufe LA, Cooper RG, DeHart GB. *Child Development: Its Nature and Course.* 3rd ed. New York, NY: McGraw-Hill; 1996
11. York S. *Roots and Wings: Affirming Culture in Early Childhood Programs.* St Paul, MN: Redleaf Press; 1991

12. Hale JE. *Unbank the Fire: Visions for the Education of African American Children.* Baltimore, MD: Johns Hopkins University Press; 1994

13. Chipman M. Valuing cultural diversity in the early years: social imperatives and pedagogical insights. In: Isenberg JP, Jalongo MR, eds. *Major Trends and Issues in Early Childhood Education: Challenges, Controversies and Insights.* New York, NY: Teachers College Press; 1997:43–55

14. Garcia EE, McLaughlin B. *Meeting the Challenge of Linguistic and Cultural Diversity in Early Childhood Education.* New York, NY: Teachers College Press; 1995

15. Zigler EF, Finn-Stevenson M. Funding child care and public education. *Future Child* 1996;6:104–121, 137–145

CHAPTER 6

Developmental Outcome of Children in Child Care

Jay Belsky, PhD, and Chet D. Johnson, MD

LEARNING OBJECTIVES

This chapter will enable the reader to:

- Become more familiar with issues surrounding parental/caregiver decisions in selecting child care.
- Understand current literature regarding child care and developmental outcomes.
- Recognize important roles in helping make high-quality care accessible.

INTRODUCTION

Should I put my child in a family child care home or center when I return to work? What will happen to my child if I do? How much does it really matter? Will having someone else care for my child make him or her insecure or more sociable by being around other children? What about intellectual functioning? Will placement in out-of-home child care promote or undermine my child's cognitive competence? Perhaps most importantly, will my child love me less and love his alternative caregiver more should I choose to have someone else provide daily care? Ultimately, am I making a mistake by letting someone else assume so much responsibility for my child during the day (or evening) while I work?

If I am going to rely on child care, does it matter whether it begins in infancy? Is it better if I wait until my child is 2, 3, or even 4 years of age? Does it make a difference if I use full-time versus part-time care? Which is best?

I hear a lot about "quality of care," but it reminds me of that phrase "quality time." Does it really matter as much as some suggest? If so, what does quality care really mean? Fundamentally, what should I be looking for when I search for a care arrangement for my child?

Any professional or paraprofessional that has advised or guided parents of young children has faced these daunting questions. And it is indisputable that different professionals provide dramatically different answers as a result of their knowledge of the scientific literature, their own personal experiences, or their ideologic beliefs about what is best for children, for families, and for women. In fact, the questions posed by parents facing the challenging tasks of deciding whether to use nonparental child care, what kind of care to use, for how long, and beginning when, are daunting because the issues are complex. Indeed, it is likely that many professionals who have been asked these questions have, on different occasions, given different answers. This is true because the circumstances facing families are different and because perspectives on these issues often change over time.

Although the questions raised above will be addressed, the reader should be aware that there is no shortage of opinion on these topics within the scientific community. Although some of this diversity in opinion reflects divergent points of view on children, families, and the role of parents in society, much of it is a function of the fact that the scientific evidence does not provide singular, clear answers to many of the issues which need to be considered. Nevertheless, current knowledge does offer guidance and it is toward that end that this chapter is directed. The chapter begins by placing child care—defined as routine nonparental care—in contemporary context and then proceeds to examine effects of child care experienced during infancy and the preschool years.

CHILD CARE IN CONTEXT

The United States is a nation deeply ambivalent about the practice of having persons other than parents care for young children, especially infants. Despite the fact that more than 60% of American mothers with children younger than 6 years are employed, the United States has no national child care policy, unlike many other industrialized countries. For the most part, the regulation of child care is left to states and local municipalities, resulting in a wide array of policies about who can care for children, how many child care providers must be available, and how many children can be included in a group. In some states, child care regulations or their enforcement are lax. In addition, much if not most child care, especially for very young children, is informal and unregulated. It is not surprising that recent studies of infant, toddler, and preschool care—provided in private homes and in centers—suggest that the average quality of care provided in America is fair, not good, and may actually be poor.[1,2] Any discussion of the effects of child care on child health and development of children, then, must be viewed in this context.

THE EFFECTS OF CHILD CARE

However complex the effects of out-of-home care on child development, one thing is clear: there are no inevitable positive or negative effects of nonparental child rearing on young children. The database that serves as the foundation of the following analysis provides evidence to support virtually any conclusion that has been advanced about child care. This occurs because the phenomenon of child care is varied and includes nanny care, family child care homes, and centers; the families using child care are diverse, including impoverished single parents and economically advantaged dual-earner couples; the children experiencing routine nonparental care are heterogeneous, ranging from newborns to 5- and 6-year-olds; and most significantly, the quality of experience that children receive spans the range from neglectful and abusive to supportive, stimulating, and affectionate care. What seems to be clear from the research is that children can thrive in care that is provided by supportive, nurturing individuals who establish enduring relationships with the children in their care and the parents of those children. This indicates, most obviously, that there are not inevitable adverse effects of nonparental care, even when it is initiated on a full-time basis in the opening months of life. But it is just as clear that care that is of low quality, defined in terms of groups that are too large, child care providers who are unresponsive and disinterested, and highly stressed settings that are crowded, dirty, and even dangerous are not in children's best interest.

Beyond these generalizations, somewhat more precise statements can be made about the effects of child care on child development. The following discussion will consider the issues of infant-parent attachment security, emotional adjustment (particularly issues of self-control), compliance, and problem behavior. Much of this discussion will focus on care initiated in the early years of life. Preschool-aged care and its effects on social and intellectual development will also be addressed.

Ultimately, quality of care, meaning the degree of attention and support children receive from their child care providers on a daily basis, appears significantly more important than the type of care setting the child experiences. Although older children approaching school age probably enjoy and benefit from group settings and children in their early years are more likely to thrive in situations with fewer children these generalizations about settings do not provide the only basis for sound decision making. Most experts would agree that an infant is better off in a group if he or she will have a greater opportunity to develop an emotional attachment to a sensitive, caring person there than he or she would be with a nanny or in a private family arrangement if comparable quality of care is unlikely to be available. Similarly, even a 4-year-old is likely to be better off in a family setting than a center if he or she will simply be lost in the crowd in the latter and receive individualized attention in the former. Ultimately, the person who is providing care—and how long they can be expected to offer care—is more important than the care setting itself.

As when buying a car, it is always a good idea to "look under the hood," that is, beyond the paint job to the engine and transmission. Metaphorically speaking, the engine and transmission in child care take the form of the adults providing care, whereas the paint job takes the form of the setting. So long as a setting is reasonably clean and meets basic standards of safety, then it is wise to disregard the bright-colored wall, the child-sized furniture, or the newness of the toys. Parents should pay attention instead to whether the child care provider seems interested and rewarded in his or her work, motivated to know each child as an individual, and capable of being sensitive and responsive to the most and least attention-grabbing children. Parents should observe the child care providers' approach to a child who is having a difficult time; is their approach sensitive and effective or merely punitive? Conversations with other parents and time spent observing in the child care milieu provide the basic means of securing such information. A glossy brochure or persuasive words from a program director are no substitute for talking with other parents and a personal, on-site assessment.

SECURITY OF ATTACHMENT

A basic developmental task of infancy is the establishment of a close relationship with one or a few child care providers. Ideally, such a relationship imparts in the child a sense that he or she can count on the fact that the child care provider will be able to read and respond in an appropriate fashion to his or her needs and desires and do so on a fairly regular and reliable basis. When such a relationship occurs, a child typically develops a secure attachment to the individual providing the care. Such bonds become a psychologic asset to the child when it comes to meeting new developmental challenges like getting along with others, coping with frustration, and finding pleasure in the everyday experience of life. Unfortunately, not all infants and toddlers develop secure attachments, principally because the routine daily care they receive is not particularly consistent, not particularly sensitive and responsive, and not particularly warm and caring. In such circumstances, infants may develop insecure attachments that lead them to doubt the availability and responsiveness of their principle child care provider, to perhaps even doubt the emotional supportiveness of the world more generally, and to be at a decided disadvantage when it comes to coping with the kinds of challenges that characterize growing up.

From the very inception of child care in this country, there have been concerns about the security of attachment of infants and young children who experience routine nonparental care. Part of this concern derived from Bowlby's theory of attachment,[3] which highlighted risks associated with separation of the very young child from his or her principal child care provider, typically the mother. Others, such as Brazelton,[4] used to note that simply the time away from the infant may undermine some mothers' ability to get to know their babies well enough to provide the kind of sensitive, responsive care that is known to foster attachment security.

A number of analyses—though certainly not all— have documented an association between insecurity and full- and near-full time nonmaternal care in the first year.[5,6] Even though such evidence revealed a significant increase in the rate of insecure infant-mother attachments among infants with more than 20 hours per week of child care experience in their first year, it was never the case that most infants experiencing early and extensive care developed insecure attachments. Rather, it was that the rate of insecurity increased among such children relative to those whose care was exclusively maternal or less extensively nonmaternal. Notable, though, the National Institute of Child Health and Development, Early Child Care Research Network[7] failed to document such an effect of quantity of care in the first year on infant-mother attachment

Efforts to promote secure attachment and emotional well-being should be directed at supporting a nurturing home environment and making high-quality child care available for every child.

security in a large-scale investigation. What this study did discover, however, was that it was principally a subset of children who were at increased risk of developing an insecure infant-mother relationship when in child care for the first year. Specifically, it was infants who received poor quality of care both at home and in their child care setting, and infants who received poor quality of care at home and more than 10 hours per week of care in their child care setting whose risk of establishing insecure attachments to their mothers was increased. Boys in care for more than 30 hours per week appeared to be at somewhat elevated risk when compared with girls. Collectively, these data indicate that security of attachment is related to factors in the child's home and his or her child care setting. Efforts to promote secure attachment and emotional well-being should be directed at supporting a nurturing home environment and making high-quality child care available for every child.

Related to parents' anxieties about whether infant child care will undermine their child's feelings of security is the concern about their replacement by the child care provider in the child's hierarchy of relationships. Simply put, the question becomes, "Will my child love and prefer his child care provider more than he loves me?" With regard to this query, the data are clear and should alleviate parental concern. In most cases, infants and young children establish stronger and preferential ties to their parents than they do to their child care providers. More importantly, perhaps, parents would be wise not to worry about the place of the child care provider in their children's hearts. It is in the child's developmental best interest to establish secure attachment to the child care provider. Children with such relationships appear to be socially and emotionally advantaged relative to agemates who establish insecure attachments to their child care providers.[8] In fact, in the same way that a child is developmentally advantaged by developing secure attachments to mother and father, rather than to just one (or neither), he or she also benefits from developing secure bonds with parent and child care provider. Parents should thus be discouraged from viewing the child's close, affectionate relationship with his or her child care provider as a source of competition and concern and be instead encouraged to regard the child-provider relationship as a source of satisfaction and comfort.

SOCIOEMOTIONAL ADJUSTMENT: NONCOMPLIANCE, AGGRESSION, AND PROBLEM BEHAVIOR

It is well established that how parents care for their infant, toddler, and young child influences the child's developing capacity to manage or regulate emotions and impulses. When parents are sensitive and responsive to their children's needs, affectionate, and firm (not harsh) and consistent in their use of discipline, young children are less likely to be disobedient and aggressive and more likely to be cooperative and agreeable. When parents are intrusive, detached, or angry and harsh in their dealings with their children's behavior, the opposite tends to be true. But it appears that however important the behavior of parents at home is, it is not the only thing that affects children's ability to manage their impulses and emotions.

Bowlby's theory of attachment led to the expectation among some child developmentalists that a history of separation from parent and especially the establishment of an insecure attachment to mother laid the foundation for the development of problems in social and emotional adjustment. Although few conceived insecurity as an inevitable pathway to maladjustment, many developmentalists regarded insecurity as increasing the probability that a child could develop behavior problems. It is interesting in this regard that for the past 2 decades, a large number of studies have chronicled linkages between early child care experience, many hours spent in child care, and multiple years of child care with noncompliance, aggression, and problem behaviors that took the form of acting out behavior.[5,9] Although early and extensive child care has not been associated with serious psychopathology, 3-, 5-, and even 8-year-olds with such child care histories have been found to be more noncompliant and aggressive than agemates with far less early child care experience.[9,10]

Certainly, not every investigation has yielded such results. However, these findings have emerged with sufficient frequency that they merit attention, even concern. For years it has been thought that it is the experience of poor-quality care that accounts for why developmental risks have been associated with full- or near full-time care initiated in the first year of life, which continues at such high levels until school entry. But the latest research reveals that this is simply not the case.[11] This is not to say that quality of care does not matter, only that it is not exclusively responsible for what happens to children in child care. The mere amount of time a child spends in care—beginning in the first year of life and continuing until the start of school—matters as well. Thus, when children spend less time in care throughout their first 5 years of life, they are less likely to be aggressive and disobedient.

Much of the work chronicling such seemingly negative effects of early care has not examined quality of care. Studies that have considered quality as well as quantity of care clearly indicate that it is not care, per se, but low-quality care that is responsible for such adverse consequences of early care. Thus, although there is reason to be alert to such negative effects, particularly when care begins on a full-time basis in infancy and continues at such intensity until entry into school, such disconcerting effects of care are certainly not inevitable. Moreover, there is increasing evidence that these adverse effects have more to do with the limited attention and insensitive care given in some child care arrangements than with simply spending a lot of time in child care. Having acknowledged this, however, the point must also be reiterated that recent evidence raises concerns about the quality of care that is typically available to most children and families in the United States today.

SOCIAL DEVELOPMENT DURING THE PRESCHOOL YEARS

Although evidence indicates that 20 to 30 or more hours of care per week beginning in the first year of life and continuing at such a high level throughout the infancy, toddler, and preschool years is associated with elevated levels of aggression, noncompliance, and problem behavior, it would be a mistake to presume that child care experience is always related to poor social development. This is simply not the case. In fact, other data indicate, especially in the case of preschoolers (ie, 3- to 5-year-olds), that child care experience can foster social competence and the ability to get along with agemates. Clarke-Stewart[12] said, "Preschool children who attend child care programs are likely to be more self-confident, outgoing, assertive, self-sufficient, more comfortable in new situations, less timid and fearful, more helpful and cooperative, and more verbally expressive" than children who lack preschool care experience. Moreover, child care experience during the late preschool years seems to increase knowledge about social rules and gender roles. Spending time in groups of other children can also promote social skills, including the ability to coordinate one's goals and desires with those of other children, the ability to be empathic and take the perspective of another, and the capacity to share.

In the case of such apparent benefits of child care during the late preschool years, quality of care seems to be critically important to understanding the conditions that foster social development. Positive social development is unlikely to be promoted when child care providers have more children than they can care for, when groups get so big that they are unruly and difficult to manage, and when child care providers fail to make themselves physically and emotionally available to the children in their charge. It is child care providers, then, who ask children to reflect on their own feelings and those of others, who offer gentle suggestions in difficult situations, who are patient in trying situations rather than hostile and controlling or detached and unavailable, and who promote the kind of social functioning that is highly valued in society. And it is child care providers who generally have more experience and training in child care who appear most likely to offer such growth-promoting care. Perhaps the best evidence of the importance of quality of care comes from a natural experiment carried out in Florida by Howes et al.[13] Assessments of child care provider behavior and children's functioning before and after new statewide regulations designed to improve quality went into effect showed that not only did child care provider responsiveness and availability increase, but so did children's prosocial interactions with their agemates.

INTELLECTUAL DEVELOPMENT

Much of our understanding of the role of child care or preschool programs on intellectual development derives from studies of intervention programs specially designed to promote the cognitive functioning of economically disadvantaged children. However informative research on the efficacy of such programs may be, there are reasons to question whether one should generalize from these special interventions to the kinds of child care programs in private homes and centers that most children have access to. For this reason, we concern ourselves here not with well-funded intervention efforts, which do seem to have positive effects on the intellectual functioning of at-risk children, but on those child care experiences available in most neighborhoods and communities.

For the most part, child care programs are not harmful to the intellectual development of preschool children and may even be beneficial. With the exception of work on some shockingly poor child care programs, most work like that of Clarke-Stewart indicates that "children in childcare programs did as well—and sometimes better—on tests of mental or intellectual development" than did children cared for at home by their mothers.[12] More specifically, children in child care programs score higher on IQ tests, demonstrate more advanced eye-hand coordination, explore and play with materials in more creative ways, know more about the physical world (eg, where rain comes from), possess more basic arithmetic skills (eg, counting, measuring) before entering school, and can understand more sophisticated language than other children.

In analyzing this work, Clarke-Stewart[12] highlights 2 important points, one of which qualifies comments made earlier about care setting. First, it appears that many of these advantages associated with preschool child care are short lived in the sense that agemates who have not had preschool experience appear to catch up with their peers soon after the beginning of formal schooling. In other words, preschool child care appears to increase the rate of early acquisition of the kinds of competencies just described rather than afford a permanent enhancement to intellectual functioning. Moreover, the benefits of child care in the preschool years appear to be associated principally with center-based care, in all likelihood because it is in such programs that more formal efforts are made to promote school-like knowledge acquisition.[11] This conclusion is consistent with that which emerges more generally from this analysis, namely, that quality of care—in this case the degree to which a child care experience is intellectually stimulating (rather than boring or simply encouraging of play)—is a major determinant of any effects that care experience is likely to have. This seems to be especially true with respect to language development and the influence of language stimulation. In child care environments in which children are spoken to frequently, encouraged to speak often, and exposed to literacy-promoting materials, language skills are enhanced.[11]

CONCLUSIONS AND RECOMMENDATIONS

Parents and pediatricians should be concerned about the state of child care in America. Unlike many European nations in which child care providers receive adequate training, living wages, and a degree of respect for the important work that they do, child care in the United States often receives less attention and appreciation than the careful parking of a car by a parking lot attendant. Perhaps that should not be so surprising in view of the fact that more time is often spent seeking a new car or computer than a child care arrangement.

Even though there is repeated indication that early, extensive, and continuous nonmaternal care in the infant years, at least as typically available in this country, is associated with increased rates of attachment insecurity in infancy and later noncompliance and aggression, it is clear that these potentially adverse effects of early care do not characterize the experience of all children receiving such care. When care is provided by dedicated child care providers who have the motivation, energy and knowledge to behave in developmentally appropriate ways with those in their care, children can and do thrive. What remains unclear, and thus a source of concern, is exactly how widely available such developmentally enhancing care is. Also of concern, given risks associated with full-, or near full-time care begun in infancy which continues until school entry, is the high levels of nonmaternal care that increasing numbers of children in America seem to be experiencing. After all, more than 50% of mothers of infants younger than 1 year are in the workforce today. This suggests that children and families may benefit from decreasing the overall amount of time a child spends in care and possibly from delaying the initiation of care through extended maternity leaves.

But it should also be appreciated that, whenever care is initiated, and for whatever amount of time it is used, there is no substitute for a careful search for high-quality care. The identification of good care should take as much work as that of a good car deal. In point of fact, it is clear that quality of care is not randomly assigned, but rather that families with the most resources—psychologic as well as economic—are more likely to secure better care. This reality underscores a most important point. At the outset of this chapter, the question was: just how much of an effect does child care have on the child's development? The answer to this question appears to be: not as much as the family. In other words, the effects of child care do not appear to be replacing those of the family, so families should not look to child care to make up for what they lack. Nor should families be worried that child care will undermine their ability to contribute to their child's development. Among the myriad of influences likely to shape the child's early development, it is the family that remains centrally important. One critical way in which such family influence is achieved is via the effort made to obtain the best quality care that a family can afford when it comes time to rely upon others to care for the child. Parents, professionals, and leaders in business and government all have an important role in helping to make such high-quality care accessible to all children.

REFERENCES

1. Whitebrook M, Howes C, Phillips D. *Who Cares? Child Care Teachers and the Quality of Care in America.* Oakland, CA: Child Care Employee Project; 1989
2. Helburn S, Culkin ML. *Cost, Quality, and Child Outcomes in Child Care Centers: Executive Summary.* Denver, CO: University of Colorado at Denver; 1995
3. Bowlby J. *Attachment and Loss: Volume II. Separation: Anxiety and Anger.* New York, NY: Basic Books; 1973
4. Brazelton TB. *Working and Caring.* Reading, MA: Addison-Wesley Publications; 1985
5. Belsky J. The "effects" of infant day care reconsidered. *Early Child Res Q.* 1988; 3:235–272
6. Clarke-Stewart KA. Infant day care. Maligned or malignant? *Am Psychol.* 1989;44: 266–273
7. National Institute of Child Health and Development, Early Child Care Network. *Infant Child Care and Attachment Security: Results of the NICHD Study of Early Child Care.* Symposium presented at the International Conference of Infant Studies; April 20, 1996; Providence, RI
8. Howes C, Matheson CC, Hamilton CE. Maternal, teacher, and child care history correlates of children's relationships with peers. *Child Dev.* 1994;65:264–273
9. Bates JE, Marvinney D, Kelly T, et al. Child-care history and kindergarten adjustment. *Dev Psychol.* 1994;30:690–700

10. Baydar N, Brooks-Gunn J. Effects of maternal employment and child care arrangements on preschoolers' cognitive and behavioral outcomes: evidence from the children of the national longitudinal survey of youth. *Dev Psychol.* 1991;27:932–945

11. National Institute of Child Health and Development, Early Child Care Research Network. *Early Child Care and Children's Development Prior to School Entry.* Symposium presented at the Society for Research in Child Development; April 19, 2001; Minneapolis, MN

12. Clarke-Stewart A. Consequences of child care for children's development. In: Booth A, ed. *Child Care in the 1990s: Trends and Consequences.* Hillsdale, NJ: Erlbaum; 1992:63–82

13. Howe C, Smith E, Galinsky E. *The Florida Child Care Quality Improvement Study: Interim Report.* New York, NY: Families and Work Institute; 1995

ADDITIONAL RESOURCES

American Academy of Pediatrics. *Choosing Child Care: What's Best for Your Family?* Elk Grove Village, IL: American Academy of Pediatrics; 2002

American Academy of Pediatrics, Committee on Community Health Services. The pediatrician's role in community pediatrics. *Pediatrics.* 1999;103:1304–1307

Berman S. Training pediatricians to become child advocates. *Pediatrics.* 1998;102:632–636

Booth A, ed. *Child Care in the 1990s: Trends and Consequences.* Hillsdale, NJ: Erlbaum Associates; 1992

Chehrazi SS. *Psychosocial Issues in Day Care.* Washington, DC: American Psychiatric Press; 1990

Fight Crime: Invest in Kids. *America's Child Care Crisis: A Crime Prevention Tragedy.* Washington, DC: Fight Crime: Invest in Kids; 2000. Available at: http://www.fightcrime.org/reports/childcarereport.pdf. Accessed March 19, 2004

Frank Porter Graham Child Development Institute. *Early Learning, Later Success: The Abecedarian Study: Executive Summary.* Chapel Hill, NC: Frank Porter Graham Child Development Institute; 2000

Head Start Bureau, Administration for Children, Youth, and Families. *Making a Difference in the Lives of Infants and Toddlers and Their Families: The Impacts of Early Head Start.* Washington, DC: Head Start Bureau; 2002

National Center for Early Learning and Development. *The Children of the Cost, Quality, and Outcomes Study Go to School.* Chapel Hill, NC: Frank Porter Graham Child Development Institute; 1999. Available at: http://www.fpg.unc.edu/~ncedl/PDFs/CQO-es.pdf. Accessed March 19, 2004

National Institute of Child Health and Human Development. *The NICHD Study of Early Child Care.* Bethesda, MD: National Institute of Child Health and Human Development; 1999. Available at: http://www.nichd.nih.gov/publications/pubs/early_child_care.htm. Accessed March 19, 2004

National Network for Child Care. *The NICHD Child Care Study Results: What Do They Mean for Parents, Child Care Professionals, Employers, and Decision Makers.* National Network for Child Care; 2002. Available at: http://www.nncc.org/Research/NICHD.ECIresponse.html. Accessed March 19, 2004

National Resource Center for Health and Safety in Child Care. *13 Indicators of Quality in Child Care: Research Update.* Aurora, CO: National Resource Center for Health and Safety in Child Care; 2002. Available at: http://aspe.hhs.gov/hsp/ccquality-ind02/index.htm. Accessed March 19, 2004

NICHD Early Child Care Research Network. Child-care structure—process—outcome: direct and indirect effects of child-care quality on young children's development. *Psychol Sci.* 2002;13:199-206

Reynolds AJ, Temple JA, Robertson DL, Mann EA. Long-term effects of an early childhood intervention on educational achievement and juvenile arrest. *JAMA.* 2001;285;2339-2346

Shore R. *Rethinking the Brain: New Insights Into Early Development.* New York, NY: Families and Work Institute; 1997

Zigler EF, Lang ME. *Child Care Choices: Balancing the Needs of Children, Families, and Society.* New York, NY: The Free Press; 1991

CHAPTER 7

Discipline for Child Care Providers

Barbara J. Howard, MD

LEARNING OBJECTIVES

- The reader will understand the 3 essential components of a system of discipline: a positive adult-child relationship, positive reinforcement of desirable behaviors, and consequences of misbehavior.
- The reader will learn different techniques for reinforcing acceptable behaviors in young children.
- The reader will learn the potential difficulties of using "time out" in the child care setting and how to solve them.
- The reader will understand strategies for working with families when a child behavior problem exists in a child care setting.

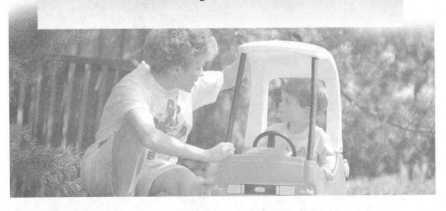

INTRODUCTION: THE IMPORTANCE OF DISCIPLINE IN CHILD CARE SETTINGS

Child care providers are in an important and unique position to help both parents and children establish healthy discipline practices. Parents look to child care providers as experts in child development and behavior, deriving expertise from their training plus intimate knowledge of the children and often of the family situation as well. Child care providers have many opportunities to observe children in group interactions, where many behaviors need to be learned and teaching can be most effective. It is estimated that 15% to 30% of preschool children have significant behavior problems, often including aggression. There is very high persistence of aggressive behaviors from this age group into adulthood. At least 50% go on to manifest serious problems later in life, so intervention at a young age is crucial.[1] It is important to distinguish between discipline and punishment. When discipline is referred to in regard to young children, what is really being discussed is teaching. In the child care setting, this teaching takes place in the context of interactions and exchanges between caregivers and children and between children, as monitored by caregivers. Throughout the child's day, the short-term goal of discipline to the young child is to provide for a safe, positive experience for the child and child care provider alone or as part of a group. It is generally achieved through methods extrinsic to the child, by means of structure provided by the child care provider. Discipline incorporates methods such as distraction, redirection, and modeling. The long-term goal is for the child to develop his or her own inner controls to help them become happy, well-adjusted, productive members of society who can build and sustain healthy relationships throughout life.

DEVELOPMENT IN PRESCHOOLERS AS RELATED TO DISCIPLINE

Preschool is an age period when children are mastering multiple skills at once. There is a huge range of normal behavior and developmental abilities at this time, leaving the children open for growth but also vulnerable to many frustrations and lapses in coping skills. Gross motor skills are quite well developed by 3 years of age, but refinement in balance, speed, and coordination of multiple tasks is still developing. Children love to practice these skills—in fact, they are developmentally driven to do so, according to Piaget. As a result, though, they get themselves into dangerous situations, because their motor skills exceed their judgment.

Fine motor skills also develop rapidly during this period. Children go from being able to stack 6 blocks at 2 years of age to building elaborate castles. They go from scribbles at 2.5 years of age to writing letters and words at 5 years of age. They watch the productions of others carefully and compare themselves without prompting. Often they become frustrated even when they have normal fine motor skills, because they can imagine more than they can produce. Children with true delays in fine motor skills may turn their frustration into aggression toward the frustrating materials or toward other children.

Language skills also fall into a broad range. Two-year-olds should be able to form sentences but may be only 75% intelligible to others. The complexity of their sentence structure is very limited. Although they may try to use words to negotiate social situations and to express emotions, they may not have the needed abilities. By 4 years of age, children can relate complex stories that often go far beyond the facts of a case. This is a time when their verbal creations may also begin to be used to avoid punishment and be labeled as lying. Children with expressive language delays are more prone to use physical actions instead of words, especially in emotionally charged moments. Aggressive patterns of interaction that develop as coping styles during the preschool period tend to persist even after language skills normalize. How these children are taught and how their behavior is managed are especially important to the child's outcome.

Moral development in the preschool years is an interesting topic. Two-year-olds are able to appreciate the suffering of others and will attempt to comfort them. When their own goals are blocked, however, they do not hesitate to use force to their own ends. By 3 years of age, children can take the point of view of others—true empathy. They don't always do so, however. By 6 years of age, children have rule-governed behavior in many parts of their lives. They still tend to bend the rules to suit themselves and even make a game of this. Six-year-olds are very interested in adult rules, however, which make them good citizens for classrooms. Moral behavior can be described in several aspects. Moral judgment has to do with being able to explain the reasoning behind decisions to act one way or another. Preschoolers will say they should act a certain way to avoid punishment. Resistance to cheating is an entirely separate dimension seeming to have more to do with impulse control, of which there is a wide range. Impulse control also has a great deal to do with the context of the situation. Greater temptation generally results in less control. Many other factors affect impulse control, including temperament, the presence of attention-deficit/hyperactivity disorder, previous experiences of deprivation or indulgence, and expectations and previous practice with self-control.

Cognitive processes during the preschool years progress from the sensorimotor learning of infants (learning and experiencing the world through all of the senses, by playing with and touching objects, imitating people, building with blocks, etc) to the preoperational thought of toddlers and early preschoolers (egocentric, prelogical, unable to take another's perspective) so that children gradually learn principles of more complex causality. Preschoolers are still unsure about transformations, for example, and can't judge multiple components at once, such as the connection between size and mass or height and volume. More importantly, perhaps, they do not understand what can change into what and which changes are reversible. This is important to their concerns about body parts and integrity and their ideas about boys and girls. They may be easily aroused to aggression when they fear for their body's safety, even if there is no objective risk from an adult's point of view.

Sexual issues emerge in child care settings in terms of differences in play styles and preferences for same-sex playmates and also sexual issues around toileting and privacy. These may present as discipline topics when sexual behaviors are overt. Sexual abuse also will be present in some children, whose sexualized behaviors in the child care setting will be the clue to a need for investigation and may present problematic behavioral interactions for the group.

School readiness is a topic of concern for parents and teachers alike in the preschool period. Signs of learning weaknesses become apparent at this age in some children, who will need special support to make optimal progress. The evidence for these developmental differences may present as distracting, out of control, or withdrawn behaviors during activities that most tap the child's area of weakness. For example, table time with writing or cutting skills may bring out behaviors as a sign that the child cannot yet perform these tasks. Although the child care setting can be an encouraging place to practice these skills, the child's difficulty needs to be respected, and the program should have tolerable, brief sessions with sufficient support. Evaluation is indicated when specific or general skill weaknesses are suspected.

There are a number of other factors that can predispose a child to behavior problems and difficulty establishing or maintaining a system of discipline. Common factors are temperamental characteristics of low adaptability, high activity level, short attention span, or negative mood as part of normal development or as part of attention-deficit/hyperactivity disorder. Developmental deviations, including mental retardation, often require adjustment of expectations and strategies to the appropriate mental age of the child. Mental health disorders of the child may require child care providers to interpret behaviors more carefully and use different approaches to behavior management.

THE 3 NECESSARY COMPONENTS OF DISCIPLINE

Discipline can be defined as a system of teaching, learning, and nurturing designed to help the child develop appropriate social behaviors and, ultimately, to attain self-control, self-direction, and caring.[2] There are 3 interrelated principles that are essential to an effective system of discipline.[3] These are: reinforcement of desired behaviors, consequences for undesired behaviors to decrease their occurrence, and an underlying positive relationship with the caregiving adults so that the child wishes to please. All 3 components must be functioning well for optimal child behavior and outcome. If positive reinforcement is offered, but there is no consequence for misbehavior other than ignoring, the misbehavior often persists. If all misbehavior is punished but there is a poor relationship between the child and the adult, the behavior is less likely to improve. When a problem is suspected in a system of discipline, all 3 components must be evaluated.

Reinforcement of Desired Behaviors

Reinforcement of desired behaviors requires noticing the desired behaviors. This is the hardest thing to do in a busy child care environment and the most valuable reinforcement itself—attention. Children inherently want and need a great deal of attention. The most important aspect of that attention is primarily its frequency, though not its duration. By preschool age, children have many interests in things and in other children. They still need to feel that adults are watching them to keep them safe as they are very aware of their own vulnerability. Frequent brief touches, smiles, and comments on their activities will make it possible for most young children to play and interact happily for hours. When those positive contacts occur selectively when the child is acting appropriately, the desired behaviors are reinforced and will occur more often. The hard part for providers occurs in a busy group of children when an individual child requires adult attention for acting inappropriately, for example, with aggression, throwing things, dangerous play, or simply whining. The adults may be work-
ing so hard at attending to all of these little emergencies that appropriate behavior may go unnoticed or is noticed with a sigh of relief that no intervention is needed. Lower child-staff ratios help make attention to appropriate behavior easier. Energetic, physically and emotionally healthy, invested providers who truly enjoy young children and are satisfied with their work situation are also more likely to have the energy needed for this kind of frequent attention giving.

Lower child-staff ratios help make attention to appropriate behavior easier.

If child care providers need to improve their attending skills or a certain child seems to need more attention because of negative attention-getting behaviors, generally out of control behavior, or withdrawn behavior, adult attending skills should be a focus. One way to do this is to practice the steps of giving "brief attention immediately." The key to brief attention immediately is for the child care provider to notice the child's first bid for attention. This may consist of a look to the adult, question or request, or simply coming near the adult. The adult should immediately turn, face the child, make eye contact, smile if appropriate, and touch the child or comment in 1 or 2 sentences on the child's situation. This is also an important language teaching opportunity, because there is something in this situation which is salient to the child. For example, if the child has noticed a broken toy, the adult might say "Oh, no, the wheel on this truck is missing. See if you can find it so we can fix it." In this way vocabulary, emotional tone, and problem solving are being conveyed as well as monitoring of the child's behavior and reinforcement of the child's appropriate concern over the broken toy. Brief attention to appropriate behaviors of quiet play without a bid for attention by the child will also gradually increase those skills over weeks of use. Attending to nonbid behavior may need to be regarded as a project for a certain child for several weeks to be done effectively by the staff. Initially, positive attention to desirable behavior may disrupt the child's quiet play. This can be disheartening to the adults unless they understand that this will lead to more quiet play over a period of weeks.

Another technique for providing positive attention to desired behaviors is that of giving more concrete approval, such as marks, stickers, tokens, or points for selected behaviors. This kind of attention to even partial performance of desired behaviors will shape behavior progressively toward the complete action desired. This is not needed routinely for children but only if there is a child or children with behaviors that have resisted requests for change or redirection. The children should be informed of the plan and ideally involved in naming the behaviors that will be rewarded. It makes them more active participants and shifts more of the responsibility to them. Each time a desired behavior is noted, the child can be interrupted, eye contact can be established, the child can warmly be told of the positive behavior, and a concrete reinforcer can be given (eg, mark made on their hand [with parental permission] or placement of a sticker or stamp). These reinforcers should be given at a frequency of 6 to 10 per hour to be effective, which implies that many positive behaviors or small approximations to positive behaviors should be acknowledged. At the end of the observation period, which could be a half-hour, several hours, or all day, the child has the marks, stamps, or other reinforcers totaled and a reward is given. The reward should be small enough so that the reward system can be practically used for weeks and should be acceptable to parents as well as staff. Examples might include an extra privilege, such as line leader, choice of a story, a snack, a special sticker, etc. After several weeks, the system can be phased out, because the staff will have developed a habit of noticing the child's positive behaviors and verbally acknowledging them to the child, and the child will have developed some more stable positive behaviors of their own. The system can be reinstituted again as needed. This same strategy is useful for very shy children when called "bravery points" to help them become aware of their own little steps in bravery and to reinforce those. This not only teaches the child what is considered desirable behavior but also helps the adults keep track of their own attending behaviors.

Parents can use this technique at home independently of the number of rewards being given at the child care center. It is preferable for child care providers to give the rewards themselves rather than to ask the parents to give rewards for several reasons. Rewards are more effective in people of all ages when given as soon as possible after the desirable behavior. In addition, parents may have their own problems with the child's behavior and may forget the reward or decide that intervening behaviors have been too negative for the child to be rewarded. Often, the whole class of children will see this game as something they want to do. It still works well when multiple children participate. Each should be rewarded on their own merits, however, with comparisons or races for the most marks avoided.

Other more concrete forms of reinforcement may be helpful for a given child. These include pats or hugs, smiley stamps, tokens, snacks, or privileges. The use of concrete reinforcers should be checked with the parents for acceptability in advance. It is a good principle to use the least that works for a given child, because most children never require such concrete measures. A tendency for a child to always expect concrete reinforcement can rapidly develop.

Even more difficult to provide in the child care setting is individual time for children. Although brief attention is a form of individual time, some children really need more prolonged individual attention to achieve behavioral control. Often, these children are the ones who act up immediately on entering the child care setting in the morning. They may also be recognized as the ones demanding attention or using negative behavior to get attention all day long. Sometimes, children for whom "time out" seems to be ineffective, as will be discussed later, will only improve when given more individual time each day. This is also a very valuable habit to teach parents of all the children attending a child care facility. Individual time should be given daily regardless of the child's behavior, have a constant but brief duration (eg, 5 to 10 minutes), be uninterrupted by others, and consist of an interactive activity of the child's choice, of which the child is in charge. Accomplishing this in a busy child care environment requires some planning. Sometimes, a child can be brought in 10 minutes early to get their special time. Sometimes it can be given by one provider while another supervises the rest of the children. Sometimes it can be given while the other children are involved in a very absorbing activity, such as watching a videotape, or are napping. When a certain child really needs special time, it is worth the effort to innovate.

Special time given by the parent is also very useful for those children who have tantrums or act up as soon as the parent arrives or as they leave at the end of the day. Children may appear to be very happy all day in child care, yet become upset when the parent arrives. It is concerning to everyone. This often represents the child's message to the parent that they were missed and that the child feels comfortable enough with them to let out their feelings. It certainly can be a genuine message that the child is angry that the parent was not with them all day, even though they had a good time. These messages are difficult for the young child to deliver calmly or even verbally, especially when the parent immediately straps them into a car seat and turns their attention to the road. Providers can suggest that the parent spend 5 minutes of special time in a corner of the center, in the office, hallway, or even in the car before driving off.

Adult-Child Relationship Component

Children are much more likely to respond to teaching of any kind when they feel connected to and wish to please the teacher. A tone of warmth and playfulness has been shown to improve child compliance at home. Even brief "prior nurturance" in an experimental situation improves child compliance and learning.[4] When children sense their own acceptance rather than irritation with them, they are less likely to react aggressively to others.

Another key to positive relationships and also positive behaviors in children comes from the way children are talked to and listened to. Children are more likely to listen to and respect someone who listens to and respects them on their own level. Children model after and treat others the way they are treated. In addition, children form opinions about themselves from what their caregiving adults say about them. If they are portrayed as troublemakers, they are more likely to be just that. Some of this comes from the expectation of the adult, not just from the words they hear. Rosenthal performed a classic experiment in which a group of children about to enter school were randomly assigned to groups described to their new teachers as "soon to bloom" or "average," although there were no real differences among them. The group predicted to do well in fact did so that year, whereas the other group had the usual behavioral and academic problems. Parental expectations work in the same ways and are often greatly influenced by what the child care providers tell them about their child, especially his or her learning potential. Children who have real learning or developmental difficulties do better when their parents hold more objective views of their true abilities. This may be because those parents adjust their level of instruction and the tasks they request of the child to a level the child can actually perform, thus producing ongoing success rather than discouragement through repeated failures. Oppositional behavior is also markedly decreased when children are asked to do things they can accomplish reasonably easily. This is not to say that children should never be challenged, but that their overall day should be one of successes. To do this, parents and providers need to understand the child's actual abilities. Sometimes, this requires formal testing by a specialist. This should be performed on any child with persistent behavior problems as well as those showing learning problems. Although adults don't want to label children, especially at a young age, nothing is as labeling as a self-perception of failure or behavior problems resulting from inability to keep up.

Talking to children effectively can be summarized as being short, simple, and specific. These principles apply to praise or encouragement as well as instruction and correction. Parents with conduct-disordered children have been found to address them in long, complicated strings of commands, charged with emotions, and often with conflicting or vague information about what is desired of them. Shorter, simpler statements are easier to remember and less likely to include those features. Specificity makes it possible for a child to comply accurately and also avoids generalizations about the child's character. An example of an "assertive instruction" might be: "David, I would like you to pick up your jacket from the floor and put it in your cubicle now." The key components of specific instructions are identification of who is making the request ("I"), what specific action they want, of whom ("you"), and the time frame in which the behavior is requested ("now"). Use of simple, specific instructions minimizes misunderstanding as a reason for noncompliance and also helps avoid generalizations, comparisons, and emotional additions that can be hurtful to the child and the adult-child relationship and interfere with compliance. An example of such negative additions might be: "Why don't you kids pick up your jackets like the other classes? You never seem to remember the rules."

Praise is optimally given in specific terms, especially for children in group settings, to avoid jealousy and comparisons, and focused on effort rather than product. Children are frequently concerned about favoritism in their child care setting just as they may be in their families. Praise can also be given to a child for not doing some misbehavior that they might do or usually did in the same circumstance previously. In situations that require a lot of self-control or effort, reinforcement may be needed every few minutes for some children to help them stay on task. Praise should be dosed appropriately to the task as a form of feedback to the child and to increase the likelihood that the child will accept the assessment as realistic. Some children respond to praise for their work by ripping up their paper or running away. This response may be attributable to low self-esteem, internal discouragement with their skills, or generally excessive praise or may be attention-getting behavior. Specific praise helps these children, although further assessment or therapy may also be needed. An example of specific praise might be: "I really like the way you painted with 3 colors in all the parts of the paper, you really worked hard on it." Having a child assess his or her own performance is an ultimately desired goal that can begin during the preschool years. Rather than telling a child how his or her performance is good, the adult could ask: "What do you think of your picture?" and confirm their impression.

Praise should be dosed appropriately to the task as a form of feedback to the child and to increase the likelihood that the child will accept the assessment as realistic.

The kind of listening that transmits empathy to a child is "active listening," which recognizes the content and feelings being conveyed. An example might be when a child is telling the adult, "Danny took my truck." The child care provider could actively listen or "echo" the child by saying, "I hear you saying that Danny took your truck (the content). You seem to feel really mad! (the feelings)." As the child care provider says these words, he or she should copy the emotional tone of the child, for example, by making their hands into fists, tensing the upper body, raising the voice, and scowling. After this brief echoing, the adult should not add any input of his or her own for at least 1 minute. Notice that no solutions or suggestions are being offered in the initial interchange. This not only avoids reprimands or teaching but also leaves an opportunity for the child to solve this situation for himself or herself. If needed, a suggestion or interpretation can be offered and role played with the child subsequently.

Routines for the day help decrease stress and help children feel a sense of security, orderliness, personal meaning, and trust in their caregiving relationships. Child care settings usually follow routines to a very great extent just to maintain order. Children become so accustomed to these routines that they even beg their families to follow them at home also. Inherent in routines are some other important components to a system of discipline. A routine implies orderliness, which is conveyed to the child explicitly: "In 3 minutes, it will be 'clean-up time'!" Children are repeatedly instructed in what to do at that clear signal each day, have the desired behavior modeled for them by staff and peers, and receive positive feedback for their participation. The children have any resistance to compliance decreased by the familiarity of the expectation, are helped to transition into the activity by adequate warning, and have many opportunities to master the task. This is an ideal way for children to learn. Families that have a high level of routine or rhythmicity have been noted to have children with higher self-esteem, competence, independence, and achievement orientation. Such a pattern is more often found in families of higher educational levels. Low rhythmicity is associated with parenting by adults with significant mental health problems and those with multiple social problems. By providing routines in the child care setting, some of the disadvantage of low rhythmicity in the home, if present, can be counteracted.

Consistency is another valuable aspect of rhythmicity. Parents of children with conduct disorder have been noted to be irritable, harsh, inconsistent, and relatively uninvolved with their children. Routines provide consistency, but consistent handling of similar situations is also important. To do this in a child care setting with multiple providers, it is essential that there be standards for behavior, planned consequences for misbehavior, and communication of these rules among providers and, ideally, to parents and children also. Young children require repeated opportunities to learn rules, and consistency makes this process more efficient. It makes testing by the child trying to find out the rules less necessary. Some flexibility is also appropriate, however, to help the child generalize rules to different situations. Some variation in response to different situations is inevitable, of course. It is also a good model for the child to experience adults adapting to different situations, especially as a response to negotiation attempts by the child, as a way of teaching flexibility and tolerance. Similarly, it is useful for children to hear and see adults admit and apologize for their mistakes and offer forgiveness to others, including to children.

One way to include flexibility in a system of discipline is to provide many opportunities for the child to choose among alternatives. Making choices is a skill that needs to be practiced. Having choices also decreases resistance in the child and ambivalence in the child care provider when the adult must dictate the plan. Choices offered should be simple, developmentally appropriate, and acceptable alternatives from the adult's point of view. Choices should not be emotionally charged or embarrassing, such as a "choice" to wear diapers publicly for a child who has had a toileting accident. Opportunities to try out different roles is an important kind of choice for learning empathy. Children should be given opportunities to be the line leader, juice server, etc and to dress up and role play different family or community personae. Children given these opportunities in their families have been found to develop higher levels of moral reasoning, presumably because they better learn to understand the points of view of others. When children experiment with the decisions and authority of adults, they learn to appreciate its difficulties.

Models of personal behavior and interpersonal interaction are important components of teaching children how to act. Even newborn infants copy adult expressions of emotion. By 3 months of age, infants regulate their emotions and actions in coordination with their caregiver. Emotional tone of the primary caregiver, even emotions offered experimentally, are echoed in the infant's mood for hours subsequently. By 15 months of age, children even copy aggression they view on television. In a 30-year study of resilience to stress, one helpful factor to good outcome was the presence of at least one positive role model for the child. Modeling of moods, how to manage emotions under stress, and how to tolerate frustration or conflict and resolve it are all as important as modeling desirable actions, especially during the preschool years, when these reaction patterns are being set. Child care providers can set a positive tone in the room, "jolly" children through minor discontent, echo strong emotions, role play solutions to interpersonal situations, read stories and ask questions about problem solving situations, and even verbalize about their own feelings when appropriate as ways of teaching these things. Children with conduct disorders have been found to have extremely limited repertoires for problem solving and interpersonal conflict as one factor predisposing them to aggressive solutions. By modeling these skills early, some of the tendency to violence may be avoidable.

Consequences of Misbehavior

Consequences after misbehavior are a necessary component of a system of discipline. As for praise or positive reinforcement, the smallest consequence that works for an individual child is preferred. For many children, simple verbal correction or a frown by a caregiving adult is sufficient. For others, greater intensity or more active consequences are needed to obtain any behavior change.

There are 2 categories of consequences: natural and logical. Natural consequences that follow directly from the child's misbehavior without adult intervention are preferable whenever reasonable, because they teach causal connections, tend to occur immediately and consistently, and are impersonal so that the child does not blame others for the result. Natural consequences, such as having no candy after eating it all at once, are reasonable to allow to happen. In other situations, natural consequences are not appropriate, as for example, jumping off the top of the jungle gym, exploring others sexually, or excessive aggression. When natural consequences cannot be used, logical consequences must be designed by the supervising adults.

It is preferable for child care providers to make consequences for misbehavior that occurs in the care setting rather than passing that job on to the parents for several reasons. Immediate consequences are better teachers than those separated in time from the offense. The adult who has seen the misbehavior can design a consequence more appropriate to the actual offense and discuss it more definitively with the child. Parents who haven't seen their child for hours should not have to strain their relationship by punishing an action they haven't seen. Perhaps most importantly, the adult who passes consequences on to someone else undermines his or her own authority with the child.

There are several important principles for designing logical consequences. Because the goal of giving a consequence is to teach, the result should be meaningfully related to the offense. Similarly, the extent of the consequence should be in proportion to the misbehavior, although smaller reactions generally work better, because they are more likely to be delivered unambivalently, promptly, and consistently by adults, and it has been found that the child is more likely to infer his own responsibility rather than feel angry at what he sees as harshness on the part of the adult. For example, a child who has grabbed crayons from a peer may have his privilege of using crayons removed for the next 10 minutes. During that time, he may well be thinking about how he could share better rather than being angry about spending an hour in a corner or having a week's restriction and, thus, forgetting about the crayons. Discussing the misbehavior and consequence should be done in a brief, respectful manner. Calmer delivery not only is a better model but also is less likely to trigger a reaction from the child of further misbehavior or escalation.[5] All consequences should be delivered as privately as possible so that the child may save face and avoid a confrontation in which the child must act defiantly to preserve status with his or her peers. Older children can be involved in deciding their own consequences. This has the effect of making the child consider the offense, showing the adult how he or she assesses its severity, and actively involving the child in the learning aspect of discipline.

Minor misbehavior, especially testing behavior, such as foul language or taunting, is often best ignored. When one goal of the behavior was an adult reaction, this response effectively extinguishes the behavior fairly quickly. Ignoring is most effective in an environment of plentiful positive attention, which provides contrast to a state of being ignored. Verbal correction alone can be effective, but in cases of sibling squabbles instead tends to increase aggression if no immediate consequence is given. At most, one warning should be given for nonaggressive misbehaviors in case the child is unaware of the rule being broken. A common behavior management mistake, however, is threatening or repeating requests, which simply cause children to disregard admonitions. Threats have the additional problems of raising tension in the child, replacing useful instruction, possibly including insults or generalizations about the child, and even precipitating misbehavior by the child to draw a punishment which will clear the air.

Prompt action is the most effective intervention, especially for preschool children, who are less moved by words alone. This action may be redirection, distraction, or removal in less serious encounters. An extremely useful intervention for noncompliant young children is what could be called "one request and then move." After gaining the child's attention, the adult makes his or her request clearly only once then waits silently for up to 10 seconds for a response. If the child does not comply, the adult leads the child to the task, remaining silent. If the child performs the task or even part of it, they are praised. If not, the adult performs the task while maintaining a hold on the child. The consequence in this case is the silence and the loss of freedom. This approach avoids the common situation of children becoming immune to adult requests, because they are repeated many times without any action. An alternative is for the child to go to "time out" until ready to perform the task and then complete it. Counting aloud with a clear statement of the number after which a consequence will occur if the task is not begun is an effective motivator for many children who are less defiant than those needing to be grasped. Setting a timer to "beat" as a race can motivate a single child or even a group with a reward of an extra story, time for free play, or other incentives. Frequently a "clean-up" song or other ritual can make this an enjoyable routine.

The most widely used consequence for changing behavior of young children is time out. Although time out has become prevalent, the details of effective administration have sometimes been lost. The definition of time out is "time away from reinforcement and attention, accompanied by disapproval of the behavior, loss of freedom, and loss of interesting things to do." Effective variations can be designed to work with different children and in different settings by keeping these principles in mind. Although time out can be used to decrease any behavior, it is most effective when only applied to 2 or 3 behaviors during any given period of time for an individual child. For preschoolers, time out is mostly needed for aggression, including biting. In the case of biting, the victim should be sympathized with and comforted first to model and to avoid secondary gain from attention to the biter.

If other more severe consequences, such as hitting, are being used for similar behaviors in other settings, such as the home, time out may be less effective. Coordination among child care providers in discipline consequences is ideal but not required. Children can adapt to different rules in different settings. Time out serves an additional educational purpose of demonstrating how individuals can deal with high emotions by withdrawing until they are able to cope. This strategy might better be given a different name, for example "cool-off time," because in this application, the child may not have misbehaved yet and they are put in control of deciding when they are ready to rejoin the group. When children have become skilled at time out, they may be given the choice of coming out when they are ready to adhere to the rules or repair any damages they inflicted. This is inadvisable in very young children, those just learning the technique, or those who have marginal emotional control, because they tend to emerge too quickly before they are able to perform better—in one study, in less than 10 seconds.

Some important components of time out follow[6]:

1. ***Warnings.*** There should be no more than one warning for a misbehavior before time out is begun. No warnings should be given for aggressive behavior, as this tends to result in additional aggression.

2. ***Instruction.*** The child should always be told in brief form (eg, 6 words or 2 short sentences) what behavior was unacceptable. Longer lectures delay the consequence and detract from the understanding of the connection between the misbehavior and the time out consequence.

3. ***Location.*** Time out should be served in a place that has a low level of interest. In child care settings, this can be difficult to arrange. Ideally, a chair within the same room allows the child to see what they are missing and requires less class disruption if the child is capable of sitting quietly. The use of a chair assists in generalizing to use of time out in other settings. The criterion of being in the chair is also clearer than for sitting in a corner, for example. This may be possible after a given child has learned the system, even if not possible initially. Children can be given the choice of sitting on a chair in the room or taken elsewhere when they are experienced. Sometimes an area behind a barrier or through a doorway will suffice. In other cases, the child may need to be escorted from the room to a hallway or the director's office to avoid disrupting the class. This obviously requires a second adult. Children should never be locked in a room, placed in complete darkness, tied in a chair, or frightened in the time out location.

4. ***Dealing with leaving time out.*** All children will try to leave the time out location at least in initial training. In the event of such an escape, the child should be returned to time out without comment and restrained there or placed in an alternative location behind a barrier from which they can see an adult, such as through use of a piece of plywood in a doorway or a Dutch door.[7,8] Restraint can be accomplished by placing hands on the child's shoulders or holding him or her on the lap. The least restraint needed should be used. Children should never be spanked, slapped, or hit by child care providers. Parents should be aware of the policy of the center regarding possible need for restraint in time out as part of their orientation at enrollment. On average, a given child may require 3 or 4 weeks before mastering time out so that they are able to sit quietly.

5. ***Age and duration of use.*** Time out has been found effective beginning before the first birthday through 10 years of age. School-aged children should rarely require time out but instead receive other logical consequences if a reasonable system of discipline and relationships have been in place. Children respond optimally to fairly brief time out; one minute per year of mental age is a good standard (ie, 5 minutes for a child of mental age 5 years). Children with atten-

tion deficits often do better with a shorter period. Very intense or labile children may need longer periods to regain emotional control. In initial training, simply requiring 15 seconds of quiet before release is effective and much easier to attain. As the child gains understanding and self-control, the time should be gradually increased to the standard length with a ticking timer placed within view but not within reach.

6. **Behavior in time out.** Initially, any behavior can be tolerated and ignored in time out as long as release occurs after 15 seconds of quiet. As the child masters the technique, quiet for the entire duration can be required. If the child is vocalizing or jumping around in the chair, the timer should be reset as many times as necessary but without speaking to the child to avoid secondary gain. Many children pretend to enjoy time out as a way to save face or to attempt to decrease its apparent power. These statements should be disregarded.

7. **Attention.** Any other children who speak to the child in time out should also serve time out once this rule has been taught. Adults should refrain from answering questions or responding or attending to the child in any way as much as possible during time out for it to be effective. Children who appear to elicit the time out consequence to get attention should be targeted for increased appropriate attention as described earlier in this chapter. Increased attention at home should also be advised. Time out is ineffective if there is no contrast with "time in" in the rest of the child's life.

8. **Release.** Once the timer rings, the adult should notify the child that time out is over and that they can come out. The child should then be redirected to some activity other than that involved in the original incident and attended to for any positive or acceptable behavior. Discussion of the offense can increase the likelihood of repeat offenses, especially in younger children. In some older children, a recitation of the rule and the offense may be reasonable. Asking a child to apologize is requesting hypocrisy unless the child truly appears sorry. Instead, the adult can apologize to the victim with sincerity for their hurt or upset. Children apologize sincerely even from a young age when they are truly sorry. They learn this aspect of humanity from sincere examples modeled before them, not from forced statements. Some children refuse to come out of time out when released. They may need reassurance that they have been forgiven but can be allowed to stay if they desire. This attitude is often displayed as an attempt to invalidate time out.

9. **Discussion of the misbehavior.** Alternative ways of expressing feelings, attaining goals, or negotiating situations should be modeled and taught continuously as described throughout this chapter. Specific role playing for the situation that resulted in the time out is best performed at least several minutes after release when the child has regained composure, pointing out the effects on the feelings of others.

There is no place for shouting, threatening, spanking, slapping, hitting, or shaking children by a child care provider. In most states, slapping or shaking are illegal. It is important to make the distinction between these assaults and the need to stop, move, or restrain young children without inflicting pain or injury as part of teaching and protecting them and other children. This is, in a way, parallel to the distinction between the comfortable holding, hugging, and patting from caregiving adults, which benefit children greatly, versus sexual misuse perpetrated for the purposes of the adult.

WORKING WITH PARENTS

Any system of discipline instituted in a child care setting is likely to differ in major or minor ways from that in the child's home. This can be a major problem if the children are harshly dealt with at home, because less severe consequences may then become relatively ineffective to alter their behavior in other settings. It makes the issue of consequences more complicated for the child care provider. Parents often have multiple concerned adults providing input on how the child's behavior should be handled. Child care providers have this tension, too, without family bonds to temper it. On the other hand, child care providers can be more objective and always have the option of requesting that uncooperative children or families remove their children from the center. The parents often feel constrained by limited options for alternatives to abide by child care center rules. Ideally, parents and child care providers will want to be consistent with each other's discipline for the sake for the child. In many states, there are rules governing discipline that child care centers can use. These apply mainly to the use of corporal punishment, however, and provide little additional guidance. It is important that the administration and the direct care providers are consistent in their philosophy as well as their use of different discipline techniques. Involvement of parents in the development of rules may enhance their knowledge of discipline principles as well as their consistency with child care center rules in their homes. As a minimum, parents should be informed of center rules before enrolling their child. There should also be regular communication between parents and providers about the child's strengths and needs for growth throughout the year so if there is an incident that needs to be reported to the parents, they are aware of the providers' good feelings and knowledge of the child and are less likely to react defensively. Because a child's behavior has meaning, it is essential for child care providers to be in communication with the family to understand the child's context and any changes or stresses that may affect his or her behavior in the care setting and vice versa.

Unfortunately, many children live in homes that do not provide adequate or appropriate discipline, or even nurturing, for a variety of reasons. Child care providers may become aware of these deficits by observation of parent-child interaction, from reports by the child, or because of patterns of the child's behavior. Ideally, the child care provider or center can be of assistance in suggesting alternative child rearing techniques by talking directly to individual parents or couples, offering handouts, distributing a newsletter, keeping a lending library of child development and parenting books and videotapes (see suggested resources), running parent groups, setting up a parent buddy system, or encouraging parents to serve as aides in the classroom to learn child management techniques. These approaches all can be effective when the parents see a need to change.

When a child has or develops problem behaviors, it is important to bring these to the parents' attention to find out about recent changes or stresses, to exchange management ideas, to inform them of interventions being tried, and sometimes to suggest referral. The best way to facilitate this communication is for child care providers to routinely exchange information with parents about the child's day, friends, activities, interests, and incidents. When a problem arises, an appointment should be made for a meeting in private to discuss the matter. Specific notes about behaviors and their context should be shared rather than generalities about the child acting up. The parents or other primary caregivers, such as grandparents, should be asked about behaviors at home and how they are managed. Stresses should be asked about, including illness of the child or other family members, changes in household composition, deaths of pets, births of siblings, changes in parental work situations or hours, or traumatic events. Often, parents are struggling with these stresses themselves but are unaware that they affect young children, too. The family can be asked what the child has been told or has asked so that approaches can be consistent. They can be asked what they would like the child care providers to do, for example, to decrease pressure on toilet training or provide more comfort. Assistance in arranging a referral or resources can also be offered,

When a child has or develops problem behaviors, it is important to bring these to the parents' attention to find out about recent changes or stresses, to exchange management ideas, to inform them of interventions being tried, and sometimes to suggest referral.

for example, for housing, social services, mediation, marriage counseling, battered women's services, protective services, or mental health counseling. Although knowledge of these resources is not necessarily within the expertise or training of child care providers, they are often the only trusted professionals involved with families of young children, and it is appropriate for them to at least keep a listing of local resources.

If the family still does not acknowledge any problem and the child's problematic behavior is not responding to strategies described in this chapter, a more serious meeting must be called. In preparation for this meeting, the relevant family members should be invited, and the child care provider should assemble notes about the child's abilities and behaviors. If child care is part of a center, the director and other staff members with knowledge of or relationships with the child and family should be organized to meet with the family together. This is especially important if hostility has developed around the issue of the child's behavior or if a protective services referral needs to be filed. Sometimes it is helpful for one staff member to be regarded as the ally while another takes a more demanding stance. It is important to begin the meeting with a description of the child's positive attributes, giving specifics so that the family can see that staff members know the child well. Then, a specific description of the problem behaviors and what has been tried should be presented. Asking "How is it for you at home?" or "How bad does it get for you?" can be helpful to find motivation for change. Finding out how the parents were raised or how similar behavior was managed when they were children may be essential to understanding their philosophy about child rearing or why they may be stuck trying to manage this problem. It is essential that the staff remain nonjudgmental and empathetic while discussing family management. Often, parents have problems managing situations for which they hold very different views than their own parents, because they disagree with how they were raised but have no model of their own to use. When such a dilemma is revealed, the family may be willing to try a strategy such as time out instead of spanking for 2 or 3 weeks to see its effects. Even if only one parent is willing to try, if they can agree not to intervene in each others' management, frequently one will be converted to the plan after observing its effectiveness over this trial period. If abuse is suspected, it must be reported to the appropriate authorities, yet a supportive relationship may still be possible with the family for the child's benefit. In severe cases in which a child's behavior is too disruptive or dangerous to be managed and the family is uncooperative, they can be asked to seek outside professional help immediately under threat that the child will be excluded from the setting. For certain children for which government contracts prohibit expulsion, professional help to the child within the setting may be a stipulation. Child care professionals can gain skills and support by establishing a relationship with a mental health professional of whom they can ask questions and to whom they can refer families. Some mental health professionals will come to observe children in the child care setting, provide in-service education to providers, and offer parent groups at the center for a fee.

CONCLUSIONS AND RECOMMENDATIONS

When child care providers truly care about children, establish and maintain good communication with families, work to build their own skills in child development and behavior management, establish an effective system of discipline, and act with compassion, children can be greatly benefited by the care they receive.

REFERENCES

1. Landy S, Peters RD. Identifying and treating aggressive preschoolers. *Infants Young Child.* 1990;3:24–38
2. Howard BJ. Advising parents on discipline: what works. *Pediatrics.* 1996;98(4 Pt 2): 809–815
3. Howard BJ. Discipline in early childhood. *Pediatr Clin North Am.* 1991;38:1351–1369
4. Parke RD. Effectiveness of punishment as an interaction of intensity, timing, agent nurturance, and cognitive structure. *Child Dev.* 1969;40:213–235
5. Blum NJ, Williams GE, Friman PC, Christophersen ER. Disciplining young children: the role of verbal instruction and reasoning. *Pediatrics.* 1995;96(2 Pt 1):336–341
6. Wilson DR, Lyman RD. Time-out in the treatment of childhood behavior problems: implementation and research issues. *Child Fam Behav Ther.* 1982;4:5–20
7. Forehand R, Roberts MW, Doleys DM, et al. An examination of disciplinary procedures with children. *J Exp Child Psych.* 1976;21:109–120
8. Roberts MW, Powers SW. Adjusting chair timeout enforcement procedures for oppositional children. *Child Fam Behav Ther.* 1990;21:257–271

ADDITIONAL RESOURCES

American Academy of Pediatrics. *Discipline and Your Child.* Elk Grove Village, IL: American Academy of Pediatrics; 1998

American Academy of Pediatrics, Committee on Psychosocial Aspects of Child and Family Health. Guidance for effective discipline. *Pediatrics.* 1998;101(4 Pt 1):723–728

Barkley RA. *Defiant Children: A Clinician's Manual for Assessment and Parent Training.* New York, NY: Guilford Press; 1997

Canter L, Canter M. *Assertive Discipline for Parents.* New York, NY: Harper and Row; 1982

Christopherson ER. Anticipatory guidance on discipline. *Pediatr Clin North Am.* 1986;33: 789–799

Christopherson ER. *Little People, Guidelines for Common Sense Child Rearing.* Austin, TX: Pro-Ed; 1982

Clarke L. *SOS! Help for Parents, A Practical Guide for Handling Common Everyday Behavior Problems.* Bowling Green, KY: Parents Press; 1985

Faber A, Mazlish E. *How to Talk So Kids Will Listen and Listen So Kids Will Talk.* New York, NY: Avon Books; 1980

Gordon T. *Parent Effectiveness Training.* New York, NY: Peter H. Wyden Inc; 1970

Howard BJ. Discipline in early childhood. *Pediatr Clin North Am.* 1991;38:1351

Howard BJ. Advising parents on discipline: what works. *Pediatrics.* 1996;98(4 Pt 2):809–815

Howard BJ, Sturner RA. Pediatric behavioral problems. In: *Home Study Self-Assessment Program.* Monograph Edition No. 186. Kansas City, MO: American Academy of Family Physicians; 1994

Hyman LA. Corporal punishment, psychological maltreatment, violence, and punitiveness in America: research, advocacy, and public policy. *Appl Prev Psychol.* 1995;4:113–130

Patterson GR. *Living With Children, New Methods for Parents and Teachers.* Champaign, IL: Research Press; 1976

Patterson GR, Forgatch M. *Family Living Series, Part 1.* (5 cassette tapes to be used with *Living With Children*). Champaign, IL: Research Press Co; 1975

Patterson GR, Forgatch M. *Family Living Series, Part 2.* (3 cassette tapes to be used with *Living With Children*). Champaign, IL: Research Press Co; 1976

Phelan TW. *1-2-3 Magic.* 2nd ed. Glen Ellyn, IL: Child Management; 1996

Straus MA. *Beating the Devil Out of Them: Corporal Punishment in American Families.* New York, NY: Lexington Books; 1994

Varni JW, Christopherson ER. Behavioral treatment in pediatrics. *Curr Probl Pediatr.* 1990; 20:639–704

Webster-Stratton C, Kolpacoff M, Hollinsworth T. The long-term effectiveness and clinical significance of three cost-effective training programs for families with conduct problem children. *J Consult Clin Psychol.* 1989;57:550–553

Webster-Stratton C. *Parents and Children: A 10-Program Videotape Parent Training Series With Manuals.* Eugene, OR: Castalia Press; 1987

Wissow LS, Roter Dr. Toward effective discussion of discipline and corporal punishment during primary care visits: findings from studies of doctor-patient interaction. *Pediatrics.* 1994; 94:587-593

CHAPTER 8

Attention-Deficit/Hyperactivity Disorder in the Preschool Child

Linda Nathanson Lippitt, MD

LEARNING OBJECTIVES

The reader of this chapter should:

- Become familiar with the *Diagnostic and Statistical Manual of Mental Disorders, Fourth Edition (DSM-IV)*[1] criteria for the diagnosis of attention-deficit/hyperactivity disorder (ADHD).

- Have an understanding of the many factors (environmental, medical, neuropsychiatric) that may cause a child to have ADHD-like behavior.

- Understand medication and psychosocial intervention modalities that may be used to assist children and families with ADHD.

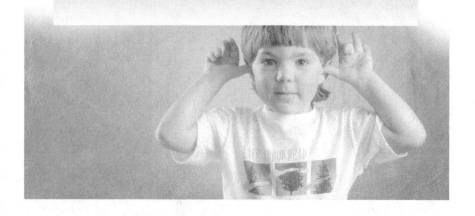

INTRODUCTION

Attention-deficit/hyperactivity disorder (ADHD) is the most common behavioral disorder diagnosed in childhood, affecting approximately 3% to 10% of all school-aged children. The features of this neurobiologically (brain) based disorder were described by a British pediatrician in 1902.[1] Until the 1960s, children with the features that we now call ADHD were given the diagnosis "minimal brain dysfunction," as it was first acknowledged that these were not bad children, but children with a structural or functional difference in their brains. The name was later changed to hyperkinetic reaction of childhood, then to attention deficit disorder (ADD) to reflect problems with attention, and finally to attention-deficit/hyperactivity disorder to include attentional and behavioral components. ADHD remains one of the most controversial childhood disorders in part because of underdiagnosis and undertreatment of true ADHD in children and misdiagnosis and treatment of children who do not have the disorder but have ADHD-like behavior. Accurately diagnosing ADHD is sometimes difficult, particularly in younger preschool-aged children, and is often complicated by other cooccurring conditions. To compound the difficulty, parents have been repeatedly confronted with media interviews and reports conveying misinformation about ADHD diagnosis and treatment, often portraying ADHD as a hoax perpetrated on the population by physicians and pharmaceutical companies. This misinformation results in increased anxiety among parents as they struggle with conflicting information from the media, well-intentioned family and friends, and their child's health care professionals. Unfortunately, this conflicting information sometimes results in children failing to receive appropriate treatment for this serious disorder. To counter these erroneous reports, a coalition of international scientists recently developed a signed consensus statement on ADHD, which references the scientific data and documents the validity of ADHD and the negative consequences suffered by those with the diagnosis.[2]

As part of the controversy, there has been concern about the national trend for increased use of all psychotropic medications in children.[3] Indeed, the use of stimulants increased almost fourfold between 1987 and 1996. This increase may be attributable to changes in diagnostic criteria as well as increased public acceptance of stimulants as part of the primary treatment of ADHD. In fact, it is likely that the prevalence and the public health impact of ADHD may have been greatly underestimated in the past. The increased use of stimulants may reflect an appropriate response to previous underdiagnosis and undertreatment.[4]

DEFINITION

ADHD is a neurobehavioral disorder in which a child's ability to function at home, in school, in child care, and in social situations or leisure activities is impaired by problems with inattention, hyperactivity, and/or impulsivity.

The *DSM-IV*[5] is a resource for mental health professionals that defines and lists the symptoms of various mental disorders in children and adults. The *DSM-IV* now recognizes 3 subtypes of ADHD: 1) attention-deficit/hyperactivity disorder, predominantly hyperactive-impulsive type; 2) attention-deficit/hyperactivity disorder, predominantly inattentive type; and 3) attention-deficit/hyperactivity disorder, combined type. There is also a diagnostic category for attention-deficit/hyperactivity disorder, not otherwise specified (NOS) for children with prominent symptoms of impulsivity or hyperactivity who do not meet criteria for ADHD. The predominantly hyperactive-impulsive type predominates among preschool-aged children.

DIAGNOSIS
The overall criteria for the diagnosis of ADHD in the *DSM-IV* are:
1. Six or more symptoms of inattention that have been present for 6 months or more to a degree that is maladaptive and inconsistent with the child's development level, or 6 or more symptoms of hyperactivity-impulsivity that have been present for 6 months or more to a degree that is maladaptive and inconsistent with the child's developmental level.
2. Symptoms of hyperactivity-impulsivity or inattention that cause impairment and were present before 7 years of age.
3. Symptoms cause impairment in 2 or more settings (home, school, work, social situations, etc).
4. Evidence of significant impairment in social, academic, or occupational functioning.
5. The symptoms do not occur exclusively as part of pervasive developmental disorder, schizophrenia, or other psychotic disorders and are not better explained by another mental disorder, such as mood disorder, anxiety disorder, etc.

Symptoms of Inattention (these symptoms must be greater than developmental level/expectations)
1. Often fails to give close attention to details or makes careless mistakes.
2. Often has difficulty sustaining attention.
3. Often does not seem to listen when spoken to.
4. Often does not follow through on instructions (although the instructions are understood) and fails to finish tasks.
5. Often has difficulty organizing tasks.
6. Often dislikes, avoids, and shows reluctance to engage when sustained mental effort is required.
7. Often loses things necessary for tasks.
8. Is often easily distracted by extraneous stimuli.
9. Is often forgetful in daily activities.

Symptoms of Hyperactivity (these symptoms must be greater than developmental level/expectations)

1. Often fidgets with hands or feet or squirms in seat.
2. Often leaves seat in situations where remaining seated is expected.
3. Often runs about or climbs excessively (may be limited to subjective feeling of restlessness in older individual).
4. Often has difficulty in engaging quietly in leisure activities.
5. Is often "on the go"; acts as if "driven by a motor."
6. Often talks excessively.

Symptoms of Impulsivity (these symptoms must be greater than developmental level/expectations)

1. Often blurts out answers before questions are completed.
2. Often has difficulty awaiting turn.
3. Often interrupts or intrudes on others.

Predominantly Inattentive Type

This subtype is used if 6 or more of the symptoms of inattention (but fewer than 6 symptoms of hyperactivity-impulsivity) have persisted for at least 6 months. Subtypes were initially envisioned as a method to better classify this heterogenous disorder. The subtypes described in *DSM-IV* were developed empirically from field trials and were not primarily derived from independent research. There has been controversy over this designation, particularly with respect to the inattentive subtype and whether it represents a distinct entity. In general, females are more likely to have the predominantly inattentive subtype of ADHD and to experience more academic impairment.[6]

Predominantly Hyperactive-Impulsive Type

This subtype is used if 6 or more of the symptoms of hyperactivity-impulsivity (but fewer than 6 symptoms of inattention) have persisted for at least 6 months and cause significant impairment.

Combined Type

This subtype is used if 6 or more symptoms of hyperactivity-impulsivity **and** 6 or more symptoms of inattention have persisted for at least 6 months and cause significant impairment.

In the preschool age group, most children diagnosed with ADHD are in the hyperactive-impulsive subtype. The symptoms must be significant enough to cause functional impairment and must occur in 2 or more settings. Therefore, it is important to interview or gather information and observations from individuals who are with the child in different settings and who may have differing observations (ie, parents, teacher, after-school care provider, coach, etc).

In October 2001, the American Academy of Pediatrics released a review of diagnostic guidelines for ADHD in school-aged children.[7] The authors stress the need to assess for the condition when appropriate, often in the context of parental or teacher/child care provider concerns regarding behavior, attention, or academic performance or physician concerns that arise during parent/child interviews in the context of well-child or other visits. Pediatricians need to recognize the need to obtain information from parents, caregivers, teachers, or other school professionals and evaluate for coexisting conditions. The authors also emphasize that much of the ADHD research has been done with elementary school-aged children and may not be generalizable to children younger or older than this age group. Recent studies of ADHD in preschool children clearly indicate that this group of children demonstrates impairment in behavioral, social, and academic functioning similar to school-aged children.[8,9]

Etiology

Although the exact etiology of ADHD is not completely defined, it probably involves an interaction between genetics and the environment that is complex and incompletely understood. In most cases, research indicates that ADHD is predominantly determined by heredity. Studies show a concordance rate of 45% to 100% (mean heritability = 0.8) among monozygotic twins who share identical genetic material.[10] Conversely, dizygotic twins, who are no more genetically alike than any other siblings, have a concordance rate of only 4% to 20%. For example, monozygotic twins would be expected to share many more physical characteristics such as height, hair and eye color, skin tones, face shape, etc than would dizygotic twins. Newer neuroimaging techniques have also identified differences in the structure and function of the brains of individuals with ADHD compared with individuals without the disorder.[11] Anatomic magnetic resonance imaging (MRI) studies have identified structural differences, and functional imaging studies (functional MRI, positron emission tomography [PET], and xenon inhalation) have shown differences in function among individuals with ADHD. Areas consistently involved have been the frontal lobes, corpus callosum, basal ganglia, and cerebellum. At this time, however, neuroimaging studies are not indicated specifically for children with ADHD and are not useful in the diagnosis of this disorder. These genetic deviations are likely to exert their effect through alterations of the neurotransmitters dopamine and norepinephrine. Dopamine is involved with risk taking and impulsivity, and norepinephrine is related to the modulation of attention.[12,13] Several studies have also identified an association between neurodevelopmental disorders and prenatal substance use, such as ADHD and alcohol and nicotine.[14-19]

DIFFERENTIAL DIAGNOSIS

It should be evident from the wording of the criteria that the diagnosis of ADHD is established primarily from parent and teacher reports of a child's behavior. The subclassifications clearly indicate that not all children who have ADHD are hyperactive. Conversely, it may also be true that not all children who are hyperactive have ADHD. In addition, at least 30% to 50% of children who do meet the criteria for ADHD have a coexisting condition that also must be identified and managed if there is to be a successful outcome.

First, conditions that could produce symptoms that may overlap with ADHD or cause symptoms that mimic ADHD will be reviewed.

A. Environmental Problems
   1. Unstable family life, including discord between parents and depressed, withdrawn, or abusive parenting figures.
   2. Impoverished environment, leading to poor nutrition and sleep.
   3. Overstimulating, chaotic, or unstructured environment. This can be characterized by a home or poor-quality child care setting with the following characteristics:
      a. The television is constantly on;
      b. There are no set hours for meals and bedtime;
      c. There is frequent arguing or physical fighting; and
      d. It is disorganized, messy, or dirty.
   4. Loss of an individual family member, as well as introductions of multiple new partners in single-parent families.
   5. Attachment disorders and multiple foster home placements
B. Medical
   1. Sensory deficits of hearing or vision.
   2. Chronic disease, including metabolic, gastrointestinal, cardiac, respiratory, or hematologic conditions.
   3. Seizure disorders.
   4. Sleep disorders.
   5. Medications, such as phenobarbital, antihistamines, theophylline, pseudoephedrine, albuterol, etc.
   6. Klinefelter syndrome and other genetic conditions
C. Psychiatric Conditions
   1. Anxiety disorders, including generalized and specific anxiety, post-traumatic stress disorder, and obsessive-compulsive disorder.
   2. Depression.
   3. Persisting effects of neglect and abuse.
   4. Reactive attachment disorders.
   5. Bipolar disorder: a controversial diagnosis in young children. Manifesting symptoms may include extreme irritability and aggressive, hyperactive-like behavior (can occur concurrently with ADHD).

6. Conduct disorder/oppositional defiant disorder (ODD).
7. Autistic spectrum disorders, including autism, Asperger syndrome, and pervasive developmental disorder NOS.
8. Nonverbal learning disorder.
9. Tourette syndrome (can occur concurrently with ADHD).
10. Degenerative disorders; Rett syndrome, HIV infection, inherited central nervous system degenerative disorders.

D. Neurocognitive Disorders
   1. Language disorders
      a. Receptive: difficulty in understanding instructions.
      b. Expressive: difficulty expressing ideas.
      c. Inner: difficulty using language to organize inner thoughts and ideas.
   2. Memory disorders
      a. Short-term memory: cannot remember things just explained.
      b. Convergent memory: cannot coordinate information from different parts of memory (visual, auditory, sensory) or different ideas.
      c. Divergent memory: difficulty associating new knowledge with other facts, a cornerstone to creativity.
      d. Sequential memory: difficulty doing things in the correct order.
      e. Active working memory: difficulty juggling 2 different types of memory and switching back and forth from one to the other (eg, remembering your good ideas and the rules for creating letters, spelling, and punctuation all at the same time).
      f. Long-term memory: difficulty easily recalling facts long known at will.
   3. Developmental Gerstmann syndrome: this is a useful concept to describe a delay in the maturation of the parietal lobe of the brain. Children with this neurologic variation have difficulty knowing what their fingers are doing without visual guidance. Their pencil hold is usually fist-like to get around this problem. Difficulty with sequential organization, body awareness, automatic writing (but not a lack of good ideas to write about), and automatic math facts (but not a problem in understanding the basic math concepts) often accompany the fisted pencil hold. A person with this challenge would appear not to follow through with instructions and would appear to lack sustained mental effort, particularly when paperwork is involved.
   4. Mental retardation: mild to moderate mental retardation in a child who is fairly adept socially can be difficult to detect in a preschooler. The child's immaturity and confusion with demands can be confused with inattentiveness and lack of ability to complete work. The immature behavior would also be appropriate for the cognitive age but not for the actual age.

All children should have an annual well-child or health maintenance visit. This gives the health care professional an opportunity to evaluate growth and development, chronic or acute medical problems, academic or behavioral concerns, psychosocial issues, peer and family interactions, and child or familial mental health concerns and to monitor the effect or necessity of prescription or over-the-counter medications.

Cognitive Style or Temperament

Much has been written concerning normal variations in temperament. The line between a high-energy, creative, enthusiastic child and a child with ADHD can be very indistinct. Often the lack of "goodness of fit" between the child and parents or teacher can determine on which side of that "line" the child is perceived. Turecki's *The Emotional Problems of Normal Children*[20] speaks to the wide range of aspects of temperament that are within the normal range. Thus, a parent who is shy and quiet and who likes predictability in her life would be poorly matched with an exuberant, impulsive extrovert who thrives on change. Imagine Pippi Longstocking as the child of Dorothy's Auntie Em from The Wizard of Oz. If Pippi's mother had been Amelia Bedelia or Mary Poppins, she would have been viewed as a delightful imaginative person. If the "fit" between the child's and parents' temperament or the child's and teachers' is not successful, the exuberance can be interpreted as hyperactivity. Birth order and parental expectations also may influence interpretation of a child's behavior.

If a child with a very intense personality, poor adaptability to change, strong negative persistence, and weak positive persistence finds himself or herself in a family with a parent of similar temperament, a diagnosis of oppositional defiant disorder with ADHD may be quickly made, because there would be a strong clash of difficult temperaments. This same somewhat difficult child might never come to a professional's attention if the parents had a low-keyed style, a low level of negative persistence, and a high level of positive persistence. Unfortunately, temperament is often inherited as surely as color of eyes or potential height. Thus, parents with the least resilience often have to raise similar children.

One might ask the parents to list specifically the objectionable characteristics of their child's behavior. These could then be evaluated one by one to determine whether they are outside the range of normal for the age or a reflection of a lack of goodness of fit.

A similar paradigm may occur in a school setting. Most school settings, even those for preschool, require adaptability to a routine, the ability to screen out nonsalient stimuli (another child whispering, the bird on the tree outside the window), and the ability to switch one's focus and interest quickly and easily. A child who does not meet these specifications might find the school or child care setting very difficult, particularly if the teacher is not a person of low-key intensity with good adaptability to change and a cooperative malleable nature with enough creativity to bring that "difficult" child along with the group.

Learning variations can also accentuate lack of goodness of fit in the classroom that would not be apparent at home. In the school setting, when confronted with demands that are beyond their level of neurologic maturation, oppositional behavior or avoidant behavior, such as excessive silliness, may occur.

Attention and Variability

Seemingly contradictory behaviors can often be frustrating to parents and teachers. Many parents and child care providers are confused by the apparent contradiction in behavior: "Johnny can watch television and play video games for hours, but when it's story time or there is classwork to do, he gets up and wanders around the room." This ability of the ADHD child to "hyperfocus" confuses teachers and parents, often leading to the conclusion that the child is lazy, unmotivated, or stupid. It is important to point out that video games constantly reinforce a child's behavior and have exciting, rapidly changing activities. These properties can easily keep the attention of even those children whose attentional systems are weak. Video games, however, do not cause ADHD. The rapt television watching is accompanied by lack of background monitoring. Thus, the child with weak attentional skills screens out everything else when he or she watches television. The parents will note that the only way to get the child's attention is to turn off the television. In a class-room in which the attention is not being constantly and intensively reinforced, the distractibility and physical fidgeting will be much more apparent. It is a rare teacher who can be as constantly fascinating as a television or video game character. It is important for the treating physician, parents, and teachers to understand the het-erogenous nature of ADHD, which results in extreme differences in presentation from child to child and also the extreme variability of performance across settings for any specific child. Too often, parents and teachers attribute these inconsistencies to motivation.

The child with weak attentional skills is very much like a car with loose connec-tions under the hood. On days when the connections are all in place, things go very well. On another day, for no apparent reason, the child will be unable to perform tasks that were done well on a previous day. This is as confusing to the child as it is to the teacher and parents. There is nothing more frustrating than the well-meant comment, "If you could do it yesterday, you can surely do it today!" or "I know you can do it if you try harder!" This is a sure course to failure and humiliation (see Treatment section).

WHAT IS NORMAL?

Some parents can estimate their child's skills almost as accurately as our psychologic tests. Observing the child in a group situation, such as child care, provides an excellent baseline with which to compare that child's behavior.

There are a few excellent scales that can be used to more formally compare competence with the norm in specific areas such as those mentioned above. The Carolina Curriculum for Preschoolers with Special Needs by Johnson-Martin, Attermeier, and Hacker[21] is one such instrument. Others include the Pediatric Evaluation of Disability Inventory by Haley et al, which is normed for children 1 to 7 years of age, and the ANSER Preschool Questionnaire, normed for children 3 to 5 years of age. The Conners Parent Teacher Rating Scales and the Child Behavior Checklist may be helpful but are not designed or normed for the preschool child. The Behavior Assessment Scale for Children (BASC)[22] is a tool commonly used by school psychologists that measures behavior and emotions in children and adolescents from 2 years, 6 months of age to 18 years, 11 months of age. Other clinic-based observational systems that are objective and empirically based facilitate diagnosis of ADHD in the preschool population.[23,24]

MAKING THE DIAGNOSIS

Children are usually referred for evaluation by a parent, teacher, or child care provider who has concerns about behavior, school failure, interpersonal relationships, or problems of attention. Children may be referred for evaluation to their pediatrician or other health care professional or to a psychiatrist or psychologist. The evaluation may take place in a private office, a specialized referral center for childhood behavioral and mental health disorders, or through the educational system.

The most important diagnostic tool is a careful history. The differential diagnoses listed above must be considered and a careful family history must be elicited or ascertained. There is a high incidence of positive family history of attentional disorders, obsessive compulsive disorder, mood disorders, and Tourette syndrome in families with a child with attentional disorders. A checklist should also be completed by parents and teachers or other caregivers. If the early education or child care setting has access to child care health consultants, they can be a valuable resource for observation and then support for the teachers/caregivers as a behavioral program is started. A careful physical and neurologic examination and, if indicated, hearing and vision screening and blood and urine tests should be conducted to rule out conditions outlined above. An electroencephalogram and magnetic resonance imaging or computed tomographic scan of the brain are not considered a routine part of an evaluation for ADHD and should be reserved for children with histories suggestive of seizures or other pathologic abnormalities on physical and/or neurologic examination that could be reflections of a structural brain abnormality. In most cases, results of imaging studies and electroencephalograms will be normal.

Environmental factors play an important and complex role in ADHD. If the parents have not developed successful strategies for coping with and capitalizing on the challenges and creativity that come with attentional disorders, their genetically vulnerable child will be raised in an unorganized, unpredictable environment that is often economically disadvantaged as well. The risk of divorce or single parenthood associated with impulsive behavior may further impoverish the environment for these children at risk. Significant prematurity, intrauterine growth retardation, hydrocephalus, malnutrition, closed head trauma, and exposure to toxins such as alcohol, recreational drugs such as cocaine, and some prescription drugs (ie, anticonvulsants) are among the many environmental factors that increase the risk of ADHD, even without a genetic predisposition.

TREATMENT

ADHD is the most common neurobehavioral diagnosis made in children in the United States today. However, research defining diagnostic criteria and treatment modalities for preschool-aged children is very limited, and recommendations are usually generalized from research involving the school-aged child. The recommendations here reflect current thinking about a treatment approach for the younger child. Children with untreated ADHD may behave inappropriately and may not respond to discipline because of their inability to control their impulses. This often leads to further disciplinary action, humiliation, and a loss of self-esteem. Severe secondary behavior disorders can be predicted with such a scenario. Children with ADHD expend far more effort than their unaffected peers do to produce the same amount of work in a given time. Such efforts should be acknowledged and rewarded.

Children with ADHD often require environmental, behavioral, and pharmacologic interventions.

Children with ADHD often require environmental, behavioral, and pharmacologic interventions. In addition, many nonstandardized treatments have been proposed over the years, and some of these will be addressed.

A National Institutes of Mental Health (NIMH) study recently reported by Jensen[25] described the multimodal treatment of combined-type ADHD among 7- to 10-year-old children ($n = 579$). The study involved 3 interventions: 1) stimulant medication; 2) behavioral treatment consisting of an intensive parent and teacher training program and a summer daytime treatment program; and 3) a combined treatment program of stimulant medication and behavioral treatment. Children were randomly assigned to 1 of the following 4 treatment groups: 1) medication management; 2) intensive behavioral treatment; 3) combination medication and intensive behavioral treatment; or 4) usual community care. Medication management was optimized during a 28-day double-blind, daily crossover titration of

3 different doses of methylphenidate (MPH) low dose (5 mg, 3 times per day), intermediate dose (10 mg, 10 mg, and 5 mg), and high dose (20 mg, 20 mg, and 10 mg for children weighing more than 25 kg; or 15 mg, 15 mg, and 5 mg for lighter children). Children received MPH treatment for approximately 12 hours per day, 7 days per week. The average total titration dose was approximately 1 mg/kg per day. Twenty-two percent of children responded best to low MPH doses, 25% responded best to moderate doses, and 30% responded best to high MPH doses.[26] Medication management was individualized and intensive for the combination and medical management groups. The study found that medication with or without behavioral intervention was more effective than behavioral treatment alone. Children in either the medication or combination groups had better overall outcome than children treated in the community. Children in the community group tended to have less frequent, less intensive follow-up and to receive somewhat lower doses of MPH. Parents and teachers were particularly satisfied with the behavioral intervention. The study concluded that combined behavioral treatment and medication, health care professional involvement, and parent and teacher training were necessary for optimal treatment of ADHD.[25]

Stimulant treatment of school-aged children has been well researched and described. Large methodologically controlled trials in the preschool age group are limited. Although less information is available for preschool-aged children, new studies of ADHD treatment in this age group are ongoing. A National Institute of Mental Health (NIMH)-funded study of treatment in 165 preschool-aged children (3 to 5.5 years of age) is currently underway at 6 sites in the United States. The Preschool ADHD Treatment Study (PATS) will provide information from a controlled clinical trial to address the issue of medication in the treatment of preschool children with ADHD. There have been more than 200 controlled trials involving nearly 6000 children, adolescents, and adults compared with only 9 studies involving just over 200 preschool-aged children.[26] Despite the lack of studies, prescription rates for this age group have increased threefold since 1990. A recent review of existing controlled trials of 3- to 6-year-old preschool children found that this age range may have a greater variability in response to stimulants but that improvement was generally noted in the areas of interpersonal interactions, hyperactive-impulsive behavior, and cognition.[26-29] Adverse effects were reported more commonly among preschoolers but were most often mild. It is also important to note that high rates of reported medication adverse effects occurred while children were receiving placebo. In fact, the reported rate of adverse effects (such as anxiety, irritability, and insomnia) was equivalent for children on placebo and those receiving 0.3 mg/kg per dose of MPH given twice a day. Some reported adverse effects improved when children were on medication. This underscores the importance of baseline behavioral assessments before the initiation of stimulant medication.

Preschool-aged children can be reliably identified who meet evidence-based criteria for ADHD. Existing studies document that these children may benefit from behavioral therapy and parent training.[30,31] It is also reasonable to conclude that carefully diagnosed preschoolers may benefit from stimulant medication administered cautiously and with intensive management to determine optimum dosage, monitor adverse effects, and support parents and caregivers. This may be particularly important for those children whose behavior puts them or others in danger or in ADHD families in which parental disorganization makes even basic behavior management challenging.

Currently, there is almost no existing research involving stimulant medication in children younger than 3 years. Because brain development continues postnatally with synaptic growth and pruning and myelinization, caution is particularly necessary when prescribing any psychoactive medication to a very young child. Until more evidence-based data are available from methodologically controlled research, stimulant medication should generally not be prescribed for children younger than 3 years.

Behavioral Interventions for the Child Care or Classroom Environment

Preschool children think concretely. They do not have sophisticated language to express their concerns and confusion about their erratic and often substandard performance. They will often attribute their difficulties to lack of intelligence or agree with adults who suggest that they are "lazy" or "bad." Sadly, this can become a self-fulfilling prophecy. The following is a list of suggestions for intervention in the child care setting. It is not necessary to implement all of these for every child, and there are undoubtedly other strategies that can be effective. Choose 1 or 2 of these and use them with consistency for 2 weeks. Remember, the first 3 to 4 days may be complicated by a deterioration in behavior. As the child becomes comfortable with the new rules, improvement will usually occur. Child care health consultants can help the teachers/caregivers implement some of these behavioral interventions. Consideration should always be given to whether a child's current early education or child care setting is right for that child and whether the school/child care center has enough resources to effectively manage the child with ADHD. Some children may even qualify for school district support of their preschool education because of their diagnosis.

1. Reduce extraneous stimulation: simplify decorations in one corner of the classroom or in the child's room. Put toys in boxes and have only 2 to 3 items out at a time. Insist on clean-up before going to another toy. For children who are distracted by sound, use of white noise, simple familiar music, or in more challenging cases, radio receptor ear phones can be helpful.

2. Organize time. Create a file of photographs, drawings, or pictures depicting the events of the day. Put a series of the next 3 or 4 events on a display board so

that the child can see what happened before and what will happen next. Allow the child to help put the schedule up. This can be particularly effective with multistep routines like clean-up and lunch or morning and bedtime routines at home. Use a simple kitchen timer to make time allotted for an activity more concrete. Set the timer so that the child gets a 2-minute warning when it goes off the first time, and then promptly move on to the next activity on the board when it goes off a second time. If the child is distracted by the ticking of a timer, consider using an egg-timer or a digital electronic timer. Further "concretize" time by having the child put a piece of adhesive paper over the picture of the completed action.

3. Reduce task size or "chunk" tasks into manageable pieces. Break tasks down into individual components ("first put your crayons back in the box," rather than "clean up the table before lunch").

4. Allow ample opportunity for physical movement; quiet wiggling or doodling may help a child to concentrate. Some work better lying prone on the floor or at a standing table rather than sitting at a desk. Allow activities such as taking notes to the office or erasing the board to permit the child to move around without embarrassment.

5. Demystification: use stories, such as those in Mel Levine's *All Kinds of Minds*, to help the child understand the nature of the problem at a level he or she can comprehend. For the very young 3-year-old, this may simply consist of the statement that, "some children who are smart and nice still have trouble sitting still and keeping their minds on one thing at a time. This makes it hard to follow rules sometimes in school, but we are going to work on a plan to make things go better. You will have to work hard, but we'll be there to help."

6. Feedback: be specific with criticism ("I know it's hard to wait, but Jim has the next turn"; "Your voice was so loud that no one could hear what Susan had to say") and praise ("I like the way you put the blocks back in the box before you took out the puzzle"). The goal is not to punish, but to modify and redirect and clarify so the child is clear about expectations. Teach children to view mistakes as opportunities to learn. Provide opportunities to practice appropriate behavior. Post photographs of the children behaving well and lavishly praise successes. Treat failures as "bad luck" and go right back to the program. If it is possible to videotape the behavior in question, a skilled adult could view a brief sample of the behavior to be modified and then use the following strategy:

Set up a "secret signal," such as a tap on the shoulder, to let the child know when the behavior is escalating. Have a "getting-it-together corner" with a bean-bag chair or rocker and a portable tape player and earphones with soothing music that can be used in a nonpunitive fashion to help the child reorganize. Never humiliate a child in front of his peers. This includes never asking, "Did you take your medicine?"

7. Be cognizant of circumstances that are predictors of unacceptable behavior. These include an overly loud, crowded, or busy environment; specific types of tasks (language based vs fine motor); sleep deprivation; poor nutrition; and physical illness, such as asthma. Try to modify the environment accordingly.

8. If it is determined that the child's ADHD is complicated by oppositional defiant disorder or an evolving conduct disorder, a much more complex behavior modification plan will be necessary.

9. Be sure that associated comorbidities are being treated or addressed simultaneously.

10. Parents, teachers, and other adults involved in the child's care must communicate regularly so that the child gets consistent messages across the different environments in his or her life.

11. Behavioral strategies should yield results within 2 to 3 weeks. Fruitless persistence beyond that point will exhaust the family and caregivers. Be sure the behavioral program is well understood by the adults involved and is viewed as a form of instruction and not punishment.

Many 3-year-olds will be managed successfully with these behavioral strategies alone, but as they get older and the environment places more demands on them, the need for medication may become evident.

MEDICATION

In the preschool-aged child with ADHD, behavioral strategies and environmental modification are often the first intervention. For the child with mild impairment, this may be the only intervention needed initially. Children who are exceptionally hyperactive and impulsive may cause injuries to themselves or others or have a severe, adverse impact on the family. These children and families may benefit most from a carefully monitored multimodal treatment plan combining behavioral and environmental modification and medication.

As many as two thirds of children with ADHD have a comorbid condition, such as bipolar disorder (previously called manic-depressive disorder), depression, anxiety disorder, obsessive-compulsive disorder, oppositional defiant disorder, conduct disorder, or learning disorders. Bipolar disorder in young children is difficult to diagnose, controversial, and sometimes challenging to treat. The disorder may manifest with symptoms of mood swings, extreme irritability, and apparent symptoms of severe impulsivity or hyperactivity. Children with comorbidities will almost always require medical intervention of their comorbid condition (as appropriate) before treatment for ADHD is undertaken. For most children who require medication for ADHD, the first drug of choice will be one of the following stimulants.

STIMULANT MEDICATIONS

Dextroamphetamine

Dexedrine (GlaxoSmithKline, Research Triangle Park, NC)
This was the first stimulant developed and in many instances remains a preferred drug for younger children. Dextroamphetamine has Food and Drug Administration approval for children as young as 3 years.

- Short-acting tablets, 5 mg, 10 mg, 20 mg; longer-acting spansules, 5 mg, 10 mg, 15 mg
- Time of onset: 20 minutes to 1 hour
- Length of action: 4 to 5 hours (short); 8 to 10 hours (long)
- Dose determination: can be performed with a reproducible test of attention in the office or by careful observation at home and school
- Dose increments: 2.5 mg; in some cases 1.25 mg
- Timing: short acting, morning and noon, possible smaller dose at 4:00 to 5:00 pm; long acting, morning and possibly short-acting 4:00 to 5:00 pm

Adderall (Shire Richwood Inc, Florence, KY)
Adderall is a combination of 4 different salts of amphetamine (75% dextroamphetamine, 25% levoamphetamine).

- Tablets: comes in a variety of doses
- Time of onset: 20 minutes to 1 hour
- Length of action: 8 to 10 hours (some rapid metabolizers only 4 to 6 hours); peak concentration occurs in about 3 hours
- Dosing determination: same as Dexedrine; increase in 2.5-mg increments
- Timing: morning; possible small doses of Dexedrine or methylphenidate at 4:00 to 5:00 pm
- *Adderall XR:* a long-acting form of Adderall
  - ~ Capsules: comes in a variety of doses
  - ~ Length of action: full day (9 to 11 hours)
  - ~ Maximum plasma concentration: 7 hours
  - ~ Dosing determination: start at 10 mg in the morning, increase by 10 mg per week. The entire capsule must be taken. Capsule may be opened and sprinkled on applesauce. The entire capsule contents should be consumed without chewing. Do not divide the dose of a single capsule.
  - ~ Timing: morning dosing
  - ~ Adderall XR has not been studied in children younger than 6 years

Methylphenidate

SHORT ACTING

Ritalin (Novartis Consumer Health, Summit, NJ)
- Tablets: 5 mg, 10 mg, 20 mg (short acting); 20 mg long-acting SR
- Time of onset: 20 minutes to 1 hour
- Length of action: 3 to 4 hours (short), 4 to 6 hours (long, but often is unreliably absorbed)
- Dose determination: increase in 2.5-mg increments
- Timing: short acting, morning and noon, possibly 4:00 to 5:00 pm; long acting, morning and 4:00 to 5:00 pm (short)

Racemic Methylphenidate

Focalin (Novartis Pharmaceuticals Corp, East Hanover, NJ)
- Dexmethylphenidate hydrochloride
- 2.5-mg, 5-mg, 10-mg tablets
- Dose morning and afternoon; at least 4 hours between doses
- This product contains only the d-threo-enantiomer (the more pharmacologically active enantiomer) of racemic methylphenidate hydrochloride

LONGER ACTING

Concerta, long acting (ALZA Pharmaceuticals, Mountain View, CA)
- 18-mg, 27-mg, 36-mg, 54-mg caplets
- 10 to 12 hours' duration for once daily dosing
- Should not be cut, chewed, or crushed

Metadate CD, long acting (Celltech Pharma Ltd, Rochester, NY)
- 20-mg capsules
- Up to 9 hours duration for once daily dosing

Safety and efficacy have not been established for children younger than 6 years.

Metadate ER
- 10-mg, 20-mg tablets
- Up to 8 hours' duration

Methylin ER (Mallinckrodt Inc, St Louis, MO)
- 10-mg and 20-mg doses
- Up to 8 hours' duration for once daily dosing

Ritalin LA (Novartis Consumer Health, Summit, NJ)
- 20-mg, 30-mg, 40-mg capsules
- Up to 8 hours' duration for once daily dosing
- Not currently approved for children younger than 6 years of age

- Capsules can be opened and the contents sprinkled on foods such as applesauce; capsules cannot be divided

New preparations and dose formulations are constantly being developed for stimulant medication. Be aware that changes may have occurred subsequent to this publication.

Adverse Effects

Individual response to stimulant medications may vary. If a child fails to respond adequately or is intolerant to one preparation, try another stimulant. All of the stimulant medications can produce adverse effects, which may include the following symptoms:

1. Appetite suppression: often disappears after 10 to 14 days. Schedule morning dose after breakfast. Supplement before bed with a healthy snack (such as Carnation Instant Breakfast [Nestle USA Inc, Glendale, CA] blended with whole milk and ice cream). Appetite suppression may be more problematic among younger children. Monitor weight.

2. Sleep disturbance: usually difficulty getting to sleep but sometimes difficulty staying asleep. Often disappears after 10 to 14 days. A small group of children benefit from a dose of stimulant given a half-hour before bedtime. Because sleep deprivation can cause symptoms similar to ADHD, change medicines if this cannot be resolved.

3. Headache: if persistent, change medication.

4. Stomachache (often avoided by taking medication with food).

5. Tics: often dose related, so lowering the dose may decrease tics. Remember, tics are frequently comorbid with ADHD even without the use of stimulant medication. Their appearance often follows typical ADHD symptoms by several years and may, erroneously, be attributed solely to medication. Currently, tics are often listed as a contraindication to the use of stimulants. A committee from the American Academy of Child and Adolescent Psychiatry is working with the Food and Drug Administration to review this listing in view of recent studies[32] that show stimulants are often well tolerated, even in the presence of tics. Medication must be used cautiously and should usually be given under the care of a psychiatrist in this situation. If the hyperactivity and inattention are impairing the child's ability to function, treating the ADHD may be the highest priority.

6. Rebound: more irritable, hyperactive behavior as the medication wears off. This may be less of a problem with the long-acting stimulants.

7. Overmedication: personality is blunted; child is too quiet and often over-concentrates and is more irritable. Learning (classification, problem solving, singing, fine motor skills) is impaired in this state, and the child may be less flexible and less creative.

A short, carefully monitored trial of a stimulant will rarely produce a catastrophic reaction. Parent and teacher checklists and daily behavioral report cards for home and school can help monitor adjustment and medication. Continuous performance tests or paired associate tests may also be useful in medication monitoring but are more commonly found in research or referral centers. Careful follow-up of observations by parents, teachers, and caregivers must be part of the treatment plan.

Stimulants should not be continued if there is less than a dramatic improvement. If there is a substantial improvement, the use of medication for the child with ADHD should be viewed in a manner similar to the use of glasses in a nearsighted child. Neither will cure the condition, but both will help to remediate the condition. The medication will enable attention; the glasses will enable vision. It is important to let the child know that this is not a medication to make him "smart" or "good." The medication will help children with ADHD pay attention and control their behavior if that is what they want to do. It is essential that the focus of control be kept in the child's hands and not in the bottle of pills. Glasses may help a child to copy material from the blackboard more efficiently, but they will not change this skill if the child is not able to decode the symbols and control his or her hand well enough to copy the work. Thus, glasses too are a facilitator, and the final factor in a successful outcome is the child's intelligence and mental health.

Other Medications

The scope of this book precludes detailed listing of all other drugs that can be useful in the treatment of ADHD and its coexisting conditions. The list may include:

- *Strattera* (atomoxetine, Eli Lilly & Co, Indianapolis, IN): nonstimulant, non-controlled medication. Can be used when stimulant medication is not tolerated or is contraindicated. Be aware of potential drug interactions.
- *Wellbutrin* (bupropion, GlaxoSmithKline, Research Triangle Park, NC): an anti-depressant that is sometimes prescribed by health care professionals for treatment of symptoms of ADHD with comorbid depression or when stimulant medication is not tolerated
- *Imipramine, desipramine, and nortriptyline,*[33] particularly when anxiety is a comorbidity. Concerns about cardiac effects with desipramine have limited its use by health care professionals.
- *Selective serotonin reuptake inhibitors,* such as Prozac (Dista Products Company, Indianapolis, IN) and Luvox (Solvay Pharmaceuticals, Marietta, GA), for circumstances in which obsessive-compulsive disorder or depression is comorbid.
- *Tegretol* (Novartis Pharmaceuticals Corp, East Hanover, NJ), Depakene (Abbott Laboratories, North Chicago, IL), other anticonvulsants, or lithium are typically prescribed for the older child with comorbid bipolar disorder. The complex nature of the diagnosis and management of this disorder in children mandates consultation with a psychiatrist familiar with bipolar disorder in children.

- *Clonidine or Tenex* (guanfacine, A.H. Robins Co, Richmond, VA) for aggression or impulsive and hyperactive behavior. Monitor for overdosing.
- *Atarax* (Pfizer Inc, New York, NY), Benadryl (Warner-Lambert Consumer Healthcare, Morris Plains, NJ), melatonin, or clonidine have sometimes been prescribed when sleep disorders occur as a comorbidity.

Although polypharmacy (the prescription of multiple drugs) is typically discouraged, it is clear that ADHD is a complex disorder that is frequently associated with comorbid conditions. Thus, many children with ADHD will require combined pharmacotherapy to adequately manage their symptoms. The more complex children can probably best be managed in conjunction with referral to a center specializing in the treatment of ADHD.

NONSTANDARD TREATMENTS FOR ADHD

The list of nonstandardized treatments is lengthy, and a full discussion of their efficacy is beyond the scope of this book. Also, there is little information from clinical research on the efficacy of these treatments.[34] Much of what is known is anecdotal. Parents are encouraged to discuss alternative treatments with their child's pediatrician before trying any alternative treatment.

1. Yeast overgrowth in the intestine secondary to multiple infections requiring antibiotics: nystatin plus antiyeast diet. Little evidence of efficacy in clinical outcome trials.
2. Elimination diets: rarely effective for ADHD but occasionally helpful for children with behavioral concerns caused or exacerbated by food allergies or intolerance. Sugar and other food additives have been studied, however, and do not appear to have a significant impact on the behavior of most children.[35] Red dye number 22 and yellow dye number 5 have been questioned.
3. Megavitamins: no evidence of effectiveness.
4. Sensory integration therapy: purported to be helpful with fine motor and sequential motor activity, tactile defensiveness, and concentration. Data to confirm efficacy in treating ADHD are not available.
5. Massage therapy: no evidence of effectiveness.
6. Chiropractic manipulation: no evidence of effectiveness.
7. Electroencephalographic biofeedback: any effect seems to be a halo effect from the intense (and expensive) treatment rather than a primary effect of the technique.
8. Eye exercises through optometrists: no evidence of efficacy.

The School-Aged Child in an After-School Child Care Program

Although parents, teachers, and health care professionals recognize the need for medication or accommodations during school hours, less thought is often given to the ADHD child in an after-school program. After a structured day of school, it is important for all children, but especially for the ADHD child, to have some time to play and interact with peers in a supervised setting that includes choices (ie, gross motor activities, board games, card games, sports, clubs, projects, homework support, etc).

Depending on the child, the program, and the type of medication prescribed, it may be necessary for a child to receive a low dose of stimulant medication after school to make this time a positive experience. Also, some children receiving short-acting stimulant preparations in the morning and at noon may experience a rebound effect in the late afternoon as the medication wears off. Less than one third of children may become irritable and inattentive to a greater degree even than their unmedicated state. These children often improve when a low dose of stimulant medication is added after school. Communication among parents, teachers, and health care professionals will be important to determine whether medication is necessary and to monitor for side effects such as insomnia and appetite suppression.

A STRATEGY TO EXTINGUISH SPECIFIC ANGRY OR AGGRESSIVE BEHAVIOR

1. If possible, videotape the child engaging in the behavior you wish to extinguish.
2. Review and select a 5-minute segment to watch with child (making no comment).
3. Ask him what he or she thought.
4. Describe the facts of what you saw.
5. Review tape again and point out these facts. If videotape was used, include facial expression, body posture, eye contact, and hand position. Talk about feelings the child or other person might be experiencing. Have the child propose possible alternatives and predict outcomes for each.
6. Work on how else the scene could have been played.
7. Role-play the way you saw it on the videotape, with you playing the child and the child playing the other involved.
8. Next, replay the scene using the "new" scenario you and the child came up with, and videotape it. Have the child play himself in this "positive solution" role-play.
9. Compare videotapes of initial behavior and the alternative scene.
10. Agree on what you both want to change.
11. Set up a signal to prevent deterioration of future situations. Cueing a child allows the child to recognize inappropriate behavior and "self-correct" before the situation escalates.
12. Have practice drills or role-plays about situations that come up frequently in the child care setting.

Occasionally, extreme aggressive behavior in children warrants treatment with medication in addition to behavior management. Although haloperidol and thioridazine are approved by the FDA for the treatment of severe aggression in the preschool-aged child, they are seldom used because of adverse effects. However, the severity of some children's aggressive behavior may require treatment with one of the new atypical antipsychotic agents, such as risperidone. Medication therapy of extreme aggression and most combined pharmacotherapy treatment should be carefully managed in conjunction with a child psychiatrist.

CONCLUSIONS AND RECOMMENDATIONS

ADHD cannot be cured, but it can be managed. Management strategies will change over time as the child grows and changes and as our knowledge of ADHD and its comorbid conditions improves. Collaboration of parents, caregivers, teachers, and therapists, together with the health care professional, is vital to a successful outcome. A knowledgeable member of this team should have the role of team leader and the responsibility for coordinating other services. Each child and family presents a unique set of challenges, but a good outcome produces a creative, energetic member of our society.

REFERENCES

1. Hallowell EM, Ratey JJ. *Driven to Distraction*. New York, NY: Pantheon Books; 1994
2. Barkley RA. International consensus statement on ADHD. January 2002. *Clin Child Fam Psychol Rev.* 2002;5:89–111
3. Olfson M, Marcus SC, Weissman MM, Jensen PS. National trends in the use of psychotropic medications by children. *J Am Acad Child Adolesc Psychiatry.* 2002;41:514–521
4. Rowland AS, Umbach DM, Stallone L, et al. Prevalence of medication treatment for attention deficit-hyperactivity disorder among elementary school children in Johnston County, North Carolina. *Am J Public Health.* 2002;92:231–234
5. American Psychiatric Association. *Diagnostic and Statistical Manual of Mental Disorders, Fourth Edition (DSM-IV).* Washington, DC: American Psychiatric Association; 1994
6. Faraone SV, Biederman J, Friedman D. Validity of DSM-IV subtypes of attention-deficit/hyperactivity disorder: a family study perspective. *J Am Acad Child Adolesc Psychiatry.* 2000;39:300–307
7. American Academy of Pediatrics, Committee on Quality Improvement, Subcommittee on Attention-Deficit/Hyperactivity Disorder. Clinical practice guideline: treatment of the school-aged child with attention-deficit/hyperactivity disorder. *Pediatrics.* 2001;108:1033–1044
8. Wilens TE, Biederman J, Brown S, et al. Psychiatric comorbidity and functioning and clinically referred preschool children and school-aged youths with ADHD. *J Am Acad Child Adolesc Psychiatry.* 2002;41:262–268
9. DuPaul GJ, McGoey KE, Eckert TL, Van Brakle J. Preschool children with attention-deficit/hyperactivity disorder: impairments in behavioral, social, and school functioning. *J Am Acad Child Adolesc Psychiatry.* 2001;40:508–515
10. Levy F, Hay DA, McStephen M, et al. Attention-deficit hyperactivity disorder: a category or a continuum? Genetic analysis of a large-scale twin study. *J Am Acad Child Adolesc Psychiatry.* 1997;36:737–744
11. Giedd JN, Blumenthal J, Molloy E, Castellanos FX. Brain imaging of attention deficit/hyperactivity disorder. *Ann N Y Acad Sci.* 2001;931:33–49

12. Levy F. The dopamine theory of attention deficit hyperactivity disorder (ADHD). *Aust N Z J Psychiatry.* 1991;25:277–283

13. Faraone SV, Biederman J. Neurobiology of attention-deficit hyperactivity disorder. *Biol Psychiatry.* 1998;44:951–958

14. Mihailescu S, Drucker-Colin R. Nicotine, brain nicotine receptors, and neuropsychiatric disorders. *Arch Med Res.* 2000;31:131–144

15. Faraone SV, Doyle AE. Genetic influences on attention deficit hyperactivity disorder. *Curr Psychiatry Rep.* 2000;2:143–146

16. Milberger S, Biederman J, Faraone SV, Guite J, Tsuang MT. Pregnancy, delivery and infancy complications and attention deficit hyperactivity disorder: issues of gene-environment interaction. *Biol Psychiatry.* 1997;41:65–75

17. Milberger S, Biederman J, Faraone SV, Chen L, Jones J. Is maternal smoking during pregnancy a risk factor for attention deficit hyperactivity disorder in children? *Am J Psychiatry.* 1996;153:1138–1142

18. Mick E, Biederman J, Faraone SV, Sayer J, Kleinman S. Case-control study of attention-deficit hyperactivity disorder and maternal smoking, alcohol use, and drug use during pregnancy. *J Am Acad Child Adolesc Psychiatry.* 2002;41:378–385

19. Ernst M, Moolchan ET, Robinson ML. Behavioral and neural consequences of prenatal exposure to nicotine. *J Am Acad Child Adolesc Psychiatry.* 2001;40:630–641

20. Turecki S, Wernick S. *The Emotional Problems of Normal Children.* New York, NY: Bantam Books; 1994

21. Johnson-Martin NM, Attermeier SM, Hacker B. *The Carolina Curriculum for Preschoolers with Special Needs.* Baltimore, MD: Brookes Publishing; 1991

22. Reynolds CR, Kamphaus RW. *The Behavior Assessment Scale for Children (BASC).* Circle Pines, MN: American Guidance Service; 1992

23. DeWolfe NA, Byrne JM, Bawden HN. Preschool inattention and impulsivity-hyperactivity: development of a clinic-based assessment protocol. *J Atten Disord.* 2000;4: 80–90

24. Merrell KW. *Preschool and Kindergarten Behavior Scales.* Brandon, VT: Clinical Psychology Publishing Co; 1994

25. Jensen P, Arnold L, Richters J, et al. 14-month randomized clinical trial of treatment strategies for attention deficit hyperactivity disorder. *Arch Gen Psychiatry.* 1999;56: 1073–1086

26. Connor DF. Preschool attention deficit hyperactivity disorder: a review of prevalence, diagnosis, neurobiology, and stimulant treatment. *J Dev Behav Pediatr.* 2002;23 (1 Suppl):S1–S9

27. Connor SCK. Controlled trial of methylphenidate in preschool children with minimal brain dysfunction. *Int J Ment Health.* 1975;4:61–74

28. Barkley RA. The effects of methylphenidate on the interactions of preschool ADHD children with their mothers. *J Am Acad Child Adolesc Psychiatry.* 1988;27:336–341

29. Musten LM, Firestone P, Pisterman S, Bennett S, Mercer J. Effects of methylphenidate on preschool children with ADHD: cognitive and behavioral functions. *J Am Acad Child Adolesc Psychiatry.* 1997;36:1407–1417

30. Barkley RA. *Attention-Deficit Hyperactivity Disorder: A Handbook for Diagnosis and Treatment.* 2nd ed. New York, NY: Guilford Press; 1998

31. Pisterman S, McGrath P, Firestone P, Goodman JT, Webster I, Mallory R. Outcome of parent-mediated treatment of preschoolers with attention deficit disorder with hyperactivity. *J Consult Clin Psychol.* 1989;57:628–635

32. Spencer T, Biederman J, Wilens T. Attention-deficit/hyperactivity disorder and comorbidity. *Pediatr Clin North Am.* 1999;46:915–927

33. Prince JB, Wilens TE, Biederman J, et al. A controlled study of nortriptyline in children and adolescents with attention deficit hyperactivity disorder. *J Child Adolesc Psychopharmacol.* 2000;10:193–204

34. Arnold LE. Methylphenidate vs. amphetamine: comparative review. *J Atten Disord.* 2000; 3(4)

35. American Academy of Pediatrics. *The Classification of Child and Adolescent Mental Diagnoses in Primary Care. Diagnostic and Statistical Manual for Primary Care (DSM-PC), Child and Adolescent Version.* Wolraich ML, Felice ME, Drotar D, eds. Elk Grove Village, IL: American Academy of Pediatrics; 1996

ADDITIONAL RESOURCES

American Academy of Child and Adolescent Psychiatry. Practice parameter for the use of stimulant medications in the treatment of children, adolescents, and adults. *J Am Acad Child Adolesc Psychiatry.* 2002;41(2 Suppl):26S–49S

American Academy of Pediatrics. *Understanding ADHD: Information for Parents About Attention-Deficit/Hyperactivity Disorder.* Elk Grove Village, IL: American Academy of Pediatrics; 2001

American Academy of Pediatrics, Subcommittee on Attention-Deficit/Hyperactivity Disorder, Committee on Quality Improvement. Clinical practice guideline: treatment of the school-aged child with attention-deficit/hyperactivity disorder. *Pediatrics.* 2001;108:1033–1044

Barkley RA. Attention-deficit hyperactivity disorder. *Sci Am.* 1998;279:66–71

Barkley RA. *Attention Deficit Hyperactivity Disorder: A Handbook for Diagnosis and Treatment.* 2nd ed. The Guilford Press; 1998

Connor DF. Preschool attention deficit hyperactivity disorder: a review of prevalence, diagnosis, neurobiology, and stimulant treatment. *J Dev Behav Pediatr.* 2002;23:S1–S9

Coyle JT. Psychotropic drug use in very young children. *JAMA.* 2000;283:1059–1060

DuPaul GJ, McGoey KE, Eckert TL, VanBrakle J. Preschool children with attention-deficit/hyperactivity disorder: impairments in behavioral, social, and school functioning. *J Am Acad Child Adolesc Psychiatry.* 2001;40:508–515

Firestone P, Musten LM, Pisterman S, Mercer J, Bennett S. Short-term side effects of stimulant medication are increased in preschool children with attention-deficit/hyperactivity disorder: a double-blind placebo-controlled study. *J Child Adolesc Psychopharmacol.* 1998;8:13–25

Goode E. Sharp rise found in psychiatric drugs for the very young. *New York Times.* 2000; Feb 23:A1, A14

Gorski PA. Racing cain. *J Dev Behav Pediatr.* 2002;23:95

Gorski PA, ed. The diagnosis and treatment of ADHD in early childhood: evidence-based controversies and implications for practice and policy. *J Dev Behav Pediatr.* 2002;23:S1–S63

Greenhill LL. The use of psychotropic medication in preschoolers: indications, safety, and efficacy. *Can J Psychiatry.* 1998;43:576–581

Rappaport N, Chubinsky P. The meaning of psychotropic medications for children, adolescents, and their families. *J Am Acad Child Adolesc Psychiatry.* 2000;39:1198–2000

State MW, Lombroso PJ, Pauls DL, et al. The genetics of childhood psychiatric disorders: a decade of progress. *J Am Acad Child Adolesc Psychiatry.* 2000;39:946–962

Tourette's Syndrome Study Group. Treatment of ADHD in children with tics: a randomized controlled trial. *Neurology.* 2002;58:527–536

Vitiello B. Psychopharmacology for young children: clinical needs and research opportunities. *Pediatrics.* 2001;108:983–989

Vitiello B, Severe JB, Greenhill LL, et al. Methylphenidate dosage for children with ADHD over time under controlled conditions: lessons from the MTA. *J Am Acad Child Adolesc Psychiatry.* 2001;40:188–196

Wender EH. Managing stimulant medication for attention-deficit/hyperactivity disorder. *Pediatr Rev.* 2001;22:183–190

Wilens TE, Biderman J, Brown S, Monuteaux M, Prince J, Spencer TJ. Patterns of psychopathology and dysfunction in clinically referred preschoolers. *J Dev Behav Pediatr.* 2002;23:S31–S36

Wilens TE, Biederman J, Brown S, Tanguay S, Monuteaux MC, Blake C, Spencer TJ. Psychiatric comorbidity and functioning in clinically referred preschool children and school-age youths with ADHD. *J Am Acad Child Adolesc Psychiatry.* 2002;41:262–268

Zito JM. Five burning questions. *J Dev Behav Pediatr.* 2002;23:S23–S30

Zito JM, Safer DJ, dosReis S, Gardner JF, Boles M, Lynch F. Trends in the prescribing of psychotropic medications to preschoolers. *JAMA.* 2000;283:1025–1030

SUGGESTED RESOURCE

American Academy of Pediatrics. *Understanding ADHD: Information for Parents About Attention-Deficit/Hyperactivity Disorder.* Elk Grove Village, IL: American Academy of Pediatrics; 2001

CHAPTER 9

Violence Prevention and Conflict Resolution

Carole Logan Kuhns, RN, PhD

LEARNING OBJECTIVES

- Identify the frequency and characteristics of children's experiences with violence.
- Describe the impact of violence on children's development.
- Identify strategies child care providers may use to support children who witness or are victims of violence.
- Identify developmental factors placing children at risk of becoming violent.
- Describe early intervention strategies to prevent violent behavior.
- Identify resources for violence prevention.

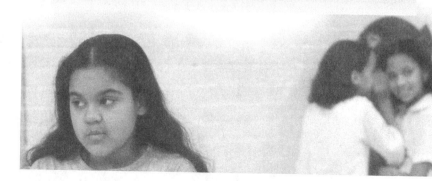

INTRODUCTION

Once the domain of the criminal justice system, childhood violence is now recognized as an important health issue for pediatric health care professionals. The American Academy of Pediatrics encourages primary pediatric health care professionals to offer parent education during well-child visits on gun safety and non-abusive discipline strategies and to assess children at risk of developing violent behavior. Specific strategies for working directly with parents are discussed throughout this chapter.

Another important opportunity for pediatric health care professionals to address childhood violence exists when providing health consultation services to child care programs. The safe and nurturing child care environment with ongoing early childhood education opportunities is a natural setting for child care providers and pediatric health care professionals to partner in addressing the violence children may be experiencing in their lives. The purpose of this chapter is to give child care health consultants the information they need to support child care providers who may be caring for children who are witnesses to or victims of violence and to assist child care providers in the prevention of violence carried out by children.

SCOPE OF VIOLENCE IN CHILDREN'S LIVES

Children Witness Violence

Children witness violence on a daily basis in their television viewing and with increasing frequency in their own homes and communities. Despite the call of health care professionals and other child advocates to decrease the amount of media violence, children continue to view violence on TV at alarming rates. Children witness 3 to 5 violent acts per hour during prime time television and 20 to 25 violent acts per hour of Saturday morning children's programs.[1] Increasingly, children's exposure to violence goes beyond TV and into their own communities and homes. Several studies report that as many as three fourths of the children living in high-risk communities have witnessed a violent incident in their neighborhood.[2,3] Within their own homes, an estimated 3.3 million children each year witness their own parent being abused by a spouse or partner.[4]

Children Are Victims of Violence

Children who are victims of violence are, unfortunately, not rare. Every 2 hours in the United States, a child dies from gun-related violence.[5] Studies found one third of the children in a high-risk community had been victims of violence.[2,3] In school yard shootings, children not only witnessed violence first-hand but became victims of violence carried out by their young classmates. Even in their own homes, children's risk of violence is high. Among the 1 million child abuse victims in 1996, 88% were victimized by their parents or another family member.[6]

Children Carry Out Violent Acts

After peaking at 26% in 1993, the rate of serious violent crimes committed by juveniles decreased to 22% in 1998.[7] Of significance to child care providers is the fact that violent youth crime is most likely to occur after school hours between 3:00 pm and 7:00 pm.[5]

CHILD CARE AS A RESOURCE TO ADDRESS VIOLENCE IN CHILDREN'S LIVES

These alarming statistics convey the urgency of health care professionals to become involved in decreasing childhood violence. An important partnership to address this health problem is that of child care providers and pediatric health care professionals. The remaining sections of this chapter provide information child care health consultants may use to assist child care providers in caring for children exposed to violence and to prevent violence by children.

Safe and Caring Environment

The child care setting should offer a safe and caring environment to support children who have experienced violence in their lives. In the child care environment, children can express their fears and describe feelings about violence they may have experienced. Child care providers can also convey a sense of safety to children by clearly setting limits for appropriate behavior in the classroom. This gives children a sense that violence is not necessarily inevitable and that alternatives exist to resolve conflict. To assist child care providers in offering a safe and nurturing environment, child care health consultants can offer training on strategies to help children who are dealing with violence in their lives.

Violence Prevention Opportunity

The early learning environment in child care programs is a natural setting for children to learn nonviolent conflict resolution skills. As discussed in later sections of this chapter, social problem-solving skills are essential for effective and prosocial interpersonal interactions. To develop social problem-solving skills, children need not only adult guidance and modeling but also free play experiences with peers. By balancing teacher directed and peer-to-peer play experiences, child care providers can give children the opportunity to learn and practice prosocial skills. Child care health consultants can support child care providers in violence prevention efforts by offering training that includes early intervention strategies to teach children social problem-solving skills.

Opportunity for Early Identification and Referral

Child care programs are an opportunity for early identification and referral of children (victims and offenders) in need of additional mental health services. Although child care professionals may have knowledge of normal growth and development, they may not always have the experience to identify the point at which a child's aggressive behavior goes beyond the upper bounds of normal and requires professional mental health counseling. Training offered by child care health consultants can include discussion of factors placing children at risk of becoming violent and the identification of community mental health resources. This will assist child care professionals to identify and refer children in need of further evaluation.

Differentiating between behavior that is challenging in a classroom setting but manageable in other contexts versus behavior that requires referral for mental health assessment and treatment is important. Some aggressive behaviors may be a child's response to a temporary environmental or situational stress, such as acute illness, parental absence, or a new sibling. For persisting behavioral concerns, child care health consultants can suggest evaluation by a mental health specialist to determine whether the child's behavior requires clinical treatment or if classroom management strategies may be sufficient to address the problem.

CHILDREN EXPOSED TO VIOLENCE

Impact on Development and Behavior

The impact of violence on child development and behavior ranges from withdrawn, fearful, depressed behavior to aggressive and hurtful behavior toward others. Erickson's theory of development suggests that a safe environment is essential if children are to progress in the early stages of development. Children in child care are usually in Erickson's initial stages of development. These include the stages of trust versus mistrust, autonomy versus shame and doubt, or initiative versus guilt. Each of these stages require that children feel safe in their surroundings to master the appropriate developmental task of that stage. Infants who experience abuse by their parent or other primary caregiver are unlikely to develop a trusting relationship with others. In contrast, infants and young children who trust their caregiver have the basis for interacting with others in a positive manner that allows successful mastery of later stages of development.

Bandura's social learning theory also emphasizes the importance of a nonviolent environment for children's social development. Children learn by observing the behavior of others, particularly the behavior of adults who are significant in their lives. When adults model aggressive and hostile behavior, children adopt this style of interacting with others.[8]

Although some have suggested that violence on TV has no effect on children or a positive effect by teaching children the consequences of violence, research has proven otherwise. Children who witness violence or aggressive behavior on TV are more likely to act in an aggressive manner.[9,10] Young children who watch violent cartoons are more likely than those watching more prosocial programs, such as *Sesame Street* or *Mister Rogers' Neighborhood*, to act aggressively in the classroom.[11,12] Repetitively viewing or hearing violent messages in the media can emotionally desensitize a child toward violence.[13-15]

Numerous studies document that even at an early age, children who experience violence, whether as victims of child abuse or as witnesses to a violent situation, are likely to respond with changes in behavior. Child abuse victims may present with nonspecific stress reactions, including depression and low self-esteem. Children may enact the violence in their play, have subdued behavior or inactivity, a more pronounced startle reaction, sleep difficulty, enuresis after previously being toilet trained, or demonstrate other regressive behavior.[16-18]

Strategies to Assist Children Exposed to Violence

Child care health consultants can provide training for child care professionals on strategies to assist children in dealing with violence they may have witnessed or by which they may have been victimized. Strategies include providing a safe, nonviolent classroom environment, assisting children to identify and discuss violent and nonviolent behaviors, and teaching children safety and self-protection measures.

Make the Classroom a Safe, Nonviolent Place for Children

Strategies to ensure that early childhood classrooms convey a sense of safety and caring are discussed within a broader context in chapters 7 and 10 through 12. The reader is referred to those chapters for a more comprehensive overview of each of these topics. Disciplinary techniques and classroom structure are 2 aspects of a safe and caring child care setting that are of particular importance in addressing childhood violence and are included in this chapter because of their significance.

Children in the United States are not protected from corporal punishment as are children in most other industrialized countries. Although the Maternal and Child Health Bureau's National Health and Safety Performance Standards for Out-of-Home Care developed by the American Academy of Pediatrics and American Public Health Association recommend against the use of physical punishment, many states do permit spanking in child care programs.* The use of physical punishment in child care programs places children at risk of being abused and does not decrease negative behavior in children. In fact, children who experience physical and hostile

---

* For information on child care regulations related to corporal punishment within a specific state, readers are referred to the following Web site of individual states' child care licensing rules: http://nrc.uchsc.edu/STATES/states.html.

discipline are more likely to become aggressive and hostile themselves.[8] Child care health consultant training and advocacy efforts to promote appropriate discipline techniques are essential to reduce disciplinary violence.

Providers can set limits on children's behavior in a proactive rather than reactive disciplinary manner by structuring their classroom to provide a safe and nonviolent environment. To proactively set limits, providers might involve the children in establishing classroom rules for behavior. This offers reassurance to children as to what behavior they can and cannot expect from their classmates. Child care providers also can decrease the potential for conflict among the children by minimizing crowding for specific play areas and equipment. Enough toys to decrease conflict and long waits should be available, but not so many toys that sharing is never required. The child care provider can make play materials and activities that offer positive social interaction available. This would include noncompetitive play in which children have a common goal, such as block building or a tire swing. When sharing is observed by the child care provider, commenting on this behavior can lead to discussion of what constitutes sharing and helpful behavior.

It is inevitable that children will at some point become angry and exhibit aggressive behavior. In the past, child care providers have been encouraged to offer children substitute aggressive play activities or targets, such as a punching bag or doll, to deal with the anger. More recent research suggests this is no longer advisable,[18] because rather than decreasing or redirecting the child's anger, it may in fact serve to increase aggressive behavior. Instead, child care providers can assist children to problem solve and resolve the conflict in an assertive but nonaggressive manner. Additional information on the importance of social problem-solving skills is discussed in a later section of this chapter.

Identify and Discuss Violent and Nonviolent Behavior

It is important that child care providers talk with children about the violence they may have observed in their own lives or on TV. In discussing the observed violence, providers should identify the behavior as violent and convey that violence hurts others and destroys things. It is also important that providers remind children that violence is punished. Too often, violence on TV goes unpunished, suggesting that violence is a successful strategy for handling a problem. The National Television Violence Study reports that 58% of all violence on TV shows no pain or injury to victims.[10] Other studies had similar findings. Portrayals of gun use showed no adverse effect or outcome (death, injury, or arrest) for the user 58% of the time.[20] Child care providers should discuss and subsequently correct childrens' perceptions of inaccurate portrayals and outcomes of violence on TV.

When talking with children about violence, child care providers should use judgment and not overdo the discussion to the point that it could frighten children. Honesty and a clear message that violence is harmful are important, but providers should refrain from describing graphic details of the effects of violence. Discussion of violent behavior should be balanced with discussion of nonviolent behavior. As children share and help one another in their play activities, child care providers can point out the positive behavior to the class. This can lead to discussions of what aspects of behavior are helpful and caring acts.

Teach Children Safety and Protective Actions to Avoid Potentially Violent Situations

The early learning environment of child care offers an ideal opportunity for providers to teach children safety measures and protective actions they can take when confronted with a potentially violent situation. The most important message to communicate to children is that they should leave a violent situation as quickly as possible, seek adult help, and not try to intervene themselves. Child care providers can lead class discussions to help children identify a safe place in their neighborhood they could go to if a potentially dangerous situation arises. Child care curricula almost always include teaching children basic emergency responses. In addition to teaching children how to dial 911 and how to state the problem and their location, children can also practice this skill frequently enough in their child care setting that they will be able to carry it out even if frightened and confused in a real-life emergency situation.

Early childhood curricula should include lesson plans for teaching children assertive behavior. Building on earlier models of substance abuse prevention curricula, children can be taught that it is all right to say "no" to hurtful behavior. Role playing opportunities are also available for child care providers to teach assertive behavior. By using pretend play initiated by children on their own or teacher-directed pretend play, such as puppet play or story telling time, child care providers can set up a story and then ask the children for suggestions on what the character in the story might do. Using the children's responses, child care providers can teach children the difference between assertive and aggressive behavior. Aggressive behavior is angry, physical, and hurtful of others. Assertive behavior is respectful, usually only verbal, and never hurtful; it is a short clear message telling the person not to hurt you.

Given the fact that 38% of families with young children keep a handgun in their home, gun safety is an important topic for child care providers to include in their curricula.[21] Parent education on the risks of keeping guns in the home and appropriate safety precautions is, of course, essential. However, research confirms that it is unrealistic at this time to expect that children's environments will be free of guns.[22] Therefore, child care providers and health care professionals must teach children basic gun safety. Children will likely need reminders that it is not always possible to tell if a gun is real or a toy. Basic safety measures should include caution not to pick up or touch a gun even if they think it is only a toy.

Bullying

Bullying among preschool and school-aged children is increasingly recognized as a problem related to child well-being and social functioning. Bullying is the repeated use of physical or verbal aggression that is intended to harm or disturb another individual when there is a power imbalance between the bully and the bullied.

Research on this issue (primarily performed outside the United States) suggests that experience with bullying (as bully, as victim, or both) is quite prevalent and is associated with a set of indicators of poor psychosocial functioning.[23] Bullies have been found to have higher levels of conduct disorders and problems with school, and victims have higher levels of depression, anxiety, loneliness, difficulty making friends, and low self-esteem. Those who experience both display particularly poor social functioning. Although this issue has been minimally studied in this country, a recently published report identifies that about 30% of sixth to tenth graders have some experience with bullying,[24] with signs of psychosocial dysfunction similar to that found in studies outside the United States; little is known about the prevalence of bullying among younger children.

Involvement with bullying is also known to have long term consequences, although work in this area is quite limited. In non-US studies, former bullies have been found to have a fourfold increase in criminal behavior by their early 20s, and formerly bullied children continue to have higher rates of depression and poor self-esteem at least into their mid-20s.[25] The relationship between experience with bullying and poten-

> *A recently published report identifies that about 30% of sixth to tenth graders have some experience with bullying.*

tial for involvement with violence in the longer term has not been studied, but the long-term psychosocial problems and anecdotal experience around more serious school violence do warrant concern about the potential link.[26]

Child care providers and pediatric health care professionals have important roles to play in the prevention of bullying and the response to those involved in bullying. Guidance on prevention strategies comes primarily from the work of Olweus in Norway, where he has documented very dramatic decreases of bullying in school settings.[23] His school-based interventions involve curricula on social skills, efforts to change social norms about bullying, establishment of clear rules and consequences that are developmentally based, increased supervision from and presence of parents, and services for those involved in bullying or being bullied. There are no evaluations of his strategies in this country, and components of his interventions need to be adapted for the cultural differences and diversities of this country.

Response to bullying and those bullied is equally important. Bullying and victimization need to be seen as red flags for problems. Although this behavior cannot be tolerated or simply dismissed, the highly associated findings of psychosocial dysfunction and the longer-term consequences clearly define a need to respond not with punishment but with evaluation and therapeutic intervention. It may be determined that punishment needs to be part of the therapeutic response, but this needs to come out of a proper psychosocial evaluation and comprehensive treatment plan, particularly for those who display chronic behaviors of bullying or being bullied.

Given the prevalence of the behaviors related to bullying, this issue does warrant attention. Forethought should be put toward this issue proactively so that child care providers are prepared to address it and health care professionals are prepared to assist parents and child care providers.

Assessment and Referral of Children Exposed to Violence

When assisting child care programs to develop health forms and conduct health assessments, child care health consultants can include assessment of a child's exposure to violence. Appropriate assessment questions include asking the parents if their child has witnessed violence first-hand in their neighborhood, asking if there is a gun in the home, and discussing the amount and type of television programming their child watches. Providing a list of community resources and assisting child care providers in identifying and referring children in need of further services will make it more likely that children obtain needed care.

Specific training topics to assist child care professionals to recognize the signs and symptoms of child abuse are discussed in Chapter 12. Health consultants can also help child care programs develop written policies and procedures to assess and respond to child abuse before the need for this action. The procedures for reporting child abuse are often complex and can vary from one community to another. By having planned procedures determined in advance, a written policy or protocol, and staff trained in the proper procedure specific to their community, the legal requirements of this process are more likely to be met and the child is more likely to receive appropriate referral and follow-up. Preferably, one child care provider or member of the administrative staff should be identified as the person to respond to and file child abuse reports for the center. This helps to ensure that procedures are consistent and formal as appropriate to the seriousness of the situation.

VIOLENCE PREVENTION

Early Childhood Development Related to Youth and Adult Violence

Adults and youth who commit violence against others are likely to have been aggressive and hostile in their early peer interactions.[27] There appears to be a cycle, in that children's early aggressive behavior results in rejection by their peers, which in turn results in even more aggressive behavior from the rejected child.[28,29] The aggressive behavior continues and often escalates into violent behavior during adolescence and adulthood. Early intervention measures to decrease aggressive behavior and promote prosocial skills in early childhood are essential to decrease children's risk of developing violent behavior in later years.

Children's ability to negotiate the give-and-take of peer interactions in an assertive but nonaggressive manner is directly related to their ability to problem solve in social situations. Social problem-solving skills are a set of discreet but interrelated skills, which include accuracy in interpreting a situation, ability to generate multiple prosocial solutions, flexibility in trying alternative strategies, accurate outcome expectations for strategies selected, and empathy and perspective taking. Children at risk of developing aggressive and violent behavior demonstrate limited ability in one or more of these components of social problem-solving skills.

To offer early intervention for violence prevention, health care professionals and child care providers need an understanding of the components of the social problem-solving process and how aggressive children who may bully or victimize others differ from their peers in each of these component skills. The discussion below summarizes findings from a series of research studies addressing differences in social problem-solving skills between aggressive and nonaggressive children.[30-32] In these studies, children were presented with pictures, videos, or drawings of various play situations. The scenes portrayed a child trying to enter a group play situation in progress (children coloring together and another child standing on the side) or a peer conflict situation (2 children both wanting the same toy). Children were asked how the child portrayed might enter the play group or resolve the conflict. Children's social problem-solving skills were determined by analyzing their responses to the questions. Children's social behavior (whether prosocial or aggressive) was measured by a teacher or observer rating of children's overall behavior in the classroom. Analysis of the relationship of children's responses to the pictured play scenes and their overall classroom behavior suggested differences between aggressive and prosocial children in their social problem-solving skills.

Accurate Interpretation of Social Situation

Clearly, how a child interprets a situation influences how he or she might respond. If a child perceives a situation to be friendly and pleasant, he or she is more likely to respond in a friendly, positive manner. In the studies referenced above, prosocial children tended to assess an ambiguous situation in more positive, friendly terms, whereas aggressive children were more likely to interpret the situation as hostile. Children's interpretation of the peer play situation is a factor differentiating aggressive children from their peers. Aggressive children are more sensitive than are their peers to hostile stimuli and less skilled in interpreting interpersonal situations accurately.

Multiple Solutions and Flexibility

The ability to identify multiple solutions to a social problem is an apparent advantage. The more options a child has available, the more likely he or she is to choose an effective strategy. Research confirms that prosocial children are able to generate 3 or more alternatives, whereas less well-adjusted children are only able to identify 1 or 2 solutions. Having alternative solutions is also helpful to children should their first attempt at resolving the problem fail. Following failure in a social situation, a child may choose to withdraw from the situation altogether, repeat the original strategy, or modify the previous strategy and try again. In comparison with more prosocial children, aggressive children are less flexible and tend to repeat their original unsuccessful strategy.

Prosocial Solutions and Outcome Expectations

In addition to the quantity of strategies a child is able to generate, the quality of the proposed strategy (prosocial vs aggressive) and the child's expectations for successful outcome are factors in developing positive social skills. As discussed in later sections of this chapter, children model the behavior they observe. Children who experience coercive and physical discipline from adults or observe adults acting aggressively learn that aggressive behavior is a successful strategy for resolving conflict. This leads a child to propose and expect aggressive strategies to be successful in peer interactions. In contrast, children who experience positive rather than negative forms of discipline and observe adults resolving conflict in assertive but friendly tones are more likely to suggest prosocial strategies and to expect the prosocial solutions to be successful. Research linking social problem-solving and social development confirms that prosocial children are more likely to propose prosocial strategies and to expect the prosocial strategies to be successful. In contrast, aggressive children are more likely to propose aggressive strategies and to expect the aggressive strategies to be successful.

Empathy and Perspective Taking

Empathy and perspective taking are important components of social problem-solving skills. Children are more likely to interpret situations accurately and to generate prosocial solutions if they can understand the perspective of other children. Developmentally, children begin with the belief that all others think and act as they do, but gradually become aware that others think differently than themselves. Initially, children can't consider their own feelings and another child's feelings simultaneously. By the end of the preschool years, most children are able to view their own and others' perspectives simultaneously but not always on a consistent basis. The consistency and degree to which a young child is able to empathize depends not only on the child's developmental level but also on the child's level of distress in a particular situation. Strategies to promote children's development of empathy and perspective taking are discussed in the next section of this chapter.

In summary, children's risk for developing violent behavior as youth and young adults is decreased when they interpret ambiguous social situations as friendly, are able to identify 3 or more prosocial strategies for resolving peer conflict, demonstrate flexibility in trying alternative strategies if their first attempt was unsuccessful, and expect assertive but friendly strategies rather than aggressive strategies to be successful and are able to consider the perspective of other children involved in the conflict. Child care programs offer many natural opportunities for children to learn and practice these component social problem-solving skills.

Early Intervention and Prevention Strategies

Although most research addressing children's development of social problem-solving skills and prosocial behavior has focused on parent-child interactions, this research has been applied to child care providers' interactions with children. Research suggests that significant adults, whether parent or child care provider, contribute to children's development of social problem-solving skills in 3 ways: by modeling appropriate behavior, by directly teaching or coaching children on how-to behavior, and by providing opportunities for children to practice skills in peer play experiences. Child care providers can use each of these mechanisms within their curricula to teach effective and nonviolent conflict resolution.

Modeling

Children's behavior is most often modeled after the behavior of significant adults in their lives. Previous sections of this chapter pointed out the importance of adults modeling appropriate behavior in discipline situations. Using hostile and punitive forms of discipline teaches children that aggressive behavior is an effective strategy for resolving conflict. In contrast, child care providers who use explanations and natural consequences in responding to children's misbehavior model assertive but nonaggressive strategies to resolve disputes. Adults also can use nondisciplinary situations, such as free play or story time, to model prosocial behavior and problem-solving skills. Using a calm, unhurried tone of voice and offering friendly comments at times when group play may become loud actively models assertive but calm and goal-directed behavior for children. Child care providers can select a story to read in which the character demonstrates effective problem-solving behavior. Similarly, child care providers can use puppet play as an opportunity to model social problem-solving skills. By setting up puppet play that presents a social problem and having the puppet think out loud, the provider can demonstrate the social problem-solving process for children and model successful nonaggressive strategies for resolving the problem.

Coaching

In addition to modeling appropriate behavior, child care providers may be more explicit by directly teaching or coaching children on social behavior. When coaching children, the concept of "scaffolding" is particularly effective to teach social problem-solving skills. In scaffolding, adults engage a child in successful problem-solving by structuring the situation to a level slightly above the child's abilities. The adult makes an ongoing assessment of the child's ability and adjusts the scaffold to support the child's increasing skill. As the child learns, the adult gradually decreases the amount of direction until the child is able to perform the task independently. Providing too little or too much direction in teaching or coaching situations does not challenge the child to higher levels of development. Coaching children without directing their behavior gives children the new information they may need and also prompts the child to think through the situation and consider alternatives. In effect, the child is problem-solving with adult guidance and reinforcement.

Child care providers may be more explicit by directly teaching or coaching children on social behavior

Child care providers can teach problem solving using scaffolding to build on the modeling examples of story time and puppet play cited previously. As the story or puppet play progresses, the child care provider can ask children what the story character or puppet can do to resolve the problem. The provider can encourage the children to think of as many alternative actions as possible to resolve the conflict. For strategies that the children propose, the provider can ask if a particular aggressive or assertive strategy is likely to be successful and what the character might do if the first strategy doesn't work. Asking the children how they think the character in story or puppet play might be feeling is an opportunity to teach perspective taking and empathy skills.

Child care providers can use free play time to coach children in problem solving. When a provider observes a child's behavior escalating, the provider can intervene before the behavior becomes overtly aggressive. Coaching the child to problem solve in this very real situation offers scaffolding for children who do not have well-developed social problem-solving skills.

Curricula and other materials are available specifically for early childhood learning professionals to teach social problem-solving skills in group settings. Sure's *I Can Problem Solve* program is a curriculum guide of 20-minute lessons for early childhood classrooms. McGinnis and Goldstein's *Skill-Streaming in Early Childhood* is designed for children who have problems with aggressive behavior. For a more complete list of curricula and other materials, see the list of additional resources at the conclusion of this chapter.

Practice Opportunities

Child care providers and other adults can model, coach, and directly teach children what is and is not appropriate social behavior, but adult-child interactions will always have one person acting in a more accommodating manner or with more authority than the other. It is only in peer play interactions that children can test the information learned with their social equals. Children are most actively learning social problem-solving skills when they are negotiating the give-and-take that occurs in peer play. The unstructured free play time in early childhood curricula is a unique opportunity for children to develop social problem-solving skills.

Child care providers can shape free-play time to promote development of social problem-solving skills by structuring the setting in which peer play occurs. The physical space should minimize crowding but bring children into proximity to promote interaction. Offering enough toys to give all children a turn but not so many that sharing is never required will decrease conflict and promote problem solving among the children. Child care providers also can provide role-playing materials that encourage social interactions, especially roles in which children can act out and respond to various helping roles, such as teacher, parent, doctor, nurse, and storekeeper or sales helper.

A balance of teacher-directed and child-directed activities is essential for children to develop social problem-solving skills. Modeling of appropriate behavior by adults helps children understand that aggressive behavior is not as effective as prosocial actions. Coaching without a high degree of direction prompts children to generate alternative solutions and to consider possible outcomes of the proposed strategies. But it is the peer play experience that is most powerful in helping children translate the information they receive from adults into self-regulated patterns of social behavior.

Parent Education

A final opportunity for child care health consultants to address childhood violence is when interacting directly with families of children in child care, whether in the course of providing primary health care services or during parent education programs held by the child care program. During these interactions, health consultants have the opportunity to reinforce the collaboration of child care providers, families, and pediatric health care professionals in decreasing violence and addressing the effects of violence on children. During primary care visits, health care professionals can offer information on the importance of children's development of social problem-solving skills and direct parents to community resources for further parent education. Specific parent education topics include: 1) promoting the use of prosocial discipline practices and discouraging the use of physical punishment; 2) teaching parents to model positive conflict resolution behavior; 3) promoting alternative play activities to decrease the amount of time young children watch television; 4) discouraging handguns in the home; and 5) screening for children at risk of developing violent behavior. Many of the strategies suggested for child care providers are appropriate for parent-child interactions. Child care health consultants can include material in this chapter in parent education programs to assist parents in developing their child's social problem-solving skills.

CONCLUSIONS AND RECOMMENDATIONS

The safe and nurturing child care environment is a natural setting for child care providers and pediatric health care professionals to partner in addressing the violence children may be experiencing in their lives. Child care health consultants should support child care providers who may be caring for children who are witnesses to or victims of violence and should assist child care providers in the prevention of violence carried out by children.

REFERENCES

1. American Psychological Association. *Summary Report of the American Psychological Association Commission on Violence and Youth.* Washington, DC: American Psychological Association; 1993

2. Richters JE, Martinez P. The NIMH community violence project: I. Children as victims of and witness to violence. *Psychiatry.* 1993;56:7-21

3. Bell C, Jenkins E. Community violence and children on Chicago's southside. *Psychiatry.* 1993;56:46-54

4. Jaffee PG, Wolfe DA, Wilson SK. *Children of Battered Women.* Newbury Park, CA: Sage Publications; 1994

5. Children's Defense Fund. Facts on youth, violence, and crime. Washington, DC: Children's Defense Fund; 2001. Available at: http://www.childrensdefense.org/education/prevention/factsheets/youth.asp. Accessed March 19, 2004

6. US Department of Health and Human Services. *Child Maltreatment 1996: Reports From the States to the National Child Abuse and Neglect Data System.* Washington, DC: US Government Printing Office; 1998

7. Federal Interagency Forum on Child and Family Statistics. Youth victims and perpetrators of serious violent crimes. Available at: http://www.childstats.gov/results.asp?field=SbjID&value=4. Accessed March 19, 2004

8. Pettit G. *Family Interaction Style and Children's Subsequent Social-Behavior Competence: A Six Month Longitudinal Investigation.* Paper presented at the Biennial Meeting of the Society for Research in Child Development; April 1991; Seattle, WA

9. Bandura A. Influences of a model's reinforcement contingencies on the acquisition of imitative responses. *J Pers Soc Psychol.* 1965;1:589-595

10. *National Television Violence Study. Executive summary.* Studio City, CA: Mediascope; 1994-1995

11. Singer JL, Singer DG. *Television, Imagination, and Aggression: A Study of Preschoolers.* Hillsdale, NJ: Lawrence Erlbaum; 1981

12. American Academy of Pediatrics, Task Force on Violence. The role of the pediatrician in youth violence prevention in clinical practice and at the community level. *Pediatrics.* 1999;103:173-181

13. American Academy of Pediatrics, Committee on Communications. Media violence. *Pediatrics.* 2001;108:1222-1226

14. American Academy of Pediatrics, Committee on Communications. Impact of music lyrics and music videos on children and youth. *Pediatrics.* 1996;8:1219-1221

15. American Academy of Pediatrics, American Academy of Child and Adolescent Psychiatry, American Psychological Association, American Medical Association, American Academy of Family Physicians, and American Psychiatric Association. *Joint Statement on the Impact of Entertainment Violence on Children Congressional Public Health Summit.* Elk Grove Village, IL: American Academy of Pediatrics; 2000. Available at: http://www.aap.org/advocacy/releases/jstmtevc.htm. Accessed March 19, 2004

16. Bell C, Jenkins EJ. Traumatic stress and children. *J Health Care Poor Underserved.* 1991;2: 175-185

17. Augustyn M, Parker S, Groves BM, Zuckerman B. Silent victims: children who witness violence. *Contemp Pediatr.* 1995;12:35-57

18. Osofsky JD, Fenichel E, eds. *Hurt, Healing, and Hope: Caring for Infants and Toddlers in Violent Environments.* Arlington, VA: Zero to Three/National Center for Clinical Infant Programs; 1994

19. Berkowitz L. *Aggression: Its Causes, Consequences, and Control.* New York, NY: McGraw-Hill; 1993

20. Price JH, Merril EA, Clause ME. The depiction of guns on prime time television. *J Sch Health.* 1992;62:15-18

21. Senturia YD, Teacher AM, Christoffel KK, Donovan M. Children's household exposure to guns: A Pediatric-Based Survey. *Pediatrics.* 1994;469-475

22. Powell E, Sheehan K, Christoffel K. Firearm violence among youth: public health strategies for prevention. *Ann Emerg Med.* 1996;28:204-212

23. Olweus D. *Bullying at School: What We Know and What We Can Do.* Oxford, England: Blackwell; 1993

24. Nansel TR, Overpeck M, Pilla RS, Ruan WJ, Simons-Morton B, Scheidt P. Bullying behaviors among US youth: prevalence and association with psychosocial adjustment. *JAMA.* 2001;285:2094-2100

25. Olweus D. Bullying among schoolchildren: intervention and prevention. In: Peters RD, McMahon RJ, Quinsey VL, eds. *Aggression and Violence Throughout the Lifespan.* Newbury Park, CA: Sage Publications; 1992:100-125

26. Spivak H, Prothrow-Stith D. The need to address bullying-an important component of violence prevention. *JAMA.* 2001;285:2131-2032

27. Dishion T. The family ecology of boys' peer relations in middle childhood. *Child Dev.* 1990;61:874-892

28. Reid J. Prevention of conduct disorders before and after school entry: relating interventions to developmental findings. *Dev Psychopathol.* 1993;5:243-262

29. Patterson G, Reid J, Dishion T. *Antisocial Boys.* Eugene, OR: Castalia; 1992

30. Crick N, Dodge K. A review and reformulation of social information-processing mechanisms in children's social adjustment. *Psychol Bull.* 1994;115:74-101

31. Dodge KA. A social information processing model of social competence in children. In: Perlmutter M, ed. *Cognitive Perspectives on Children's Social and Behavioral Development. The Minnesota Symposium on Child Psychology.* Hillsdale, NJ: Erlbaum; 1986:77-125

32. Crick N, Dodge K. Social information-processing mechanisms in reactive and proactive aggression. *Child Dev.* 1996;67:993-1002

ADDITIONAL RESOURCES

Center to Prevent Handgun Violence. *Pediatrician Firearm Prevention Counseling Materials.* Washington, DC: Center to Prevent Handgun Violence; 1993

Kaiser B, Rasminsky J. *Meeting the Challenge: Effective Strategies for Challenging Behaviors in Early Childhood Environments.* Ontario, CA: Canadian Child Care Federation; 1999

McGinnis E, Goldstein AP. *Skill-Streaming in Early Childhood: Teaching Prosocial Skills to the Preschool and Kindergarten Child.* Champaign, IL: Research Press; 1990

Salby RG, Roedell WC, Arezzo D, Hendrix K. *Early Violence Prevention Tools for Teachers of Young Children.* Washington, DC: National Association for the Education of Young Children; 1995

Sandall S, Ostrosky M. *Practical Ideas for Addressing Challenging Behaviors.* CO: Sopris West; 1999

Shure MB. *I Can Problem Solve: An Interpersonal Cognitive Problem-Solving Program for Children (Preschool).* Champaign, IL: Research Press; 1992

CHAPTER 10

Child Care as a Resource and Support System for Families

Douglas R. Powell, PhD

LEARNING OBJECTIVES

This chapter will enable the reader to:

- Describe the diverse needs of families that must be addressed when choosing a child care arrangement (flexible hours, proximity to home, willingness to accept children with disabilities, etc).

- Become familiar with the role of child care in:

  ~ identifying special needs of the child or family and making appropriate referrals;

  ~ providing respite care to families of children with special needs or single parent families; and

  ~ parenting education.

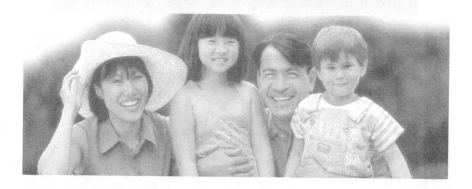

INTRODUCTION

Historically, children have been viewed as the primary client of child care services in the United States. In general, parents have been an ancillary focus of child care programs; in some child care traditions, the program has been viewed as compensating for the limitations of inadequate parents. This pattern has been undergoing change in the past decade as a growing body of evidence indicates a high-quality child care arrangement is one of the most important family support systems for working parents of young children. Research suggests that performance in the workplace, parent-child relations, and other key aspects of individual and family functioning are influenced by the quality of child care.[1] At the same time, child development is increasingly approached from an ecologic perspective that emphasizes connections between child functioning and characteristics of the family, community, and societal systems surrounding the child.

This chapter examines the ways in which child care centers and family child care homes can support families living in diverse circumstances. Families and child care programs vary considerably in the availability of resources. Consideration of child care as a family support system requires an understanding of how family characteristics and child care quality are related. This chapter reviews briefly what is known about connections between family resources and child care quality, identifies and describes the roles of child care in supporting families, and concludes with recommendations for pediatricians.

FAMILY CHARACTERISTICS AND CHILD CARE QUALITY

Quality child care is not equitably distributed across families of different socioeconomic status in the United States. Research indicates that child care centers predominantly serving children from upper-income families provide the highest quality of care, and centers predominantly serving children from middle-income families often provide the poorest quality of care. Many centers that serve children from low-income families mostly do not differ significantly in quality from centers serving children from upper-income families.[2] Perhaps middle-class families are at a disadvantage, because they lack the financial resources to purchase high-quality care or cannot receive government subsidies that often provide some assurance of quality. Centers providing higher-than-average overall quality have been found to receive in-kind donations or extra funding that is used to improve quality. These relationships between center quality and family income have not been found in studies of care provided in family child care; in this type of setting, children from lower-income families generally are in lower quality care than their higher-income counterparts.[3]

What are the implications of these patterns for children? Poor-quality child care can contribute to cumulative developmental risk for very young children from high-risk circumstances. In one major study, for infants whose mothers were relatively insensitive in interactions with them, the incidence of insecure attachment was further elevated when the quality of observed child care was poor or the arrangement was unstable or when care was used for more hours.[4] On the other hand, participation in a high-quality child care center from 3 months of age has been found to have a positive effect on the intellectual functioning of children from socioeconomically disadvantaged families.[5] A large probability sample study found that initiation of child care attendance before the first birthday was associated with higher reading recognition scores at 5 or 6 years of age for children from more impoverished home environments but with lower reading recognition scores for children from higher-quality home environments. Also, center-based child care was associated with higher scores in mathematics comprehension for children from impoverished backgrounds and with lower mathematics scores for children from more stimulating home environments.[6] In summary, the effects of child care on a child may depend on the extent to which the child care program provides growth-enhancing opportunities that are equal to, better, or worse than those provided in the child's home.

ROLES OF CHILD CARE IN SUPPORTING FAMILIES

Six roles of child care programs in supporting families are identified and described in this section. Typically, each role is not enacted independent of the other roles; supportive child care combines these roles in ways that are responsive to the needs of individual families. Moreover, family-supportive child care providers expend considerable energy learning about the interests, needs, and preferences of families before carrying out a role intended to be of assistance to a family.

Accommodate Family Logistics

Supportive child care needs to be responsive to the logistics of family life. Location, hours of service, and flexibility in entry and exit times are important factors in determining whether a child care service successfully accommodates parents' work or job training schedules and transportation patterns. To this end, a diverse range of child care options should be available to parents. For instance, welfare mothers' ratings of their child care on quality, convenience, dependability, and cost showed that no particular arrangement was superior across all of these dimensions; each type had strengths and weaknesses.[7]

Flexible child care arrangements may be of particular interest to parents of children with disabilities. Mothers of children younger than 3 years with disabilities have been found to enter the workforce at approximately the same rate as the general population of women with children younger than 3 years, but a greater proportion of mothers with children with special needs have been found to be employed part-time.[8] Family child care homes are viewed by most parents of very young children with special needs as more appropriate setting for their children than is center-based child care, because family child care homes provide greater opportunity for individualized attention, continuity of caregiver, decreased risk of infections because of small numbers of children in the setting, and flexible hours.[9]

Promote Healthy Child Development

Although flexible program hours and convenient location are important elements for responding to adult needs, it is essential for child care programs to support families through the provision of high-quality work with children. Characteristics of high-quality care are described in other chapters in this manual.

Stimulating and nurturing child care environments for children are the starting point of family support. Poor-quality child care not only has direct negative effects on children's development but also can contribute to difficulties in the parent-child relationship and patterns of interaction within the family system. For instance, a child's reluctance to go to a child care arrangement because it is chaotic or stressful and a child's troubling behavior at the end of the child care day may trigger strained interactions within a family and heighten parental guilt about the use of child care. Conversely, when a child care program enables children to learn new skills that positively impress their parents, the type and amount of stimulation in the home environment may improve as parents accommodate a new appreciation and understanding of their children's abilities.

Coordinate With Parents

Child care providers support families by contributing to the continuity of children's experiences between home and child care program. Continuity entails congruence between family and child care program regarding similarity in child-rearing values, goals, expectations, language and language codes, and the nature of adult-child interactions and relationships. Continuity also includes linkages between the family and child care program maintained through frequent and preferably personal communication, including regular parental presence at the child care program.

Families and child care programs constitute different social environments for children in terms of behavioral expectations, patterns of adult-child interaction, and sometimes child-rearing values. Although appropriate levels of incongruence can be beneficial to children's development, extreme differences are likely to be an educational or developmental risk for children whose parents have limited formal education or are of cultural or racial backgrounds not reflected in the program.[10] Accordingly, it is recommended that child care programs communicate with families in their home language and ensure that practices of the home and expectations of the program are complementary; linguistic and cultural continuity between the home and child care program supports children's social and emotional development.[11]

A frequent flow of information between parent and child care provider enables parents to elaborate on and extend at home the curriculum activities of the child care program (eg, a nutrition lesson) and allows child care staff to acknowledge or incorporate family events or developments (eg, a relative's visit) into a child's experiences at the program.

Coordination with parents also is important for facilitating children's transitions to a child care program. Provisions for child visits to a child care program before entry and for a sustained period of parental presence on the first several days after a child enters a new setting are among the ways child care programs can support parents in helping their children adjust to new relationships and physical surroundings. Because parents' provision of information to their young children about an impending transition to a new setting has positive effects on child separation behaviors, a useful role for child care programs is to inform parents about the value of giving concrete information to their children about how the leave taking will work and what the setting will be like.

Supportive child care programs recognize that separation anxiety is not limited to children. Research shows that parents can experience a sense of displacement, including anxiety and tension, regarding the child's relationship with the child care provider. Parents' separation anxiety can include feelings of sadness, worry, or uneasiness about being away from the child as well as

Parents' anxious feelings may be decreased through a strong sense of trust in their child's caregivers.

guilt about not being at home with the child. Parents' anxious feelings may be decreased through a strong sense of trust in their child's caregivers. Thus, it is potentially helpful for a program to emphasize the competence and commitment levels of providers regarding the care of children.

Parents' relationships with early childhood program staff can be a training ground for acquiring skills that contribute to effective relations with their children's teachers in elementary and secondary school. A 10-year follow-up study of the effects of a family support program that included child care for children of low-income families found that program mothers were more self-initiating in contacts with their child's teacher than were control-group mothers.[12]

Enhance Parent Knowledge and Skills

The traditional role of early childhood programs in supporting parents is formal education in child development and care offered to parents through lectures, workshops, discussion groups, 1-on-1 consultation, and opportunities for parents to volunteer in classrooms. This tradition is stronger in half-day nursery schools and early intervention programs, such as Head Start, than in child care centers; for instance, one national study found that less than half of child care centers but 91% of Head Start programs and 64% of school-sponsored early childhood programs offered workshops to parents.[10] Nonetheless, there are important model programs in which child care centers serve a major parent education role. For instance, a Vermont initiative aimed at adolescent parents involves a parent training component that places adolescent parents in a child care center for 20 hours per week for 1 semester to gain prevocational skills, such as punctuality, responsibility, and managing relations with others in the workplace.[11]

In recent years, there has been movement away from professionally driven parent education offerings and a growing interest in parent support efforts that are designed through collaborations between parents and program staff. Illustrative of this approach is the Parent Services Project model, which originated in California child care centers serving low-income, at-risk families. Joint planning between parents and staff enables services to be tailored to the interests and needs of a specific population. These include parent education classes, adult outings, skill-building classes for parents, peer group discussions, mental health services, leadership training, English-as-a-second-language classes, cardiopulmonary resuscitation training, and recreational activities for families.[15]

Informal exchanges between parents and child care providers may be a significant program support of parents' child-rearing knowledge and skills. Providers in center and family child care home settings have been found to use an active helping response in dealing with parents' questions and concerns about their child; they ask questions, offer alternatives, and share personal experiences in response to parents' interests. These discussions may alter parents' perceptions of their child, prompt self-examination of child-rearing practices and beliefs, and enhance skills in relating to their child.[10]

Child care programs also contribute to parents' child-rearing knowledge and skills by modeling appropriate practices with young children. The modeling role transcends adult-child interaction. Communication to parents about the nutritional component of a child care program, for example, provides practical guidance on nutrition as well as examples of food items that are healthy for children. Children also may influence the type and quality of food at home by requesting parents to serve items similar to those found at the child care program.

Serve as a Respite for Parents

Child care serves as respite care for parents of children with special needs, providing temporary relief from the constant care demands. Respite care has the potential to decrease stress levels and improve the quality of life in a family; one of its important functions is to enable a family to be more socially active and connected. Family child care is a promising form of respite care; in addition to flexible hours, the neighborhood location of family child care provides geographic proximity to a family and the potential to extend a family's informal support network within a neighborhood. A model respite care demonstration project is the Delaware FIRST (Family/Infant Resource, Supplement, and Training) Program, which uses an individual family service plan to provide an appropriate match between a family and child care provider. A case study involving a medically fragile infant in the Delaware FIRST Program found there were developmental gains for the child and that the mother was able to strengthen her life skills by taking driving lessons and securing a part-time job.[8]

Child care programs also can provide needed relief for parents in abuse-prone families, in which research indicates the demands of child rearing are among the greatest stresses of family life. The preventive value of child care includes the opportunity for families to decrease their reliance on informal care from extended kin, which may add stress to relationships with extended family members, and on ad hoc arrangements with live-in companions or neighbors who may not provide a reliable or quality service.[16] High-quality child care also can be a valuable source of social support for maltreated children by promoting secure attachments to alternative caregivers for maltreated infants and by fostering preschoolers' social competence in relating to peers and adults. Caregivers in high-quality settings have been found to become a young child's attachment figures and the source of emotional support.

Identify and Refer to Sources of Assistance

Child care providers are among the first nonfamilial adults to interact with very young children on a sustained basis and, therefore, are in a good position to identify developmental delays or other disabilities that may not be detected by family members or professionals who have limited contact with a child. The potential to identify mild or moderate delays, particularly in language development, is especially high in a child care setting because of frequent and sustained adult contact with children. This potential is realized most readily through the systematic training of providers and the provision of current and detailed information about available resources within the community.

Child care providers also are in a good position to monitor the health and general functioning of children in terms of potential abuse or neglect and have a unique window on the family via the child and periodic interactions with parents.

Family-supportive child care programs maintain close relationships with health clinics, human service agencies, schools, and other sources of family support for the purpose of making adequate referrals to services and securing periodic consultation with children and families enrolled in a program. Clearly, an important role of child care is to help families make good use of community resources.

CONCLUSIONS AND RECOMMENDATIONS

1. Pediatricians should provide parents with information about the components of high-quality child care settings. Optimal child care environments for children are a foundation of program support for families.
2. Pediatricians should encourage parents to maintain frequent communication with their child care providers. Children's experiences in child care and at home are improved significantly when parents and child care providers share information about the child, family, and their goals for the child.
3. Pediatricians should advocate for quality child care services in the community, including policies that support a range of child care options and practices that enable child care programs to be responsive to the diverse needs of families.

4. Pediatricians should offer to be health consultants to child care programs on a number of health-related issues, including the care of children with special needs. High-quality child care requires well-trained staff who can work effectively with a range of children.

REFERENCES

1. Perry-Jenkins M, Repetti RL, Crouter AC. Work and family in the 1990s. *J Marriage Fam.* 2000;62:981–998
2. Phillips DA, Voran M, Kisker E, Howes C, Whitebook M. Child care for children in poverty: opportunity or inequity? *Child Dev.* 1994;65:472–492
3. Kontos S, Howes C, Shinn M, Galinsky E. *Quality in Family Child Care and Relative Care.* New York, NY: Teachers College Press; 1995
4. National Institute of Child Health and Devlopment, Early Child Care Research Network. The effects of infant child care on infant-mother attachment security: results of the NICHD Study of Early Child Care. *Child Dev.* 1997;68:860–879
5. Burchinal M, Lee M, Ramey C. Type of day-care and preschool intellectual development in disadvantaged children. *Child Dev.* 1989;60:128–137
6. Caughy MO, DiPietro JA, Strobino DM. Day-care participation as a protective factor in the cognitive development of low-income children. *Child Dev.* 1994;65(2 Spec No):457–471
7. Sonenstein FL, Wolf DA. Satisfaction with child care: perspectives of welfare mothers. *J Soc Issues.* 1991;47:15–31
8. Landis LJ. Marital, employment, and childcare status of mothers with infants and toddlers with disabilities. *Top Early Child Special Educ.* 1992;12:496–507
9. Deiner PL. Family day care and children with disabilities. In: Peters DL, Pence AR, eds. *Family Day Care.* New York, NY: Teachers College Press; 1992;129–145
10. Powell DR. *Families and Early Childhood Programs.* Washington, DC: National Association for the Education of Young Children; 1989
11. National Association for the Education of Young Children. Responding to linguistic and cultural diversity—recommendations for effective early childhood education. *Young Child.* 1996;51:4–12
12. Seitz V, Rosenbaum LK, Apfel NH. Effects of family support intervention: a ten-year follow-up. *Child Dev.* 1985;56:376–391
13. US General Accounting Office. *Early Childhood Centers: Services to Prepare Children for School Often Limited.* Washington, DC: US General Accounting Office; 1995
14. Link G, Beggs M, Seiderman E. *Serving Families.* Fairfax, CA: Parent Services Project; 1997
15. Galinsky E, Weissbourd B. Family-centered child care. In: Spodek B, Saracho O, eds. *Yearbook in Early Childhood Education, Vol. 3: Issues in Child Care.* New York, NY: Teachers College Press; 1992:47–65
16. Thompson RA. *Preventing Child Maltreatment Through Social Support: A Critical Analysis.* Thousand Oaks, CA: Sage Publications; 1995

CHAPTER 11

Emotional Health in Child Care

Peter A. Gorski, MD, MPA, and Susan P. Berger, PhD

LEARNING OBJECTIVES

After completion of this chapter, the reader will be familiar with:

- Key components of infant-toddler child care that support the very young child's emerging self-concept and development of relationships with others.

- Current research and perspectives on the relationship between child care attendance and infant attachment security.

- Key components of child care programs that support positive self-esteem and social competence in preschoolers.

- The role of child care in responding to the emotional needs of children experiencing family crises or disruption.

- The role of child care in identifying and referring children who may be experiencing mental health challenges.

INTRODUCTION

One of the major developmental tasks for young children is the establishment of a positive identity—a vision of oneself as cared about, competent, and able to meet life's challenges and enjoy its pleasures. For infants, toddlers, and preschoolers, experiences in relationships are central contributors to the emerging sense of self. Childhood emotional well-being is fostered in environments that provide security, protection, and intimacy with others. As younger and greater numbers of children spend significant portions of their days away from home, child care programs become extensions of family life. As such, program staff assume a significant measure of responsibility for supporting healthy emotional development of the children in their care. The day-to-day challenge in group care for young children is to create a setting in which children are treated as individuals, caregiving is responsive to developmental as well as uniquely individual needs, and relationships among children, their caregivers, and their families are nurtured. Under such circumstances, children become confident in themselves and trusting of the world in which they live—attitudes they carry forward into future relationships and school experiences. A complementary challenge for the pediatric health care professional lies in providing anticipatory guidance to families as to characteristics of child care that represent a high quality environment supportive of children's emotional health and well-being.

In this chapter, the interpersonal characteristics of the child care setting that facilitate the development of a positive and effective sense of self are highlighted. Although it is acknowledged that some young children may receive out-of-home caregiving on a 1-on-1 basis, the focus will be on the group care environment, because it is that type of setting for which guidance is often sought from health care professionals. Interpersonal attributes of group care that support positive emotional adaptation during childhood vary somewhat depending on the age of the child in care. Therefore, the preliminary discussion of day-to-day components has been divided into 2 sections; 1 for infants and toddlers and another for preschoolers. The last portion of the chapter addresses how child care can be responsive to young children's needs under special circumstances that may threaten emotional security.

SUPPORTING EMOTIONAL HEALTH AMONG INFANTS AND TODDLERS IN GROUP SETTINGS

Key Components

Child care environments that are designed to encourage the development of relationships and to support the emotional security of very young children have several characteristics in common. The following components are adapted and expanded from a description by Lally et al[1]:

Group Size

Although the ratio of adults to children is an important feature of child care for children of all ages, the size of the group is particularly significant for very young children. Infants and toddlers have a difficult time developing relationships when there are too many different people to get to know at one time. Recommended group sizes are 6 or fewer for infants who are not yet mobile; 9 or fewer for children who are crawling through approximately 18 months old, and 12 or fewer for children between 18 months and 3 years of age.

Primary Caregiving

For very young children, relationships are built on repeated experiences with others that foster expectations that needs will be met and signals will be understood. In group settings, assigning specific adults who have principal responsibility for the care of particular children is an effective method for promoting responsive caregiving. Primary caregiving does not mean that all caregivers do not interact with the infants in a group to some extent. Rather, it ensures that families and child care staff know who is responsible for each of the children in a group and that every infant or toddler has a special adult with whom to develop a close relationship. Parents also are supported by a primary caregiving arrangement, because they have someone specific with whom to exchange important information about their child on an ongoing basis.

Continuity of Care

If the very young child's positive sense of self is encouraged through relationships, then continuity in caregiving is an important component to the interpersonal quality of the child care setting. Two aspects of continuity of care should be considered in evaluating any child care program. First, how long have the adults who provide direct care to the children been employed by the child care program? Staff turnover in child care can be the result of a number of issues, including low salaries, lack of benefits, and poor working environments. Regardless of cause, losing an important caregiver can be difficult for very young children, whose sense of self-confidence is tied to their security with others in their environment. When a child care setting has a significant amount of staff turnover, children are repeatedly required to rebuild and question their trust in others. As a general rule, parents should be advised to seek child care settings in which caregivers have been employed for at least 1 year but preferably for a period equivalent to the amount of time they expect their child to be attending the program.

Second, how long do children stay in the care of a particular provider, and how are transitions to new providers undertaken? In child care programs in which the emotional security of infants and toddlers is truly encouraged, continuity with the primary caregiver over an extended period of time is the norm. In some cases, children actually stay with the same provider throughout their time attending a particular child care site, as can often be found in family child care homes and centers that use a family (rather than age-based) grouping strategy. In others, children have access to previous caregivers even when they no longer spend most of their day with them and are given significant opportunities to get to know new caregivers gradually in a formal transitioning process. Further, the timing of a child's transition from a younger to an older developmental group should be based on individual readiness, not an arbitrarily determined cut-off point.[2]

Individualization Within the Group Setting

Every child comes to the child care setting with a unique set of rhythms and an individual temperament. A baby begins to build a positive self-concept when his characteristics are recognized by others and when they are treated as important enough to be responded to in an individualized manner. Programs that use a flexible scheduling model which can accommodate needs for sleep, food, stimulation, and comforting among individual infants when they are very young support early self-development. In addition, caregivers who accept each child's temperamental traits (even those that are challenging) and strive to find individualized ways to help children manage difficult situations encourage healthy emotional adaptation. Finally, child care that values and tries to nurture the unique qualities in each child looks to parents as the experts about their child's needs and characteristic responses. In such settings, parents are encouraged to provide staff with their perceptions about their child as well as any special caregiving techniques used at home. Health care professionals can advise parents to take time to observe ways potential child care providers respond to particular infants and handle routine caregiving. Asking questions from direct observations about why a strategy might have been used with a child then can illuminate how well child care providers know and respond to children as individuals.

Supporting Peer Social Skills

One aspect that makes the child care setting unique from a home environment for the young child is the continual presence of a similarly-aged group of children special peer relationships. Learning to get along with other agemates is often thought to be a developmental task of preschool and older children. Yet, anyone who has spent time in a toddler classroom is aware of the familiarity in interactions among particular children as well as how important belonging to the group can be to an individual child's emerging sense of self. As notable as finding one's place in a group can be in child care, 1- and 2-year-olds need help from significant adults to develop peer social skills. For example, because toddlers have difficult time sharing, an important feature of a child care program that supports young children in their bids to interact with agemates is adequate (and multiple identical) numbers of toys and equipment for all participants. More importantly, caregivers can help young children learn the following 4 sets of skills that result in positive interpersonal exchanges[3]: 1) how to enter a group play situation; 2) how to sustain a play episode with another; 3) how to recognize a friendly peer overture; and 4) how to respond appropriately to the friendly bid for play of another child.

Continuity With Home

Even for young children who spend long hours in group care, the strongest emotional ties most often remain at home. Emotional security can be best supported in child care when children are permitted some continuity with the people and things that have meaning for them in their lives outside the child care setting. In the previous section, we have already mentioned the significance of including methods parents use in the daily caregiving routines of individual children within the child care setting. Keeping parents' images "alive" for young children, especially during developmental periods when separations from significant others can be most challenging (especially 8 to 10 months, 18 to 21 months, and any time the child experiences a sudden loss or change in the family or home environment), is a crucial element in quality care. Child care environments in which children are allowed to bring special objects from home (eg, a blanket or stuffed toy), where family pictures are posted at toddler eye level in accessible locations, and at which children's questions about parents' whereabouts are met with reassurance about parental return coupled with emotional support by a child care provider all encourage young children to feel as though there is a connection between home and child care. Similarly, when child care staff come from a variety of communities and cultures, an added measure of cultural diversity and communicative continuity is available to the children.

Emotional security is further enhanced when child care providers and parents of children in their care develop their own supportive and noncompetitive relationships with each other in which each respects the other's roles and has a genuine concern for the other as a person. Whether or not this happens consistently in particular child care settings may be difficult for parents to ascertain from site observations. When discussing prospective child care options, health care professionals might advise parents to speak with other parents whose children are currently enrolled in a given program for feedback from a family perspective. Sometimes parents are hesitant to become closely involved with their children's child care providers because of their own feelings or concerns about being away from their child for extended periods of time. In such cases, the health care professional can serve as a source of accurate information about infants, parents, and attachment relationships to alleviate any expressed or unexpressed fears parents might have about their own importance to their child vis-a-vis an alternate caregiver. The following section offers the health care professional the background necessary to fulfill this role.

Child Care and Infant Attachment

By reported statistics alone, nearly 60% of mothers of infants are currently in the workforce in this country and rely on some form of alternative child care during the hours that they work.[2] Reports in the popular press have raised awareness among families with young children about issues surrounding the relationship between child care attendance and mother-infant attachment. As a result, health care professionals, often asked about such issues, must be knowledgeable about what is currently known regarding child care and attachment to effectively provide guidance and information to families in their practices. As background, variations in infant attachment security have been studied for nearly 3 decades by observing infant behavior during a series of brief separations from and reunions with the mother in a standardized laboratory protocol called the Strange Situation.[4] Three major patterns of attachment demonstrated by infants between approximately 12 and 18 months of age were initially identified (secure, insecure-avoidant, and insecure-ambivalent),[4] and a fourth pattern (insecure-disorganized/disoriented)[5] has also been identified. The significance of these patterns stems from abundant research demonstrating that children who were securely attached as infants appear better than those who were insecurely attached in a variety of subsequent emotional and behavioral areas, such as persistence, frustration tolerance, cooperation with others, task enthusiasm, social competence, and self-esteem.[6-12]

On the issue of child care, findings from a series of studies conducted several years ago stirred debate when they appeared to indicate that early (eg, before 12 months of age) and extensive (eg, 20 or more hours per week) nonmaternal care increased the risk of insecure (particularly insecure-avoidant) mother-infant attachment.[13-15] Yet, not all infants with such child care experience were found to have insecure attachments with their mothers, thereby giving rise to a number of questions. Is the methodology for studying attachment appropriate for child care infants who experience repeated separations and reunions from parents on a daily basis and who may be less stressed by the Strange Situation than their home-reared counterparts? Are there characteristics of the families of insecure infants in child care that differed from secure infants in child care? Are there characteristics of child care itself that supported infant attachment security or insecurity?

Recently, members of the research network constituting the National Institute of Child Health and Human Development Study of Early Child Care published the findings addressing these issues.[16] This project is notable for its prospective, longitudinal approach to the study of a large sample of children from 10 diverse geographic locations around the country. With a sample size greater than 1000 infants, investigators were able to explore the validity of the Strange Situation for assessing attachment in children with extensive, early child care experience as well as effects of and interactions between family (demographics, employment status, maternal sensitivity, and psychologic adjustment), child (temperament, gender), and child care (type, amount, age of entry, frequency of care changes, quality of care-giving) variables hypothesized to influence infant attachment security. Results can be summarized as follows.

1. Neither infants with extensive child care nor those with minimal child care during the first year of their lives could be differentiated by the amount of distress they exhibited during the separation episodes of the Strange Situation; therefore, researchers concluded that the Strange Situation was as equally valid an assessment for infants having spent extensive time in child care as it was for those with little nonmaternal care.

2. Compared with insecurely attached infants, infants who were securely attached had mothers who were more sensitive and better adjusted psychologically independent of child care experience.

3. None of the features of the child care experience were independently related to attachment security or insecurity.

4. Low-quality child care, unstable care, and more than minimal hours in care were each related to increased rates of insecurity for infants whose mothers were relatively insensitive. In other words, children in "dual risk" conditions are most vulnerable to insecurity.

5. Extensive care for boys and limited care for girls were associated with somewhat elevated rates of insecurity; infant temperament was not.

What are the practical implications of these findings? When the quality of an infant's relationship with his mother is secure, child care attendance is unlikely to disrupt or change the trajectory of that relationship. Alternatively, however, for the parent and infant already experiencing difficulties in their interactions, extensive early child care, multiple changes in child care settings, or child care that itself is insensitive to the infant's needs may contribute to ultimate attachment insecurity. Notably, the National Institute of Child Health and Development study failed to show high-quality child care (as opposed to lower-quality care) to be associated with less insecure mother-infant attachment for children with insensitive mothers. Yet, there is reason to believe such settings may have a different compensatory value.

Infants' sense of themselves and their future interactions with others are influenced by components from all of their relationships. Studies of vulnerable but resilient children completed outside the child care arena indicate that relationships beyond one's family of origin can positively impact overall adaptation.[16-19] The very young child who is able to establish a secure relationship with an alternative caregiver in child care despite an insecure parent-child attachment may be able to carry forward a positive sense of himself or herself with others, even in the absence of any changes in the quality of the parent-child relationship. Although all children deserve daily experiences that are nurturant and respectful of their individual needs for care, the previous discussion of key components defining interpersonal quality in child care might be most crucial in helping avoid situations that might put young and vulnerable children at dual risk.

SUPPORTING EMOTIONAL HEALTH OF PRESCHOOLERS IN CHILD CARE

Achieving a sense of self-mastery is a salient developmental task during the early childhood years. The preschooler who feels comfortable and secure in his environment will actively explore and interact with others, thereby gaining confidence in himself and his abilities. In collaboration with families, child care can facilitate healthy affective development and promote mastery motivation by assisting children in managing separations, coping with feelings, and getting along with peers and by encouraging each child's positive self-image on a day-to-day basis. Although these areas overlap in practical application, each will be considered separately in this section.

Managing Separations in Child Care

For the child who has not attended child care as an infant or toddler, the transition to spending days away from home requires careful attention. Even the child who has been in early out-of-home care but who is changing sites as a preschooler needs time to separate from previous child care providers and adjust to new surroundings. Young children rely on direct experience to build mental images and expectations of people and events. The more children (and their parents) know about a particular child care site before daily attendance begins, the smoother the transition is likely to be.

In preparation for initial separations, it is recommended that families take children to visit the child care center, see the classroom in which they will be enrolled, and meet their teachers several weeks before starting regular attendance. After the visit, discussions about the activities observed and people met should occur frequently between parent and child as a context for helping the child remember what he has seen and anticipate positively what he will experience himself at child care. When possible, parents can pass by the child care center with children when out on errands and family outings, promoting the connection between child and child care by using terminology such as "your school." As with younger children, the transition to child care is easier for preschoolers when they have a particular adult to support them on-site initially. Parents can be advised to ask whether a child care program uses a primary caregiving model and to invite the child's main caregiver to their home before the start of child care. Finally, parents should be encouraged to take advantage of a variety of developmentally appropriate children's books focusing on going to school (some specifically about child care) for the first time that are available from the public library.

When the time arrives for child care to begin, most programs recommend that a parent stay on-site initially and be flexibly available for the first week or 2. Also suggested are abbreviated days, for example, beginning at the regularly scheduled hour of the morning but ending earlier in the day during the transition period than might eventually be the case. For parents who may be planning to enter or return to the workforce when their child begins child care, the practical implication of these recommendations is that child care attendance should be initiated, when possible, a week or 2 before parents' full-time employment commitments begin.

The importance of saying "good-bye" to children when parents leave them at child care needs to be included in anticipatory guidance. Even parents who are confident about their selection of a child care program can have trepidations about how their child will react to being away from them. Many adults believe children will be less distressed if they escape unnoticed while the child is engaged in some activity. In fact, quite the contrary is true over the long run. Many children do protest a parent's departure early in the child care experience. But families who develop a routine for saying "good-bye," which includes reassurance about the timing of reunions (eg, "Mommy will pick you up after your nap") help children understand that the separation is temporary. Repeated good-byes coupled with parental returns at the expected time of day builds a child's trust in his parents and confidence in his child care setting to care for him in the interim, therefore minimizing separation distress.

Children require some continuity between home and child care to feel most secure. To ease transitions between sites, children should be permitted to bring to child care some objects from home that may be comforting for them, such as stuffed animals or favorite blankets. Younger preschoolers often need concrete reminders of important family members as well. In such cases, family photographs can be displayed in classrooms or within an individual child's storage area or cubby, and tape recordings of parents' voices can be available. For some children, an object of the parents'

Children require some continuity between home and child care to feel most secure.

with which they are identified can be reassuring, as can scheduled phone calls from parents at regular and predictable points in the day. Finally, a child who is having a particularly difficult time with separations will feel much more secure if he or she has the support of 1 special caregiver during the most difficult times (eg, when first arriving, at nap time) in child care.

Most preschool-aged children begin to adjust to a child care setting within the first 2 weeks of attending. It should be noted, however, that some children only start to protest being away from home after a few weeks, when the excitement of the new setting, people, and activities begins to wear off. Children who, by nature, resist change and adapt slowly to new circumstances may feel unsettled for longer. A consistent, caring staff person can greatly facilitate the adjustment process. A child who continues to be seriously distressed or inhibited at child care for longer than 2 weeks during the initial adjustment period may be manifesting internal stress (eg, developmental disorder), or external conflict (with the child care environment, outside life events and stressors, or his family experiences and relationships). When working with families initiating child care when their children reach preschool age, health care professionals should encourage parents to check in with them by telephone during the third week of the child care experience. If adjustment concerns are evident, a consultation can be scheduled with the parents to discuss current circumstances and provide guidance around ways to alter the situation before the child's self-confidence is seriously affected.*

Helping Children Handle Feelings

Before children enter their preschool years, they will have experienced a wide range of feelings related to internal states and external circumstances. For the very young child, positive and negative emotions are played out physically, often appearing to be out of the child's control, as in a toddler temper tantrum. As children approach 3 years of age, their newly developing facility with language allows them to reflect on and discuss their experiences in a manner that permits a greater understanding of themselves and the world around them. The new world of child care and its expectations for behavior engenders a myriad of feelings for preschoolers. Yet, a surprising number of children enter child care without words to express emotional states. Without words for feelings, children are compelled to continue to demonstrate their emotions physically often in aggressive, overactive, or withdrawn ways. Such immature behavior prevents children from having positive interactions and forming affiliations with peers, perhaps leading to social isolation and a loss of self-esteem.

When evaluating a child care program, parents might be advised to watch for the ways staff respond to children when they get upset, angry, frustrated, scared, excited, and happy. Do they recognize children's feelings and use words that are developmentally appropriate to describe the underlying events? Are they affectionate toward the children? Opportunities for making such observations frequently occur in the context of children's interactions with one another. For example, if an altercation occurs because one child takes a toy from another, an astute adult might respond to the offender with a statement such as, "I know it's hard for you to wait when someone else has the toy you want, but Joey will give you a turn when he is done," and redirect the child to something else enjoyable in the meantime. To the child whose play was interrupted, the response might be, "You're angry because Dinah took your toy. Tell her it makes you mad when she does that." With such actions, the child care provider identifies both children's feelings, validates their experiences, and provides alternatives to physical actions for coping with the event. In quality child care programs, discussions about feelings occur spontaneously

---

* See the *Diagnostic and Statistical Manual for Primary Care. (DSM-PC) Child and Adolescent Version* coding for primary care counseling. Suggestions include V62.3 (educational challenge—this may be a stretch). If a child is having anxiety problems, there are a series of applicable codes (eg, V65.49 [sadness]).

around emergent events for individual children as well as for the group as a whole. In addition, conversations about emotions should be a part of positive and negative experiences. Finally, child care providers must be good models for the management of their own emotions. Rather than implying that child care providers should not demonstrate any emotions, being a good model suggests that child care staff also are able and willing to express their pleasure and distress verbally with others in socially appropriate ways.

By putting emotions into words for children consistently, it helps them understand and relate current feelings with previous experiences. It permits children to have a common reference point for sharing what is going on inside them and for beginning to recognize and empathize with the feelings of others. With challenging feelings identified, the child can begin to consider what to do to alleviate or overcome current circumstances. Thus, verbalizing emotions becomes the first step toward their control and mastery.

Relating to Peers

Most of our lives will be spent in the company of agemates. Our earliest experiences with acceptance and rejection, belonging and isolation, and empathy and insensitivity with peers influence how we come to think about ourselves among others. For many children, child care provides the first consistent and regular experience within a peer group from which this sense of emotional competence with others can be shaped. Yet, the preschool-aged child's cognitive egocentrism limits his ability to think about the needs and feelings of others. This highlights the importance of supporting young children as they venture into the broader social world.

Aggression and shyness are 2 characteristics that can impede a child from interacting successfully with peers in a classroom setting. Managing aggressive behavior is discussed in a separate chapter in this volume and will not be addressed here. Children who are shy or slow to warm up in new situations may take longer to adjust to child care initially and may need extra support moving into play with others. When thrust too quickly into expectations of participation with others, these children can feel so uncomfortable that they begin to withdraw consistently from new experiences. If encouraged gently, on the other hand, such children can thrive socially and emotionally. Some suggestions for supporting healthy development of children who are shy or slow to warm up include the following:

1. If possible, arrange for the child to be in a classroom with someone he or she knows and plays with at home. Alternatively, have the school provide the name of a child who will be in the same classroom with whom to spend some time before beginning child care.

2. Have a consistent time to arrive at child care and a routine for how to begin the day there. It is helpful, at least initially, for a special teacher to be there to greet the child daily and to guide him into ongoing activities. Sometimes, children are

less reticent to enter a room before all the other children have arrived and to interact with others who approach them rather than having to make overtures themselves.

3. Sometimes, shy children need to watch others over an extended period before they are willing to join in play. Watching from a distance should be noted but not always assumed to mean a child is ready to move into the action. Sensitive child care staff take time with such a child, knowing when to give the child the option to participate and when to let the child remain an observer.

4. Child care staff can help the shy child select particular other children to join in play who may be most receptive to the new child. In addition, child care providers should accompany new children in their initial overtures with others, only gradually removing themselves from the scene and remaining available if needed.

5. Shy children need opportunities to demonstrate what they know, yet sometimes have a difficult time taking the initiative in group activities. When child care providers allow comfortable opportunities for such children to tell their stories or be leaders in games, they support the development of self-confidence.

Promoting Positive Self-images for Children

Successfully negotiating being away from parents while enjoying time in child care, developing close relationships with child care providers and peers, and learning to manage the strong feelings that are a part of early childhood all contribute to the child's beliefs in his or her own self-efficacy. Day to day, the child care program that respects a child as an individual while supporting his or her emerging skills as a member of a group helps provide the foundation for emotional security and control that a preschooler requires. Calling children by their names, listening to them when they have something to say, respecting their feelings, providing some opportunities for children to make choices and participate in decision making, providing places for personal belongings, and planning activities in which children can succeed are relatively small aspects of a day in group care. Yet, they represent everyday ways that child care demonstrates to each child his importance and value and should be components parents are recommended to seek out when exploring child care alternatives.

Finally, on a broader level, positive self-esteem is derived from acceptance of all the characteristics that make a person who she is. In addition to responding to unique styles of individual children, child care staff who truly advocate for children's emotional health respect cultural diversity. Quality child care programs employ a culturally representative staff. They encourage children and families from different backgrounds to share their experiences and are open to incorporating aspects of the cultures of the families in the child care community into caregiving practices. Familial and cultural continuity in child care provides the child with the sense of wholeness and acceptance that fosters self-esteem and emotional maturity.

Supporting Young Children Through Especially Stressful Circumstances

Children experience loss differently at each stage of development. Loss itself occurs in many forms, including death, divorce, prolonged separation, depression, hospitalization, and chronic illness. Child care providers have an important opportunity to understand and support children's emotional reaction to such dispiriting crises.

As an example, infants, toddlers, and even preschoolers have no ability to conceive of death as an irreversible biologic process. For them, the disappearance of a primary caregiver is grieved as a physical and emotional rupture. They certainly feel the acute pain of sudden separation. Even infants act in ways that communicate their sense of bereavement. Young babies may turn inward to seek consolation through gaze avoidance, weepiness, apathetic muscle tone and inactivity, inexpressiveness, or hyperexcitability and inconsolable irritability. Toddlers may demonstrate developmental regression, seemingly losing skills of standing, walking, and vocalizing. They may refuse to eat and drink or they may revert to constant oral stimulation. Anxiety states may appear as sleep refusal and nightmares. Their activity levels may wax and wane to extremes. Three- to 5-year-old children often appear to lose their imaginative play behavior and grow more outwardly aggressive, excitable, or sullen. They are very likely feeling bewildered as well as abandoned.

Although not quite mature enough to be overwhelmed with the guilt that 6- to 10-year-olds commonly feel on experiencing physical or emotional separation or loss, the preschool-aged child's cognitive egocentrism leaves him or her feeling desperately alone and exceptionally needy of close, continuous affection and oversight. In response, child care staff must increase their vigilance on behalf of creating a stable commitment for the bereaved child. Expectable waves of uncontrollable grief may crash into play as sudden fits of rage, inconsolable crying, frozen apathy, or constant movement. Such behavior should be anticipated and must be expressed and understood. At first daily, and over time weekly, conversations with family members can help interpret the child's feelings and coordinate supportive responses at home and at child care.

The glue that cements every child's emerging sense of personal safety and social opportunity is the security of emotional relatedness to parents and primary caregivers. Therefore, the reactive depression of very young children always reflects a family crisis. Just as no baby can grow healthy and develop normally unless reared by a reliable, loving caregiver, no young child can weather the emotional storms of profound sadness unless caregivers patiently rebuild a lost feeling of protection, guidance, and unconditional love.

CONCLUSIONS AND RECOMMENDATIONS

The young child's first experiences with peers and caregivers outside the family set an emotional tone and cognitive expectancy for later social and educational opportunities and challenges. Pediatricians, together with early childhood educators and child care providers, can offer vital support and guidance to families who strive to give their young children a positive emotional base. In so doing, they will help secure the foundation for lifelong health, development, and well-being.

REFERENCES

1. Lally JR, Torres YL, Phelps PC. Caring for infants and toddlers in groups: necessary considerations for emotional, social, and cognitive development. *Zero to Three.* 1994;14:1-8
2. US Bureau of the Census. *Who's Minding the Kids?* Washington, DC: US Bureau of the Census; 1984
3. Honig AS, Thompson A. Helping toddlers with peer group entry skills. *Zero to Three.* 1994;14:15-19
4. Ainsworth MD, et al. *Patterns of Infant Attachment: A Psychological Study of the Strange Situation.* Hillsdale, NJ: Erlbaum; 1978
5. Main M, Solomon J. Procedures for identifying infants as disorganized/disoriented during the Ainsworth strange situation. In: Greenberg MT, Cicchetti D, Cummings EM, eds. *Attachment in the Preschool Years: Theory, Research, and Intervention.* Chicago, IL: University of Chicago Press; 1990:121-160
6. Arend R, Gove FL, Sroufe LA. Continuity of individual adaptation from infancy to kindergarten: a predictive study of ego-resiliency and curiosity in preschoolers. *Child Dev.* 1979;50:950-959
7. Lieberman AF. Preschooler's competence with a peer: relations with attachment and peer experience. *Child Dev.* 1977;48:1277-1287
8. Londerville S, Main M. Security of Attachment, compliance and maternal training methods in the second year of life. *Dev Psychol.* 1981;17:289-299
9. Matas L, Arend RA, Sroufe LA. Continuity of adaptation in the second year: the relationship between quality of attachment and later competence. *Child Dev.* 1978;49:547-556
10. Sroufe LA, Fox NE, Pancake VR. Attachment and dependency in developmental perspective. *Child Dev.* 1983;54:1615-1627
11. Troy M, Sroufe LA. Victimization among preschoolers: role of attachment relationship history. *J Am Acad Child Adolesc Psychiatry.* 1987;26:166-172
12. Waters E, Wippman J, Sroufe LA. Attachment, positive affect, and competence in the peer group: two studies in construct validation. *Child Dev.* 1979;50:821-829
13. Belsky M, Rovine M. Nonmaternal care in the first year of life and the security of infant-parent attachment. *Child Dev.* 1988;59:157-167
14. Clarke-Stewart KA. Infant day care. Maligned or malignant? *Am Psychol.* 1989;44:266-273
15. Lamb ME, Sternberg KJ. Do we really know how day care affects children? *J Appl Dev Psychol.* 1990;11:351-379
16. National Institute of Child Health and Development, Early Child Care Research Network. Child care and family predictors of preschool attachment and stability from infancy. *Dev Psychol.* 2001;6:847-862
17. Werner EE, Smith RS. *Overcoming the Odds: High Risk Children From Birth to Adulthood.* Ithaca, NY: Cornell University Press; 1992

18. Rutter M. Protective factors in children's responses to stress and disadvantage. In: Kent M, Rolf JE, eds. *Social Competence in Children*. Hanover, NH: University Press of New England; 1979:49-74

19. Bryant BK. *The Neighborhood Walk: Sources of Support in Middle Childhood*. Chicago, IL: University of Chicago Press; 1985

CHAPTER 12

Issues of Child Abuse and Child Care

Randall C. Alexander, MD, PhD

LEARNING OBJECTIVES

This chapter will help the reader to:

- Gain a better understanding of the scope of the problem of child abuse.
- Learn how to recognize signs of child abuse.
- Become familiar with primary, secondary, and tertiary prevention efforts.
- Understand reporting requirements for health care professionals who have knowledge or suspicion of child abuse.

INTRODUCTION

Child abuse is a common occurrence, with approximately 4.6% of all children reported each year as being abused.[1] For the year 1999, this meant that more than 3.2 million children were reported for suspected child abuse. Of these reports, about 33% (1 million or 1.5% of all children) were confirmed victims of maltreatment. These numbers, however, considerably underestimate the actual incidence of abuse. Evidence gathered from interviews of adults indicates that about 8% to 10% of the population experienced moderate to severe physical abuse during their childhood. Approximately 1 in 4 women and 1 in 6 men have had some form of childhood sexual mistreatment.[2] Significant neglect is even more common. Because these types of child abuse often overlap, the proportion of children who will experience some type of child abuse is probably 20% to 25%. Often, this abuse never comes to the attention of authorities.

After birth defects and perinatal conditions are accounted for, the leading cause of death during the first 6 months of life is sudden infant death syndrome (SIDS). Most of the 3000 to 3500 annual cases of SIDS occur before 6 months of age. Between 6 and 12 months of age, child abuse is the leading cause of death. From 6 months to 14 years of age, child abuse is the second leading cause of death, with only accidental death being more common. Nearly all child abuse deaths occur in children who are younger than 4 years. Most child abuse deaths occur in the home of the child and at the hands of caregivers. After 4 years of age, child abuse deaths are much less common, because children are physically larger and have increased opportunities to be in the care of others. Males are responsible for about 60% of all cases of fatal physical abuse, and females are responsible for about 60% of all deaths by neglect.[3] Note that many child care programs that provide respite child care and parenting education are targeted toward women and not men.

Despite the large number of child abuse deaths, the actual fatality rate is very low, because child abuse is so common. However, it is the emotional rather than the physical consequences of child abuse that are usually most devastating. Approximately 70% of adult psychiatric outpatients and more than 90% of prison inmates give histories of child abuse. Many adults are emotionally crippled by the consequences of incidents that occurred years or decades earlier, when they were children. Many more have intermittent and recurrent memories that interfere with their optimal emotional health and development. In this sense, child abuse may be best considered an emotional developmental disability. The modeling provided in some child care programs helps parents to overcome patterns of mistreatment by demonstrating more appropriate parent-child interactional patterns and, thereby, helping to break the cycle of abuse.

CHILD ABUSE IN CHILD CARE SETTINGS

Notorious cases of child abuse in child care centers periodically have captured media attention. Parents have subsequently expressed fears that their own children, in a similar setting, might be at high risk of abuse. Yet, cases in which an entire large center is alleged to be involved in systematic abuse are infrequent and have been difficult to prove. The key issue for parents and health care professionals counseling parents about child care is the actual risk of child abuse in a child care setting and which types pose the greatest danger.

Only 2% of all confirmed cases of child abuse occur in child care or in a foster home.[1] Thus, most child abuse occurs outside the child care setting. When time spent in child care is considered, it appears that center-based care may be statistically as safe or safer, with respect to serious unintentional injuries or abuse, than may family child care homes or even the child's own home setting.

Chadwick and Salerno[4] examined records of children from birth to 6 years of age brought to a trauma center for serious head trauma resulting from unintentional trauma or abuse. Motor vehicle crashes were excluded. Because child care centers usually have multiple caregivers (hence, multiple witnesses), they wondered whether there might be a protective effect of such settings. Of the 338 seriously injured children, only 1 occurred in a child care center (and that case was not among the most serious). On the basis of calculations of population and hours spent in child care, it was determined that the risk of serious head injury in center-based child care was 19 children per million per year, compared with the general population risk of 227 children per million per year. Thus, child care centers are about 12 times safer in terms of serious head injuries than are family child care homes or home-based care. Certain types of inflicted head trauma, such as shaken baby syndrome, are rare in center-based care.

In a national survey, 270 cases of sexual abuse (involving 1639 victims) were identified in 1 year as occurring in center-based child care.[2] Most sexual abuse centered around toilet training and consisted of fondling and touching. Cases of reported sexual abuse were seen at a rate of 30.7 per 10 000 centers, compared with 15.3 per 10 000 family child care homes in the United States. However, centers have more children present at any given time than do family child care homes. With this correction, children were reported as sexually abused at a rate of 5.5 per 10 000 children enrolled in centers versus 8.9 per 10 000 children cared for at home or in family child care homes. Thus, in this national survey, sexual abuse was also less commonly seen in center-based care.

Despite negative publicity about child care centers, they are a relatively safe form of child care with respect to physical and sexual abuse and serious head injuries. The presence of multiple providers in a center has the potential to create an atmosphere of mutual support, oversight of child care practices by the group, and the availability of respite if a caregiver is feeling frustrated or overwhelmed. Also, because most centers are open to parents at all hours of operation and parent visits are likely to be unannounced, the expectation of parental observation of center-based child care providers may serve as an additional protective measure. However, family child care homes[1] and, theoretically, in-home care by a nanny, sitter, or au pair pose similar child abuse risks to those of a child cared for at home.

SELECTING CHILD CARE TO MINIMIZE THE RISK OF CHILD ABUSE

Many considerations go into the decision about whether to place a child in child care. In many states, center-based and registered family child care homes are required to undergo checks at the state child abuse registry and/or police registry. This helps to screen out previously detected abusers before employment. However, some abusers may have moved from another state for which records are not accessible or may have yet to commit their first known abusive incident. In contrast, caregivers providing unlicensed family child care or relatives providing less formal care have not received even this modest screening and have, therefore, unknown risk levels.

When selecting a child care center, a key indicator of quality is whether the children already enrolled appear to be happy. This sign is nonspecific but may indicate whether there is sufficient attention and nurturance being provided. Are there noticeable safety hazards? What is the policy regarding parents dropping in unannounced any time of the day? If there are restricted visiting hours, child care should be sought elsewhere. Before choosing a particular child care situation and periodically after a child is enrolled, the parent should make unannounced visits at different times of the day to see how providers interact with children, how discipline is handled, and how social skills are modeled. Obviously, meals should be adequately safe and sanitary, especially for infants, whose growth is so dependent on satisfactory intake. Supervision should be continuous, with children never unattended. Neglect of children through inadequate staff-child ratios can lead to injuries and low-quality custodial care. Centers should have written policies about how they screen potential employees for previous abuse, how they handle any suspected abuse situations that may arise, and what they teach their employees about child abuse identification and reporting, discipline, and behavior management practices. Parents should determine whether such policies exist and review them.

Spanking is a controversial subject for the public and within the American Academy of Pediatrics (AAP). Many states have banned spanking in public schools, and some do not allow it for children in foster care. Because children in foster care may have experienced violence that may or may not be known to foster parents and because spanking may inadvertently resurrect emotionally traumatizing memories, a policy forbidding corporal punishment makes developmental sense. Although spanking is considered to be abuse in all Scandinavian countries and Austria, no state in the United States considers spanking to constitute child abuse. However, if a child is physically punished and an injury occurs (eg, bruise), then the incident is considered physical abuse. The difference in interpretation is that spanking does not leave a physical injury, but a child with a bruise or other evidence of physical injury is considered to have been beaten. Sometimes, children will reflexively put their hands behind them to protect from being spanked. If an injury occurs, this is not unintentional, but physical abuse. Even if spanking is not considered to be physically abusive, it is humiliating and ineffective and does not foster emotional or developmental growth. This is particularly relevant in light of the recent research on early brain and child development and the knowledge that adult caregivers are important role models for young children learning to deal with conflict, frustration, and the expression of anger. Because of the negative consequences of spanking, the AAP[5] and other professional organizations recommend alternative forms of discipline. In addition to the fact that any corporal punishment is developmentally inappropriate, child care centers are legally vulnerable if they practice spanking as a method of discipline. A parent may object and file charges or bring suit, an unintentional injury may occur that will legally constitute child abuse, and other unforeseen liability issues may arise. Determine the center's policy in this regard. Parents should be discouraged from enrolling their child in any setting that allows spanking or any other form of corporal punishment or physical restraint (except in the case in which limited restraint is needed to protect the child or other children [see Chapter 7]). Health professionals should advocate for policy change, education, and greater awareness of more positive and developmentally supportive approaches to discipline.

Regardless of the type of child care, it provides one of the few opportunities for young children to be seen by someone other than the family. Physicians, dentists, and other professionals have very limited exposure to the preschool child. Unless a child is in child care, only when the child attends grade school is there regular exposure to a professional outside the family. Sometimes, the child care setting provides an educational opportunity to assist parents to make changes in caregiving practices that are dysfunctional or that arise from lack of knowledge or experience. Programs that involve child abuse or violence prevention or a strong child development focus often include a framework of support or mentoring for parents and other caregivers. Pediatricians and other health care and educational professionals can be of considerable assistance by promoting such efforts in general (eg, Healthy Child Care America, Healthy Families America, Head Start) and specific programs in their own community.

Less commonly, observations of the child or insight into parenting practices may reveal an instance of abuse that then must be reported to child protective services (ie, the state department of social services or the equivalent). In addition to child physical abuse, sexual abuse, emotional abuse, and neglect, observations by child care providers may reveal evidence of substance abuse by a caregiver or some other subtle form of child maltreatment.

RECOGNITION OF CHILD ABUSE

Neglect

Neglect is the most common form of child abuse and one of the most deadly. Although officially, neglect accounts for approximately 60% of all child abuse reports, it is often unrecognized and, therefore, underreported. In many instances of physical and sexual abuse, there is concurrent neglect by the perpetrator or someone else in the environment. In addition to accounting for about half of all child abuse deaths, neglect is often a component in many unintentional deaths, such as drowning, motor vehicle crashes (ie, children were not properly restrained), or burns. Perhaps the greatest harm resulting from neglect is the failure of the caregiver and the caregiving environment to nurture, support, and stimulate the developing brain and by emotionally crushing the spirit and potential of the child. Whereas perpetrators of physical and sexual abuse know they have committed a crime and frequently lie or try to hide evidence of the abuse, perpetrators of neglect commonly believe that they are good parents and do not perceive any wrongdoing or possible injury to the child. Remediation is very difficult in view of this often profound resistance.

Failure to thrive is one of the most common forms of neglect in the infant and young child. Although often equated with failure to grow, "failure to thrive" refers to the child's entire developmental process. For example, one of the potential long-term dangers of failure to thrive is a lack of stimulation in early childhood, impairing the development of language skills. If not identified early, such language impairments may present as problems later in childhood or even into adulthood, long after physical growth has ceased to be a problem. Similarly, microcephaly may be a long-term outcome of failure to thrive even if other growth parameters have normalized. By robbing the rapidly developing brain of adequate nutrients and nurturing during the first several years of life, even mild neglect may result in lower intellectual functioning. Frequently, child protective workers and the legal system fail to appreciate the substantial developmental impairment that may result from even mild protein-calorie malnutrition. A perception too often exists that once linear and body mass growth is eventually achieved, all will be well. This often leads to delays in effective treatment of this condition and ignores the impact on development. It is imperative that the health care professional recognize the seriousness of failure to thrive and the need for rapid assessment and intervention.

The growth component of failure to thrive can be attributed to 3 basic problems: insufficient intake of calories, unusually high metabolism of calories, and/or abnormal caloric loss. Most failure to thrive is the result of inadequate caloric intake. This may be secondary to parental ignorance (eg, thinking 3 meals a day is sufficient for a young infant), feeding difficulties (eg, problems with breastfeeding), poverty, or neglect. Usually, parental education is sufficient intervention to correct the problem of inadequate calories. If the starvation is severe or the caregivers fail to comply with medical recommendations, neglect has occurred and a child abuse report should be made. Failure to thrive, on the basis of a high metabolic rate, is actually quite rare (eg, hyperthyroidism) and should manifest with additional symptoms besides weight loss alone. Failure to thrive attributable to high caloric losses is usually the result of a physiologic problem, sometimes with a serious prognosis. A child may lose calories through the urine (eg, diabetes) or stool (eg, cystic fibrosis).

By regularly monitoring growth parameters, health care professionals are able to detect growth problems that may not be obvious to casual inspection. Health care professionals and experienced child care providers can also identify the mother and infant with impaired attachment behaviors that commonly accompany failure to thrive (lack of eye contact between mother and baby, lack of cuddling and holding, lack of interest in the infant, etc). Early intervention and support for the family and referral for any needed services is essential. Careful dietary histories are especially important for the child with multiple caregivers, such as the child attending a child care center or family child care home. At times, communication problems between the different settings result in meals being missed.

Other forms of neglect that may be identified by child care providers or health care professionals include supervisory neglect, denial of medical care, dental neglect, and failure to obtain necessary vision and hearing care (Table 12.1).

Failure to obtain necessary immunizations may or may not legally be considered neglect, depending on state standards. However, when immunizations are missed because the child is not taken for routine health maintenance visits or when immunizations are refused without careful and informed parental choice, it may be a symptom of other more subtle forms of inadequate parenting.

Emotional abuse and neglect broadly refer to actions or inactions by the caregiver that may lead to a mental injury or are potentially traumatizing to the child. In many states, emotionally destructive actions or inactions by the child care provider would be considered neglect, and a separate category of "mental injury" is reserved for those children with a demonstrable mental health problem caused by the child care provider. Such mental health problems might include behavior disorders, adjustment disorders, or depression. In many cases in which a child has been identified as having behavior problems, close examination reveals that a parent-child interaction problem, poor parenting skills, or a dysfunctional lifestyle or family is the underlying cause or contributes to the problem.

The presence of illegal drugs may confound the development of a child. Studies indicate that approximately 4% of newborns and 3% to 5% of older children have a cocaine metabolite in their urine.[6] After birth, the most common way in which a child is exposed to cocaine (or methamphetamine) is by passive inhalation of smoke from adults in the environment who are using the drug. The presence of symptoms is a poor indicator of whether children have been exposed to cocaine. A history of possible exposure or specific behaviors by the child that indicate drug exposure (eg, child demonstrating how to roll a joint) warrant drug testing.

TABLE 12.1. Types of Neglect	
Supervisory neglect	• Leaving children alone • Failure to safeguard from injury within the environment (eg, swimming pool safety) • Failure to safeguard from injury from other persons • Inappropriate confinement • Use of drugs to inappropriately sedate or confine the child
Dental neglect	• Failure to seek treatment for visual untreated cavities, oral infections, or oral pain or a failure to follow through with treatment once informed the conditions exist
Medical neglect	• Failure to follow medical advice • Failure to provide needed eyeglasses • Failure to provide hearing care • Misuse of prescription drugs
Emotional neglect	• Substantial emotional abuse or neglectful behaviors (eg, chronic belittling, punishment of bedwetting) • Denial of necessary mental health care
General neglect	• Inadequate food, clothing, or shelter

However, most state child protective service systems have no specific procedures to deal with this increasing problem.

Physical Abuse

The most common type of physical abuse involves skin injury. Those who care for a child are in the best position to view the child's body and identify suspicious or unusual injuries. Teachers in elementary school and beyond are much less likely to view areas of the body hidden by clothing compared with child care providers, who typically perform multiple diaper and clothing changes daily. Visual identification of skin injuries attributable to abuse depends on the type, location, and magnitude of the injury and the experience and training of the observer. The AAP has published an especially useful slide set for identification of such injuries.[7] High-quality reference books also address identification (eg, *Child Abuse: Medical Diagnosis and Management*[8]).

Toddlers and young children are prone to burns, which may be severe, from pulling over containers filled with hot liquids from above (eg, table, stove). These may be difficult to distinguish from intentional burns inflicted by adults. Immersion burns often involve toilet training mishaps and usually have well-demarcated waterlines that would not occur if the burn occurred unintentionally. Cigarette burns are usually explained as happening when a child runs into a lit cigarette. In a certain sense, it is no coincidence that cigarette burns occur primarily in households in which someone smokes. Multiple cigarette burns (unless they are back-to-back burns in skinfolds or creases) strongly suggest abuse. It is a normal developmental milestone for children 3 to 5 years of age to be inquisitive about fire. If matches or lighters are accessible, children will play with them. Verbal warnings or admonishments are insufficient and are not a replacement for careful supervision.

Hair loss may indicate nutritional neglect, autoimmune disease, fungal infection, trauma, or other conditions. If it is traumatic in origin, hair shafts will be broken off at different lengths, and there may be physical findings (eg, bruises) on the scalp. Sometimes, referral to a dermatologist is needed to clarify a specific situation. If another child is reportedly responsible for causing substantial hair loss through hair pulling, then it is the child care provider's responsibility to protect the child, or else neglect should be considered. Alternatively, a child care provider pulling a child's hair out would be committing physical abuse. Some children pull their own hair out (trichotillomania), which can be a sign of emotional problems.

Human bites are another common childhood injury. Examination of the suspected bite mark by a forensic dentist or forensic pathologist may establish whether it represents an adult-sized mouth, and sometimes a match can be made to a specific individual. High-quality 35-mm photographs with a ruler or some other scale in the picture can suffice in many cases in which immediate examination by a forensic dentist or pathologist is not possible.

Typical, healthy children engage in play activities that may sometimes create soft tissue or bone injuries. For example, clavicle injuries are almost always unintentional and are most common among preschoolers. Femur fractures in infants are sometimes detected when a child care provider moves the leg during a diaper change and notices the child is in pain. Sudden disuse of arms and legs is another sign of possible bone injury. Rib and skull fractures, however, are almost never suspected unless there is significant external trauma over the site of injury. The child may seem fussy or irritable, but the fractured bone is not one that is moved actively by the child or passively by the caregiver.

Sexual Abuse

Sexual abuse is a diagnosis that is made primarily by history. Children who are verbal may confide to their parents, child care provider, teacher, or health care professional about inappropriate sexual activities. Children who are verbal and those who are not yet verbal may engage in sexual acting-out behavior, raising the question about possible exposure to sexual activities. Sexual acting out may take the form of excessive masturbatory activity or engaging other children in sexual play. In rare situations, preschool children have been known to combine sexual behaviors and aggression toward other children. Although sexualized behaviors may indicate sexual abuse, this is not always true. Of concern are occasional efforts by child care providers to use various checklists of behavioral problems, totaling the scores, and then reporting for sexual abuse if the score is high enough. Invariably, such lists identify nonspecific stress symptoms (eg, death of a relative) and do not necessarily indicate sexual abuse.

Armed with a specific indicator or statement about possible sexual abuse, further interview and physical examination are appropriate. Many cities and states now have specialized regional centers for forensic interviewing of children who may have been sexually abused. However, children may not relate their story in such settings, preferring to share with someone they know. Staff at child care centers or family child care home providers should not attempt to interview the child. However, it is important to document anything that the child spontaneously discloses. Therapy is the best method of eventually achieving as complete a story as possible. Even with special equipment (eg, colposcope) and a knowledgeable health care professional, only 20% of girls who are believed to have been sexually abused will have physical findings.[9] For boys, the proportion is even lower.

The purpose of a physical examination is first to ensure the health of the child and second to gather evidence of possible sexual abuse. The primary care pediatrician can help to screen children by regularly examining the genitalia of all children when conducting a complete physical examination. This includes spreading the labia majora of girls and identifying the hymen and other structures. Children younger than 3 years tend to equate such examinations with diaper changes and are cooperative. Older children who are accustomed to the genital examination as a routine part of their overall evaluation tend not to single this out. Children should be referred to a specialist or a specialized center for acute (forensic) interview and examination when key conditions are met and sexual abuse is suspected (Table 12.2).

Although vaginitis is a common, nonspecific finding most often related to poor hygiene, any significant discharge should be examined via bacteriologic culture, because certain pathogens are associated with sexual activity (Table 12.3).

REPORTING

Most states require that only a reasonable or credible suspicion of child abuse exists before a child abuse report should be made. The intent is for further investigation into the suspicious circumstance to be launched, not for the reporter to have conclusive proof at the start. Health care professionals are required to report suspected child abuse to appropriate state authorities. In some states, all citizens are mandatory reporters. In others, mandatory reporters consist of professionals who examine, attend to, or treat the child, and anyone else is a permissive reporter having no

TABLE 12.2. Indicators for Sexual Abuse Examination	
Children to be seen as soon as possible:	• Assault occurring within 72 hours • Evidence of trauma, genital bleeding, pain, or discharge • Potential for immediate return to unsafe environment
Children to be scheduled reasonably soon:	• History of more remote abuse • Sibling who was abused • Children in care settings in which another child was abused

TABLE 12.3. Possibility of Sexual Abuse or Activity

Diagnostic	Highly suspicious	Suspicious	Inconclusive
Sperm in vagina or anus Pregnancy Gonorrhea*† Syphilis* HIV infection§ Chlamydia*	*Trichomonas vaginalis*	Condylomata* (anogenital warts) Genital herpes‡	Bacterial vaginosis

HIV indicates human immunodeficiency virus.
* If not perinatally acquired
† Use culture as definitive test
‡ Unless there is a clear history of autoinoculation. Herpes 1 and 2 are difficult to differentiate by current techniques.
§ If not perinatally or transfusion acquired

Adapted from American Academy of Pediatrics Committee on Child Abuse and Neglect. Guidelines for the evaluation of sexual abuse of children: subject review. *Pediatrics*. 1999;103:186–191.

obligation to report. In some states, child care providers are mandated to report. Immunity laws in all states and the military protect the reporter from criminal or civil penalties. Often, failure to report such suspicions is punishable as a misdemeanor. State licensing boards have also punished health care professionals for failure to report child abuse. Thus, legal mandates encourage reporting of suspected cases and penalize failure to do so.

Once a report is made, a process is set in motion that varies somewhat between states. Key elements, however, are similar in all states (Table 12.4).

A common complaint from mandatory reporters is that they receive insufficient feedback about the child abuse report they have made. Sometimes, the reporter

TABLE 12.4. What Happens After a Child Abuse Report is Made?

Child Protective Services	• Intake to determine whether report meets criteria for investigation • Response to the child's location (often within 24 hours or sooner depending on the perceived risk) • Coordination with police if meets criteria for joint investigation • Data gathering • Determination as to whether report is substantiated • Placement in foster care if child is deemed unsafe in his or her environment • Placement on state child abuse registry if meets criteria • Provision of services or referral for prosecution if case warrants
Prosecutor	• Review of information sent by police or child protective services • Determination whether case meets criteria for juvenile court • Determination whether case meets criteria for criminal court

may disagree with the determination of child protective services. Mechanisms may exist to effectively address this disagreement (Table 12.5). Even if there is an inadequate or incorrect response to the child abuse report, it is important to continue to work with the system and not give up on reporting suspected child abuse in the future.

TABLE 12.5. What if the Report is Unsubstantiated (and You Disagree)?	
Child Protective Services	• There may be a formal appeal process • Talk to the supervisor of the investigator's supervisor (the immediate supervisor was probably part of the decision making)
Legal	• Prosecutor has different rules on how to proceed and is responsible for effective juvenile or criminal intervention • Judge may appreciate hearing directly from a professional
Therapeutic	• Continue to support the family and child • Continue to make additional child abuse reports when circumstances warrant

Reporting is only one step in helping a family and child in a crisis situation. A child abuse incident is a symptom of an often larger problem and is an opportunity to aid the family. The main function of reporting is to access needed services for the child's safety and well-being. Even when child abuse is substantiated, most cases are dealt with through the social services system, with only a small portion that go to court. The therapeutic relationship is important in that many children will remain in the home, and most who are temporarily removed will return home. Responsibility for child abuse does not rest only with the child protective services system, but is a community concern. Legal intervention does not heal a bone or counsel a child or family. Thus, educational and therapeutic issues accompany any professional relationship involving the child or the family.

When constructing a case plan for working with the family, protective child care is one area in which professionals can be of additional assistance. By providing respite care, the parent may better learn how to cope with the stresses of life and caring for children. It is a time in which the parent may be engaged with his or her own concerns, such as mental health or substance abuse counseling or parenting classes. The child may gain valuable exposure to peers and a greater degree of stimulation than they have at home. Specialized developmental services may be more easily accessed in some cases. Parents may also benefit from the informal modeling of positive behavioral approaches to discipline, stimulation, support, and nurturing provided by skilled child care providers.

PREVENTION

All states have child abuse prevention programs. Prevention is considered to be primary when it is directed at entire populations. Secondary prevention exists when at-risk populations are identified for intervention. Once child abuse has actually occurred, further prevention efforts are said to be tertiary.

One example is Healthy Families America, an intensive, voluntary home visitation program beginning prenatally or at the birth of a child and extending for at least the first 1 to 2 years of a child's life. More than 400 sites exist in the United States, and the number of programs is rapidly expanding. The programs screen for high-risk families to be enrolled with a professional or paraprofessional (secondary prevention). In some states (eg, Georgia, Iowa), a concurrent program of volunteers to work with low-risk families ensures that every child born has some intervention regardless of risk (primary prevention). Goals of such home visitation programs include identification of a health care professional for every child, enhancement of parent-child interactions, and referral to services. Child care is one of the services frequently recommended as a peer-enhancing experience or as protective child care. A combination of respite child care, coupled with parenting education, may be valuable child abuse prevention. This may provide the opportunity to engage in violence prevention programming (see Chapter 9) and developmentally appropriate safety programming (including sexual abuse prevention education).

ROLE OF THE HEALTH CARE PROFESSIONAL OR CHILD CARE HEALTH CONSULTANT

The primary role of any health care professional working with children is to recognize when the child's safety is threatened by illness or circumstance. As a leading cause of childhood death, even "minor" abuse should be taken seriously. Recognizing child abuse is even more likely to avert the physiologic trauma all forms of mistreatment entail. Although no simple list can be constructed as to what physical findings necessarily imply child abuse or what factors indicate neglect or sexual abuse, listening to the child and having an appreciation of normal childhood development is very helpful in deciding what is abnormal.

Protocols for child care homes and centers are helpful in deciding how to respond once child abuse is suspected. With high staff turnover in some centers and the relative infrequency of recognized abuse in settings with low numbers of children, the sequence of responding to a case of suspected child abuse may not be familiar to all. The state child protective services or the licensing board may have some helpful examples.

A procedure for screening of staff members should also be developed. In some states, applicants for child care jobs can be assessed against the state child abuse registries. In many states, newly enacted sexual abuse registries have been constructed to track known offenders. In addition to preemployment checks, a protocol should be developed to deal with staff who might be accused of child abuse (on or off the job) and those found to have committed child abuse.

The health care professional or child care health consultant should support efforts to help staff in child care centers with the emotional consequences that staff members face in becoming involved with cases of suspected child abuse or in the background search required for prospective employees. Child care providers may find themselves treated with hostility or threatened (incorrectly) with lawsuits or, in turn, be accused of child abuse for their actions in protecting children. Emotional support is crucial in difficult cases.

CONCLUSIONS AND RECOMMENDATIONS

The child care health consultant should be available to address or refer any child abuse concerns that might arise. The consultant can reassure parents that center-based care is actually the safest child care setting with respect to child abuse and delineate additional steps a center may take to ensure the children's security.

REFERENCES

1. Peddle N, Wang C. *Current Trends in Child Abuse Reporting and Fatalities: The 1999 Fifty State Survey.* Chicago, IL: National Committee to Prevent Child Abuse; 2001
2. Finkelhor D, Moore D, Hamby SL, Straus MA. Sexually abused children in a national survey of parents: methodological issues. *Child Abuse Negl.* 1997;21:1-9
3. US Advisory Board on Child Abuse and Neglect. *A Nation's Shame: Fatal Child Abuse and Neglect in the United States.* Washington, DC: US Government Printing Office; 1995
4. Chadwick DL, Salerno C. Likelihood of the death of an infant or young child in a short fall of less than 6 vertical feet [letter]. *J Trauma.* 1993;35:968
5. American Academy of Pediatrics, Committee on School Health. Corporal punishment in schools. *Pediatrics.* 2000;106:343
6. Rosenberg NM, Marino D, Meert KL, Kauffman RF. Comparison of cocaine and opiate exposures between young urban and suburban children. *Arch Pediatr Adolesc Med.* 1995; 149:1362-1364
7. American Academy of Pediatrics and C. Henry Kempe National Center for the Prevention and Treatment of Child Abuse and Neglect. *The Visual Diagnosis of Child Physical Abuse.* Denver, CO: The C. Henry Kempe National Center on Child Abuse and Neglect, University of Colorado School of Medicine and Health Sciences Center; 1994
8. Reece RM, Ludwig S. *Child Abuse: Medical Diagnosis and Management.* Philadelphia, PA: Lippincott Williams & Wilkins; 2001
9. Adams JA, Harper K, Knudson S, Revilla J. Examination findings in legally confirmed child sexual abuse: it's normal to be normal. *Pediatrics.* 1994;94:310-317

ADDITIONAL RESOURCES

Dubowitz H, ed. *Neglected Children: Research, Practice, and Policy.* Thousand Oaks, CA: Sage Publications; 1999

Giardano AP, Christian CW, Giardano ER. *A Practical Guide to the Evaluation of Child Physical Abuse and Neglect.* Thousand Oaks, CA: Sage Publications; 1997

Helfer ME, Kempe RS, Krugman RD. *The Battered Child.* 5th ed. Chicago, IL: The University of Chicago Press; 1997

Helfer RE. *Childhood Comes First: A Crash Course in Childhood for Adults.* East Lansing, MI: Ray E. Helfer; 1978

Hobbs CJ, Wynne JM. *Physical Signs of Child Abuse: A Colour Atlas.* London, England: WB Saunders Co; 1996

Kleinman PK. *Diagnostic Imaging of Child Abuse.* 2nd ed. St Louis, MO: Mosby; 1998

Ludwig S, Kornberg AE. *Child Abuse: A Medical Reference.* 2nd ed. New York, NY: Churchill Livingstone; 1992

CHAPTER 13

Nutrition

Catherine Cowell, PhD

LEARNING OBJECTIVES

The goal of this chapter is to help the reader to:

- Understand the important role of child care in providing clean, safe, age-appropriate, nourishing food to meet a child's daily nutritional requirements.

- Learn how to integrate food and eating into the comprehensive care of children in the child care setting.

- Recognize special nutritional needs and issues and how to counsel parents and caregivers around these topics.

- Gain knowledge of and learn how to form partnerships with community nutrition resources designed to improve the nutritional status of young children and their families.

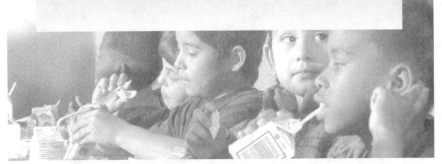

INTRODUCTION

There is growing interest in the food intake of young children on the basis of emerging evidence linking early eating habits and other factors with increased risk of developing certain chronic diseases later in life.[1-2] Scientific evidence relates dietary excesses and nutrient imbalances to chronic diseases. Current pediatric dietary recommendations are based on evidence documented by the *National Health and Nutrition Examination Surveys* II and III, the *Nationwide Food Consumption Surveys,*[3-5] and *Healthy People 2010.*[6] Joining in strategies to promote healthy diets among the young population are national groups, such as the American Academy of Pediatrics (AAP)[7] with the publication, *Guide To Your Child's Nutrition,*[8] and the National Heart, Lung, and Blood Institute with their *Report of the Expert Panel on Blood Cholesterol Levels in Children and Adolescents.*[9] The AAP, for example, recommends that healthy children older than 2 years decrease their intake of dietary fat to about 30% of total calories, saturated fat to less than 10% of calories, and dietary cholesterol to 250 to 300 mg per day. In addition to promoting a prudent diet, the AAP supports a healthy lifestyle for young children.

Regular physical activity is linked with a healthy diet to improve the well-being of children and adults. A moderate level of age-appropriate physical activity by all is recommended in *Physical Activity and Health: A Report of the Surgeon General.*[10] For young children, physical activity is important, because it promotes their growth and development and helps decrease their risk of developing a range of health- and nutrition-related problems. Recent publications reinforce this linkage between healthy eating and physical activity as they relate to health.[11] *The Food Guide Pyramid for Young Children* (2- to 6-year-olds) recently developed by the US Department of Agriculture illustrates the food groups and physical activities recommended for the pediatric population (Fig 13.1).[12] Daily servings of a variety of foods to meet the nutritional needs of children are colorfully depicted along with suitable physical activities, all sending the message that lifestyle habits of children begin to form early in life.

Food provides energy and nutrients for the physical growth and development of infants and young children. A primary responsibility of child care is to serve food that is clean, safe, nutritious, and age appropriate. Nourishing food is important to young children to:

- meet their nutritional needs to support physical growth;
- introduce new foods, reinforce culturally accepted foods, and aid in developing appropriate eating habits;
- develop and refine eating skills (oral, fine, and gross motor);
- promote social and emotional development during mealtime.

Food, the environment in which children eat, and the eating dynamics between young children and child care staff and parents lay the foundation for developing eating behaviors. These behaviors are reinforced each time children are fed; therefore, staff who are knowledgeable about the important role of food and the

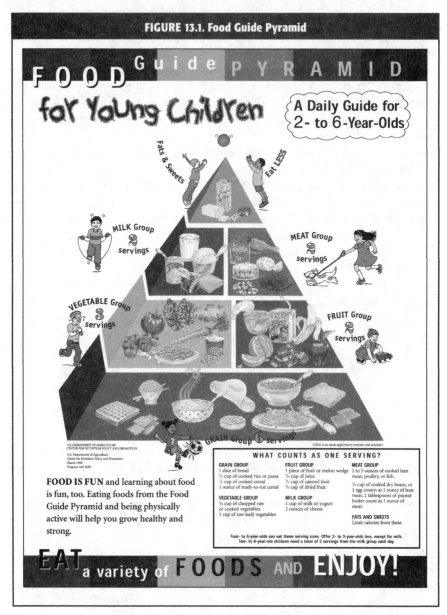

FIGURE 13.1. Food Guide Pyramid

Reprinted from US Department of Agriculture, Center for Nutrition Policy and Promotion. *Food Guide Pyramid for Young Children.* Washington, DC: US Department of Agriculture; 2000. Available at: http://www.usda.gov/cnpp/KidsPyra/LittlePyr.pdf.

nurturing of children in their care can make a significant contribution to the growth and development of those children.

PROMOTING HEALTHY MEALS AND SNACKS

Child care settings should serve healthy meals and snacks (Table 13.1) that provide essential nutrients and energy for growing, active young children.[10-13] Meal and snack times should be pleasant, relaxing and unhurried, with children and adults sitting and eating together while interacting socially. These times, as well as play times, offer a unique opportunity to integrate food learning experiences into child care, which together promote the cognitive, language, social, and emotional development of children.

NUTRITION GUIDANCE FOR FEEDING

Guidelines for feeding children in the child care setting include:

- Provide children with a variety of clean, safe, nutritious, and age-appropriate foods, including ethnic choices.
- Create a pleasant and relaxing environment for meals and snacks.
- Integrate food and nutrition into the total child care program, including food learning activities.
- Provide appropriately sized furniture (table, chairs) and eating utensils.
- Modify diet, eating utensils, and furniture for correct positioning of children with special health care needs.
- Train staff to implement pediatric dietary guidelines.
- Encourage family-style meal service to promote socialization and support appropriate eating practices among children and staff.
- Strengthen and support nutrition component of child care program that promotes the physical, dental, mental, and emotional health and well-being of children.

TABLE 13.1. Suggestions for Healthy Snack Foods	
Plain yogurt	Carrots (strips)
Milk	Celery
Cottage cheese	Green, red, or yellow pepper
Tuna	Broccoli
Hard boiled egg	Cauliflower
Whole grains—bread, cereal, cracker	Tomato
English muffin	100% vegetable or fruit juice
Pita bread	Cabbage
Bagel	Apple, pear, peach, plum, nectarine
Tortillas	Banana, papaya
Plain muffin	Orange, tangerine, mango, or grapefruit
Plain cookie (vanilla, oatmeal)	Melon slices
Pudding (plain, rice, bread)	

See text on foods to avoid for children younger than 4 years to prevent choking; hard, raw fruits and vegetables may need to be cooked and cut into small pieces before serving.

The Child and Adult Care Food Program (CACFP) sponsored and directed by the Food and Nutrition Section of the US Department of Agriculture, encourages child care programs to meet the *Dietary Guidelines for Americans*.[14,15] The CACFP provides federal funds, donated foods, or cash in lieu of food commodities to child and adult care centers, child care homes, and after-school care programs to promote serving nutritious meals and snacks. The CACFP distributes recommendations addressing which foods and how much to feed children from infancy to school age.

The frequency of serving a meal or a snack (supplement) is based on the length of time young children spend in child care. *Caring for Our Children: National Health and Safety Performance Standards*[16] recommends the following schedule:

● Children in care for fewer than 8 hours shall be offered at least 1 meal and 2 snacks, or 2 meals and 1 snack.
● Children in care for more than 8 hours shall be offered at least 2 meals and 2 snacks, or 1 meal and 3 snacks.

Young children should be fed every 2 to 3 hours with a meal or snack. Meals should be fed at least 2 hours apart and not more than 3 hours apart unless sleeping. Very young children may need to be fed at shorter intervals. For children who may not have eaten in the morning and have a snack before arriving at child care, breakfast foods should be available and should be offered. On occasions when young children stay late at the program or staff members are aware of a child who will have a late dinner after arriving at home, additional snacks should be offered.

FOOD AND FEEDING GUIDANCE FOR THE FIRST YEAR OF LIFE

Breast milk is the ideal first food to feed an infant, on the basis of the known advantages, including health, nutritional, environmental, psychosocial, immunologic, safety, developmental, and economic benefits.[17,18] Child care providers should promote and provide emotional support for breastfeeding by reaching out to mothers and encouraging them to continue to breastfeed their infants after they return to work or school. Once new parents are registered, child care providers have the opportunity to make the child care setting breastfeeding friendly. For breastfed infants, breast milk can be collected, placed in a clean ready-to-feed bottle by the mother, and properly stored in the refrigerator with the infant's name and the date collected. Having the mother bring breast milk in ready-to-feed bottles decreases the chance of spills and exposure of the child care provider to body fluids. Breastfed infants should be fed on demand. The nutritional needs of infants not breastfed can be met with iron-fortified infant formula recommended by the infant's physician or primary health care professional. The child care provider or parent should prepare bottles with only the smallest amount they think the infant will consume at a feeding, then refill the bottle as necessary. Any milk left in the bottle after feeding should be discarded. Breast milk can be stored in the refrigerator (40°F or colder) for 48 hours or frozen at 0°F for up to 3 months.[16] Bottles and infant foods should be warmed under running warm tap water or by placing in a container of warm water no warmer than 120°F. Never warm bottles for more than 5 minutes. Bottles and infant foods should not be warmed in the microwave. Shake bottles and infant foods carefully to distribute heat evenly.[16]

Fresh whole cow milk is strongly discouraged during the first year of life, because it may cause blood loss from the intestinal tract and anemia. Skim milk and 1% or 2% cow milk are also not recommended for children younger than 2 years, because rapid growth during this time requires the additional calories contained in whole milk.[19]

Dry, iron-fortified single-grain cereal, such as rice cereal, is usually the first food added to an infant's diet at approximately 4 to 6 months of age. Feeding an infant solid foods before approximately 4 to 6 months of age is not advised, because an infant is not developmentally ready to eat and digest solid food before that time. Cereal should be mixed with breast milk or infant formula before feeding and is usually not introduced until an infant is about 4 to 6 months old. Place cereal in a small bowl and feed using a small, rounded spoon. Do not feed cereal from a bottle unless directed to do so by the infant's health care professional. Small amounts of cereal (1 to 2 teaspoons) should be offered initially.

After the introduction of cereal, 1 or 2 weeks should be allowed before adding another solid food. This spacing gives an infant the chance to adjust to a new taste, texture, and flavor before the introduction of another solid food. Using this pattern of introducing a single solid food at a time will help to identify any reaction the infant may have, such as a sensitivity, allergic reaction, or discomfort from a food. If an infant is fed from a bottle, no other food should be added to the bottle. Also, never prop a bottle (in a crib or place bottle on a pillow) or allow an infant to fall asleep while sucking from a bottle to avoid contributing to the development of ear infections or the development of baby-bottle tooth decay.[20]

Finger foods herald an infant's emerging independence in eating. Beginning as early as 6 months, infants may show interest in picking up food with their hands, because they are developmentally able to grasp and bring food to their mouths. This is an important developmental process to foster oral motor skills (chewing) and to provide the first stages of feeding independence and self-feeding. First finger foods are typically small, soft, round, dry cereals such as Cheerios (General Mills, Minneapolis, MN) or hard toast like zwieback, both of which quickly liquefy in the infant's mouth so it can be munched. The next solid food usually offered is fruits or vegetables. Home-prepared or commercially prepared jars of strained or pureed fruits or vegetables are of a texture and consistency that are appropriate for an infant. Nutrition labels on jars of baby food should be read carefully to check the "use by" date to make certain they have not expired and to check for added sugar, salt, food dyes, and other additives. When choosing fruit or vegetable juices, select only 100% fruit or vegetable juice. Place juice in a cup for feeding.

After strained or pureed food, the next level of food consistency offered includes foods with a coarser texture. Chopped or commercially prepared junior foods are appropriate around 9 months of age or toward the end of the first year of life, as are some family or table foods. Among family (table) foods suitable for infants are plain yogurt, mashed potatoes, canned and drained boneless fish (tuna, salmon), and well-cooked and finely ground lean meat or poultry. Near the end of the first year, the typical infant is developmentally ready to sit in a child-sized chair at a table of an appropriate height and eat with the family.

Clean drinking water should be provided, even though the amount needed is relatively small in infancy. Young infants usually get all the water they need from breast milk or infant formula. For the older infant, excessive water intake may be associated with decreased intake of milk, which may affect growth patterning. The need for water increases later in childhood, but by then, older children are able to ask for water when they are thirsty. Water, which may be served at room temperature, can be placed in a clean cup with or without a spout or served from a clean bottle with a clean nipple. Fruit or vegetable juice, soda, and punch are not substitutes for water when a child is thirsty.

Child care providers should always be present to give guidance when an infant or young child is eating or drinking. Seating young children in age-appropriate chairs at a suitable table height while eating is a way to prevent food from lodging in their throat and causing them to choke. Children should never eat while walking, running, or playing.

FEEDING GUIDANCE FOR THE YOUNG CHILD

A variety of food should be properly prepared and served attractively to young children. Servings of food should be small, with the availability of an additional serving if desired. Meals should be carefully planned in advance in consultation with a professional dietitian or nutritionist, because the food served may be a significant contribution toward meeting the daily nutritional needs of children. Taste, texture, color, flavor, shape, and method of preparation contribute to making meals and snacks appealing and appetizing. Other factors to take into account in meal planning are food likes and dislikes of the children and their families. By incorporating ethnic foods into meals, some children may more readily accept foods offered. Food preferences are sometimes transient, because children may begin to exert their independence by indicating what foods they will eat. Offering a variety of food or offering some of the same food previously rejected after a period of absence can address this issue.

Cost and availability of food, time spent in food preparation, and costs for labor are also factors in planning meals. The number of children enrolled, the level of training of food service personnel, the physical space, and equipment all influence the kind of meals and snacks served. Appropriate serving and eating utensils are essential to help children develop their eating skills. Continuous on-the-job training of food service personnel will build onto their skills, which will help ensure their ability to meet pediatric dietary recommendations.

Because young children are still developing their independent eating skills and behavior, family-style meal service is encouraged. This kind of meal service supports and helps children to continue to refine their fine and gross motor skills by serving themselves. The concept of family-style meals can be carried into the home. Spooning food from a serving bowl or platter onto their plate, pouring from a pitcher to their bowl or cup, and taking a fork to serve themselves a piece of chicken from a platter are practical ways children grow developmentally. Staff and parents need to understand the importance of family-style meals by first, planning for the kind of meal service that consists of adults sitting with children at the table; second, giving guidance throughout the meal; and third, ensuring that food is properly and safely handled. When spills occur, which is likely, staff or parents should assist in cleaning up. Spills and mistakes should be viewed as another learning experience.

Young children imitate adults in their environment, including child care providers. Adults sitting with children at mealtime and socially interacting with them can also set limits of behavior. There are polite ways for children to learn how to refuse a food without causing total turmoil during mealtime. Also, food is not used as a reward or punishment. For a number of reasons,

Young children imitate adults in their environment, including child care providers.

appetites of children vary, so this should be considered. The setting of family-style meals also creates an opportunity to discuss appropriate portion size with children.

Young children require something to eat at least every 2 to 3 hours. Snacks are an important component of a child's diet and should be planned to complement nutrient intake. Foods served as snacks or meals should include a variety of foods, all of which should be consumed in moderation. Child care providers have an important role that doesn't stop with just the feeding of children but includes nutrition education to teach young children and their parents about appropriately sized servings of recommended foods. Greater flexibility in food choices is possible when any food served is eaten in moderation.

CHILDREN WITH SPECIAL DIETARY NEEDS

Children with a written documentation for a modified or special diet require that all staff, especially a professional dietitian or nutritionist, work together in consultation with parents, physicians, and other health care or nutritional specialists to meet the needs of the child. Special dietary needs might include food allergies; food sensitivity; vitamin, mineral, or other supplements; prescribed medication; or altered food textures that may require special feeding equipment and feeding schedules. Children from families who are vegetarians are also among those needing special dietary attention. Any special diets or foods should be planned by a trained dietitian or nutritionist who consults with parents, staff, and others. A written record of special diets should be posted to inform staff, especially food service and classroom staff, of what foods are to be avoided to protect the child's health. Most food sensitivities or intolerances produce minor, mostly annoying symptoms like diarrhea. True (medically diagnosed) food allergies, however, can be serious, even life threatening. Children with known food allergies should wear medical-alert bracelets with the offending food identified. For severe or potentially severe allergies, discuss with the parents the advisability of keeping medication on hand and with written procedures along with designated staff trained to administer medication at the center in case of a reaction. Written instructions for a special diet from a physician or other health care professional should be on file at all times to protect the child and the child care program. On the basis of these instructions, the dietitian is uniquely trained to develop an individual nutrition plan. Procedures for following special diets or any food brought from home may vary depending on the official city, county, or state regulations and policies, so it is important for child care staff to check with the appropriate child care licensing personnel or health agency responsible for child care.

FOOD SAFETY

Cleanliness begins with the practice of frequent and proper handwashing by all children, including staff washing the hands of infants, and by all staff the entire time children are in care.[21] For staff, there is a need for them to always wash their hands before and after changing diapers and using the bathroom. Before and during the preparation of a meal or snack, it is important for staff to wash their hands frequently. Tables, including high chair trays or any other eating surfaces, should be sanitized with a diluted bleach solution consisting of a quarter cup of household bleach in 1 gallon of water before and after children are fed. All food cans, bottles, and packages should be thoroughly washed before opening, and fresh fruits, vegetables, meat, fish, and poultry should be thoroughly washed before using. As a constant reminder of the importance of handwashing, posters should be prominently displayed in the kitchen, bathroom, and classrooms.

Food service personnel must understand the importance of safely handling and storing food. Only fresh and clean food should be purchased, and anything else should be rejected on delivery. Perishable food, like milk, cheese and other dairy products, meat, fish, poultry, or eggs, should be stored in the coldest section of the refrigerator that registers a temperature of 40°F or less. The temperature of a freezer for storage is 0°F or less. To avoid bacterial growth, food should be served immediately after preparation or maintained at 40°F or less for cold food and not less than 140°F for hot food.[16] The refrigerator and freezer should be clean and free of frost and should have working appliance thermometers to denote current temperatures at any given time. Thermometers should be visible and in working condition and should be checked at least once a month to ensure the appliance is functioning properly.

Cooked food should be placed in a clean, covered container or completely wrapped and stored immediately in the refrigerator. Cooked foods stored in the refrigerator should be served within 24 hours to protect the health and well-being of children. It is most economic to use standardized recipes to cook an adequate amount of food to feed children and staff and avoid an excess of leftover food.

Boxes of cereals, rice, or pasta; canned fruits or vegetables; jars of infant food; or cans of infant formula should be stored in a clean, dry pantry or closet that is ventilated to prevent deterioration and eventual spoilage. Opened cans of liquid formula must be refrigerated and discarded after 48 hours if not used.[16] All foods should be stored at least 6 inches from the floor in clean, tightly covered containers. When large quantities of dry food are delivered for storage, dates should be marked on boxes and containers so newly delivered food is moved to the back of the storage area and food already stored is moved to the front. Records kept by food service personnel are useful for preparing a food budget, because they track the costs of food, quantities of food ordered and delivered, amount of food stored and used, and the amount of food remaining.

Immediately discard food that doesn't smell right. Remember, however, that unsafe food may not have a bad smell. Milk, formula, infant food, and other food remaining in a bottle, cup, bowl, or plate should be thrown out and not reused. Do not purchase or use home-canned foods; cans that are dented, bulging, or rusted; or food with any packaging that is not intact.

PREVENTING CHOKING FROM FOOD

Young children are at high risk of choking from food that becomes lodged in their throats. There are steps child care staff can take to prevent choking.

PREVENTION TIPS

Encourage young children to:
- Eat only while sitting.
- Chew food well before swallowing.
- Eat slowly and eat small portions.
- Take only 1 bite at a time.

For infants, food should be cut into pieces no larger than one-quarter-inch cubes or thin slices. For toddlers, food should be cut into pieces no larger than half-inch cubes.

Foods to avoid for children younger than 4 years include foods that are smooth, slippery, round, hard, small, thick, or sticky—for example:
- nuts
- popcorn
- pretzels
- chips
- seeds

- whole grapes
- hard candy
- raw peas
- dried fruit
- marshmallows
- hot dogs (whole or cut into rounds)
- cherries with pits
- spoonfuls of peanut butter or other nut or seed butter
- hard, raw vegetables
- chunks of meat larger than can be swallowed whole.

Favorite foods of children that can be served safely if the form is changed include:
- hard fruit or vegetables cooked until slightly soft, then cut into bite-sized pieces for infants and toddlers or thin sticks for preschool-aged children
- thinly spread nut butters on crackers, bread, or toast
- hot dogs cut into thin strips lengthwise
- seedless grapes or cherries without pits cut into small bites.

CONCLUSIONS AND RECOMMENDATIONS

Child care providers should provide clean, safe, age-appropriate, nourishing food to meet a child's daily nutritional requirements. Health care professionals should recognize special nutritional needs and issues and counsel parents and child care providers about these topics. Health care professionals and child care providers should gain knowledge of and learn how to form partnerships with community nutrition resources designed to improve the nutritional status of young children and their families.

REFERENCES

1. US Department of Health and Human Services, Public Health Service. *The Surgeon General's Report on Nutrition and Health.* Washington, DC: US Department of Health and Human Services; 1988. Publication No. 88-50210
2. American Academy of Pediatrics, Committee on Nutrition. Cholesterol in childhood. *Pediatrics.* 1998;101:141–147 [reaffirmed April 2001]
3. Abraham S, et al. *Dietary Intake Source Data: United States, 1971–74.* Hyattsville, MD: US Department of Health, Education, and Welfare; 1979. Publication No. PHS 79-1221
4. *Dietary Intake Source Data: United States, 1976–80.* Hyattsville, MD: Department of Health and Human Services; 1983. Publication No. 83-1681
5. *Nationwide Food Consumption Survey, Continuing Survey of Food Intakes by Individuals.* Hyattsville, MD: US Department of Agriculture; 1988
6. *Healthy People 2010.* Washington, DC: US Department of Health and Human Services; 2000
7. American Academy of Pediatrics, Committee on Nutrition. Prudent life-style for children: dietary fat and cholesterol. *Pediatrics.* 1986;78:521–525

8. American Academy of Pediatrics. *Guide to Your Child's Nutrition*. Dietz WH, Stern L, eds. Elk Grove Village, IL: American Academy of Pediatrics; 1999

9. National Education Program. *Report of the Expert Panel on Blood Cholesterol Levels in Children and Adolescents*. Bethesda, MD: National Heart, Lung and Blood Institute, 1991

10. Centers for Disease Control and Prevention, National Center for Chronic Disease Prevention and Health Promotion, and President's Council on Physical Fitness and Sports. *Physical Activity and Health: A Report of the Surgeon General*. Atlanta, GA: US Department of Health and Human Services; 1996

11. Story M, Holt K, Sofka D, eds. *Bright Futures in Practice: Nutrition*. 2nd ed. Arlington, VA: National Center for Education Maternal and Child Health; 2002

12. US Department of Agriculture, Center for Nutrition Policy and Promotion. *Tips for Using the Food Guide Pyramid for Young Children 2 to 6 Years Old*. Washington, DC: US Department of Agriculture, Center for Nutrition Policy and Promotion; 1999

13. Head Start Performance Standards and Other Regulations, Administration for Children and Families, Administration on Children, Youth and Families, Head Start Bureau. Washington, DC: Department of Health and Human Services; 1998

14. *Child and Adult Care Food Program*. Washington, DC: US Department of Agriculture, Food and Nutrition Service; 1991

15. *Dietary Guidelines For Americans—Aim For Fitness. Build a Healthy Base, Choose Sensibly...For Good Health*. Hyattsville, MD: US Department of Agriculture and US Department of Health and Human Services; 2000

16. American Academy of Pediatrics, American Public Health Association, and Maternal and Child Health Bureau. *Caring for Our Children. National Health and Safety Performance Standards: Guidelines for Out-of-Home Child Care Programs*. 2nd ed. Elk Grove Village, IL: American Academy of Pediatrics; 2002

17. American Academy of Pediatrics. Work Group on Breastfeeding. Breastfeeding and the use of human milk. *Pediatrics*. 1997;100:1035-1039

18. Trahms CM, Pipes PL, eds. *Nutrition in Infancy and Childhood*. 6th ed. New York, NY: McGraw-Hill; 1997

19. Lifshitz F, Tarim O. Considerations about dietary fat restrictions in children. *J Nutr*. 1996;126(4 Suppl):1031S-1041S

20. American Academy of Pediatrics. *Pediatric Nutrition Handbook*. Kleinman RE, ed. 5th ed. Elk Grove Village, IL: American Academy of Pediatrics; 2003

21. Cowell C, Schlosser S. Food safety in infant and preschool day care. *Top Clin Nutr*. 1998; 14:9-15

COMMUNITY NUTRITION RESOURCES

There are a range of community nutrition resources that child care providers can link with. Often, local agencies employ a public health nutritionist or a dietitian who may be available to provide technical assistance. The following is a list of some agencies and organizations that might be useful.

- Local health department
- Regional office of the US Department of Health and Human Services, Public Health Service

- Special Supplemental Nutrition Program for Women, Infants, and Children (WIC)
- Regional office of the US Department of Agriculture, Food and Nutrition Service
- Local university or college with programs in nutrition, allied health, human ecology, or maternal and child health
- Local chapters:
  ~ American Academy of Pediatrics
  ~ American Dietetic Association
  ~ American Diabetes Association
  ~ American Heart Association
  ~ American Cancer Society
  ~ Society for Nutrition Education
  ~ March of Dimes
  ~ American Dental Association
- Local department of education—office of school food service or nutrition education and training
- National Office of Food and Drug Administration
- National Center for Education in Maternal and Child Health
- Food safety hot lines:
  ~ US Department of Agriculture, Meat and Poultry Hot Line: 1-800-535-4555 (weekdays 10:00 am to 4:00 pm, Eastern Standard Time)
  ~ US Food and Drug Administration, Seafood Hot Line: 1-800-332-4010 (weekdays 12 pm to 4:00 pm, Eastern Standard Time)
- **Best Start**
  1-813-971-2119 or 1-800-277-4975

INTERNET RESOURCES

Academy of Breastfeeding Medicine
http://bfmed.org

American Academy of Pediatric Dentistry
http://www.aapd.org

Bright Futures
http://brightfutures.aap.org/web/

Centers for Disease Control and Prevention
http://www.cdc.gov

Child and Adult Care Food Program Sponsors Association
http://www.cacfp.org/

Child Care Nutrition Resource System, CACFP-Talk
http://www.nal.usda.gov/childcare/Cacfp/subscribecacfptalk.html

Child Care Resource System
http://www.nal.usda.gov/Childcare

Cooperative State Research, Education, and Extension Service
http://www.reeusda.gov

Eat 5 A Day
http://www.5aday.com

Federal Citizen Information Center
http://www.pueblo.gsa.gov

Healthfinder—Gateway to Reliable Consumer Health Information
http://www.healthfinder.gov

LaLeche League International
http://www.lalecheleague.org

National Center for Education in Maternal and Child Health
http://www.ncemch.org

National Center for Nutrition and Dietetics
http://www.eatright.org/ncnd.html

National Food Service Management Institute
http://www.nfsmi.org/

National Heart, Lung, and Blood Institute
http://www.nhlbi.nih.gov

National Information Center for Children and Youth With Disabilities
http://www.nichcy.org

National Parent Network on Disabilities
http://www.nphd.org

US Department of Agriculture, Child and Adult Care Food Program
http://www.fns.usda.gov/cnd/care/cacfp/cacfphome.htm

US Department of Agriculture, Food and Nutrition Information Center
http://www.fns.usda.gov/fns

US Food and Drug Administration
http://www.fda.gov

WIC Works
http://www.nal.usda.gov/wicworks/index.html

CHAPTER 14

The Health Care Professional as a Consultant to Child Care Programs

Karen Sokal-Gutierrez, MD, MPH, and Mary Dooling, RN, MSN

LEARNING OBJECTIVES

- To understand the role and qualifications of the health care professional as a consultant to child care programs.
- To identify strategies for developing relationships between health care professionals and child care providers.
- To review the consultation services that health care professionals can offer child care providers.

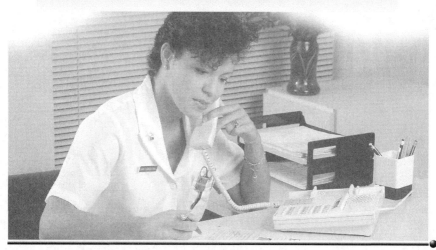

INTRODUCTION

"Having a health consultant for my child care program helps me give accurate information to parents, prevent infections, and get answers about my concerns. It is an important part of offering a high-quality child care program for families."

~ Marlene Levine, Executive Director
Southside Day Nursery
St Louis, Missouri

THE ROLE OF THE CHILD CARE HEALTH CONSULTANT

To become a consultant to a child care program, the health care professional must first understand the consultant's role in relation to the program.[1] The consultant's role must be distinguished from the roles of other health care professionals who care for children and their families and child care staff. Each child and family and staffperson should have his or her own primary health care professional who coordinates that individual's health care. The essence of the role of a health consultant for the child care program is advising the program on health issues that apply to the children, families, and staff as a group. The health consultant should regard the entire child care program as the "patient" or "client." For health care professionals whose experience is only in a clinical setting in which the focus is on an individual child, parent, or family, serving as a health consultant to a child care program may require a shift in approach.

Group health questions for which child care providers may request consultation include:

- What infection control measures are necessary to prevent the spread of disease in the child care program?
- What are important safety features of equipment used in playgrounds and indoor active play areas to prevent injuries to children?
- What snacks are nutritious and interesting for children at different developmental levels?
- What toilet training and discipline practices are developmentally appropriate?
- What measures should be taken to prevent back injuries and job-related infectious diseases among staff members?
- How can the program provide support for children and families affected by substance abuse, mental illness, or family violence?

Although the child care health consultant's focus is on group health issues, the health consultant can also help the program meet individual children's special health needs while attending child care. For a child who has no primary health care professional, the health consultant could offer referrals to the local public health department, community health clinic, or private health care professional. For a child recovering from an acute condition, such as a broken leg, the health consultant can help the program plan accommodations for the child's activities. For a child with a chronic medical condition, such as asthma or allergies, the health consultant could help facilitate communication among the program, family, and the child's primary health care professional and specialists and assist in developing health protocols and training for the child care staff. A health consultant to a child care program might also be the primary health care professional for some children in the child care setting.

Health consultants must recognize their professional limitations and seek the advice of other experts and use community resources. If several health consultants are involved with the child care program, they should coordinate services. When necessary, health consultants should also coordinate their efforts with the government agencies that oversee child care. For example, the department of public health might be involved for communicable disease outbreaks, and children's protective services and child care licensing agencies might be involved for suspected child abuse or neglect.

The health consultant must respect certain limits to his or her role. The child care program engages the health consultant to make observations and provide information and recommendations. The consultant is an "outside expert" and has no authority within the program to make decisions and ensure that the recommendations are followed. However, the consultant's recommendations are more likely to be implemented if there is a trusting relationship with the program director and effective program management. In addition, staff and families are more likely to accept the recommendations when they are involved in the planning process.[1] Ultimately, the health consultant's role is to increase the child care program's capacity to gather health information, to access resources for the program, and solve the program's health-related problems (Table 14.1).

QUALIFICATIONS OF THE CHILD CARE HEALTH CONSULTANT

Health issues in child care can range from simple to complex. Most child care programs can handle routine health matters, such as caring for a child's scraped knee, on their own. However, when programs face more complex health concerns, such as caring for a child with chronic medical conditions, consultation with trained health care professionals can greatly improve the quality of care.[1-5]

Health care professionals from a variety of educational backgrounds can offer valuable consultation to child care programs. Depending on their training and experience, they can provide consultation on a single health issue or cover a broad range of topics. Health consultants may be physicians with training in pediatrics, family practice, public health, or preventive medicine; nurses or nurse practitioners with training in pediatrics, family practice, public health, or community health; mental health professionals; dentists; nutritionists; or health educators.[1-4]

Because child care health consultants work at the interface of 2 fields—health and child care—they need expertise in health and early childhood education issues. Training and experience is necessary in child health and development and public health principles, such as health promotion and disease and injury prevention.

TABLE 14.1. Examples of Activities of Child Care Health Consultants		
Goal	**Activities Focused on the Child Care Environment**	**Activities Focused on Caregivers' Practices**
Promote early brain development	Observe child care equipment and materials and recommend equipment and materials suitable to the developmental needs of children.	Support caregivers in providing warm, positive, continuous relationships with children.
Prevent child injuries	Check playgrounds and indoor play areas and make recommendations for safe equipment, surfacing, and fall zones under and around equipment as well as adult supervision.	Observe staff safety practices, provide staff training on child injury prevention, and encourage regular safety checks and monitoring of safety practices.
Prevent the spread of infectious disease	Check the facilities and make recommendations for sufficient sinks, sanitary diapering and toileting areas, supplies for hand washing and sanitizing, and easily sanitized toys.	Observe staff infection control practices, provide staff training, and encourage monitoring of hand washing practices, hygienic diapering and toileting, and cleaning and disinfection of surfaces and toys.
Promote routine well-child preventive health care (checkups)	Check that the facility has a place to collect and protect the confidentiality of health information about each child.	Help staff interpret and use information from children's health records to accommodate special health needs, and help staff set up a system to identify children who are overdue for routine checkup services, such as immunizations or screening tests, to ensure children are up-to-date.
Promote appropriate care for children with special health needs	Help staff plan to adapt the facility as needed for children with special needs, such as allergies, asthma, and developmental or motor disabilities.	Help staff work with the child's family and health care professional to develop special care plans for use during the hours the child is in the child care facility, including plans for routine care and emergencies.

Consultants should understand the health and safety implications of different types of child care. Facilities may be child care centers, family child care homes, Head Start programs, or preschools. Programs of all types may have part-day, full-day, weekday, weekend, or nighttime hours. Children in child care may be infants, toddlers, preschool-aged children, and school-aged children in before- and after-school care. All programs care for mildly ill children (eg, those recovering from a colds), but child care programs differ in their exclusion practices, using their own criteria in addition to whatever restrictions are set by state regulation.

Health consultants must know the laws and regulations that apply to child care programs (see section on legal issues in this chapter). They should also be familiar with community health resources and key professional networks and materials available through organizations involved in child care health, such as the American Academy of Pediatrics (AAP), American Public Health Association (APHA), and the federally supported National Resource Center for Health and Safety in Child Care. In addition, the health consultant should be familiar with the leading organizations for child care center and family child care home providers, administrators, trainers, and regulators. Many of these organizations have Web sites and local affiliate organizations. Some nationally recognized organizations can be accessed through the Web site of the National Child Care Information Center.

DEVELOPING AND SUSTAINING RELATIONSHIPS BETWEEN HEALTH CARE PROFESSIONALS AND CHILD CARE PROVIDERS

There are many different ways that child care providers and health care professionals can link with each other to coordinate health consultation services to child care programs.

For Health Care Professionals Interested in Providing Consultation to Child Care Programs

- *Learn about families' experiences with child care.* Ask patients' parents, colleagues, and friends where their children attend child care and how they made the choice. Ask about their experiences with different types of child care programs, particularly how the programs worked with children of different ages, temperaments, and special needs.
- *Visit local child care centers.* Contact different types of child care programs and ask to observe their program and learn about their experiences and concerns with health and safety. Schedule observations to include low staffing periods (usually during arrivals and departures) and at peak activity and meal times. Try to observe children and caregivers involved in a range of activities, including quiet and active play, food preparation and meals, and diapering and toileting. Plan discussions at times that are convenient for caregivers to talk, such as during children's naptime.
- *Participate in early childhood professional organizations and conferences.* Attend conferences sponsored by the local child care resource and referral (R&R) agency, child care regulatory or subsidy agency, local office of the National Association for the Education of Young Children (NAEYC), Head Start, or family child care associations. Attend workshops on health issues to meet child care providers and listen to their concerns about health and safety in child care.

- *Present workshops on health issues.* Contact the coordinators of early childhood conferences to offer workshops or question-and-answer sessions on "hot topics" in child health. Local community college or university early childhood education courses might welcome a guest speaker, and child care programs may need staff training or parent workshops on health and safety.

- *Write articles on current health topics for child care.* Contact the publishers of child care journals and offer to write articles on health. Local child care associations, child care R&R agencies, and university extension offices may have newsletters for child care providers.

- *Offer health consultation to local child care programs.* Health care professionals can start by offering consultation to the child care programs their own children or patients attend. The local child care R&R agency might recommend child care programs that need health consultation. Infant centers, programs for children with special needs, facilities that provide care for ill children, and large child care centers may have a particular need for health consultation. Offer to serve on child care advisory boards, such as the health services advisory committee for a local Head Start program. Family child care home providers also need health consultation. Some parents who bring their own children for clinical care and who work as family child care home providers may want advice about caring for children in their home. All states have had federal funding to stimulate development of health consultation infrastructure as part of the Healthy Child Care America Campaign. Check with the national AAP or with AAP chapters to identify state activities in the Healthy Child Care America Campaign. Some NAEYC-accredited programs, university child care, corporate child care, Head Start, and state-funded child care quality improvement programs may have funding and materials for health consultation and training.

- *Offer health consultation to agencies providing technical assistance to child care.* These include child care R&R agencies, child care licensing agencies, and family child care home associations. Particularly when there are new health recommendations, such as immunizations, it is important to inform these agencies so they can disseminate up-to-date health information to child care programs.

For Child Care Programs Seeking a Qualified Health Consultant

- *Ask other child care programs for recommendations.* Ask colleagues how they found health consultants, whom they have used, the kinds of consultation involved, and their opinions about the strengths and weaknesses of the consultants.

- *Attend health workshops at child care conferences.* Health care professionals who offer workshops might also provide health consultation to child care programs. The workshop format can provide the opportunity to get to know the consultant's skills and style of interaction.

● *Contact local organizations to ask for referrals.* The local child care R&R agency might know local health care professionals that have worked with child care programs. In addition, health professional organizations such as the AAP, APHA, National Association of Pediatric Nurse Practitioners, public health departments (especially maternal and child health services), school health departments, state Healthy Child Care America campaigns, pediatric departments of medical schools, community health sections of nursing schools, and schools of public health may provide contacts for locating child care health consultants.

COMMUNICATION BETWEEN THE HEALTH CONSULTANT AND CHILD CARE PROGRAM

Health consultation is most effective when it is provided in the context of a respectful, trusting, and consistent relationship among health care professionals and child care providers and parents. Effective communication between the health consultant and child care provider is essential. The key to effective communication is that all the partners in child care—child care providers, families, and consultants—recognize and respect each others' unique knowledge, experience, and concerns. It is important to listen carefully, ask questions, and clarify the issues involved. Communication can be challenging because health care professionals and child care providers may have different styles of communication, terminology, office procedures, schedules, time constraints, and approaches to problem solving.[6]

In establishing the relationship between the health consultant and the child care program, it can be helpful to discuss some practical guidelines for contacts.[6] For example:

● Who is the contact person at the child care program—the director, a designated health coordinator or advocate, or any staff person or parent?

● How and when are contacts made—on a spontaneous basis, only during specified hours, or on a scheduled basis?

● What is the most effective way to present observations, questions, and recommendations?

ASSESSING THE NEEDS OF A CHILD CARE PROGRAM

Health consultation must be tailored to the needs of the individual child care program. Although some health and safety issues are common to most child care programs, each program has unique characteristics, health needs, and resources. To ensure that the health consultation meets the program's needs, an initial needs assessment should be done with the child care program director in person, by telephone, or in writing. The needs assessment should acquaint the consultant with the program's general characteristics and specific health needs and resources.

Program Characteristics

- What is the philosophy of the program?
- How long has the program been in operation?
- How many children attend?
- What are the ages of children?
- How are children grouped and how many children are in each group?
- What special health needs do children have?
- How many staff members are there? What special health needs do they have?
- What are the program hours?
- Is the program accredited?
- Are there any special features of the program, children, or families served (eg, ethnic backgrounds, languages, low income, teen parents, migrant workers)?

Program Health Needs and Resources

- How are health issues currently addressed?
  ~ Health policies?
  ~ Health training for staff?
  ~ Health education for parents?
  ~ Health education for children?
  ~ Health consultation?
- What are the health problems that the program has faced over the past few years? Are any health problems becoming more common? At the last licensing visit, were any health and safety issues noted? If so, what has been done about them? What are the health issues that are of most concern?
- What are the program's needs regarding:
  ~ Health policies?
  ~ Health training for staff?
  ~ Health education for parents?
  ~ Health education for children?
  ~ Health consultation?

The initial needs assessment process should also allow the child care director to get to know the health consultant and his or her areas of expertise, style of interaction, and availability. The child care director and the health consultant, together, should identify what the child care program wants and how much time is needed and determine whether that matches the health consultant's expertise and availability. Some programs might need only a brief or limited consultation; other programs might want an ongoing relationship with a health consultant to address a broad range of health needs. The work involved in developing and implementing a plan for health consultation is analogous to the familiar problem-oriented approach to patient care: the health consultant collects subjective and objective data about the child care program (including concerns and chief complaints) and collaborates with the child care staff to develop an assessment and plan.

PROVIDING HEALTH CONSULTATION SERVICES

Health consultants can offer a broad range of services to child care programs. Consultants should first respond to the questions or needs that programs have identified. In addition, consultants can alert child care providers to health issues about which they were not previously aware, such as concerns identified at site visits, emerging health issues, and new regulations and recommendations that affect child care practices.

Consultants should always try to demonstrate an appreciation for the unique features of the child care program, its strengths, and its challenges. It is important to prioritize the health concerns to address the most critical issues first and avoid overwhelming the program with too many issues at once. Recommendations should reinforce and build on the programs' positive characteristics and attributes that already exist. They should be clear and simple, cost-effective, easily implemented, and outlined verbally and in writing, if possible.

When the health consultant and child care program have the opportunity to work together over an extended period of time, a quality improvement plan can be developed that proceeds at a reasonable pace from addressing the most critical to less critical health concerns. A long-term consulting relationship also allows the opportunity to follow up and evaluate progress, to revise the action plan if needed, and to achieve steady quality improvement over time.

Visiting the Child Care Site and Observing the Facilities and Health Practices

Site visits help the health consultant understand the individual child care program and identify the health concerns of the staff, parents, and children. A site visit can be requested for a particular concern, such as observing infection control practices associated with a disease outbreak, or for a comprehensive observation. Depending on the size of the child care program, a comprehensive site visit could last up to a full day. The consultant should have a chance to inspect the facilities and observe the children and staff engaged in a full range of activities. The consultant should observe how well the child care program meets key standards for infection control, safety, nutrition, and developmentally appropriate practice. Resources are available[5,7,8] to help the health care consultant assess a child care program but should be used with care to avoid intimidating child care providers and parents. After the site visit, the health consultant should meet with the program director to summarize the program's strengths, identify the most important health concerns, and discuss plans for improvement.

Developing and Reviewing Program Policies on Child and Staff Health

Every child care program needs written health policies that cover a broad range of child and staff health concerns.[1,2,5,7,8] The health policies should be consistent with *Caring for Our Children,* the national standards published by the AAP, APHA, and the Maternal and Child Health Bureau (MCHB)[2]; federal regulations such as the Americans With Disabilities Act[9] and bloodborne pathogens regulations from the Occupational Safety and Health Administration[10]; and state licensing regulations and medical and nurse practice acts. A model health policy serves as a useful basis for developing new health policies or for reviewing and revising existing health policies.[8]

Assisting With Health Screening and Assessment for Children

The health consultant can help the child care program ensure that all children receive screening, diagnosis, and treatment of special health needs. For children who lack a "medical home," the consultant can provide referrals to primary health care professionals in the community. Although best practice is for children to receive health care in their medical home, for cases in which such arrangements cannot be made, the health consultant might provide child health screening, such as physical examinations, developmental screening, and vision and hearing tests (see section on legal issues in this chapter). The health consultant also can help the program interpret the results of health assessments and their implications for the care of children.[4]

Developing Plans for Children With Chronic Medical Conditions

On the basis of results of children's health assessments, the health consultant should work with the child care program, family, and health care professionals and, in the case of school-aged children in before- and after-school child care, with school health personnel, to ensure appropriate care of children with chronic conditions in the child care setting. The health consultant can help the program identify and understand information needed from the family and health care professionals to care for the child's routine and emergency health needs in child care. Specific health forms can clarify the accommodations needed in activities, nutrition, medications, health procedures, equipment, and facilities.[5,8] The health consultant can also provide staff education and training about the child's condition and care needs.[4]

Conducting Health Education for Staff, Parents, and Children

The health consultant can work with the program director to identify the program's health training needs. The training topics can be based on state licensing requirements, specific health concerns that the program has experienced, and problem areas identified by the health consultant at the site visit.[1,3,4,11] Common topics for staff health education and training include:

- Child growth and development
- Mental health promotion
- Communicable disease prevention and management
- Injury prevention, emergency preparedness, first aid, and cardiopulmonary resuscitation
- Nutrition and food safety
- Caring for children with chronic conditions
- Child abuse prevention and response
- Communicating with parents about health and safety issues
- Emerging health issues

The health consultant can provide the education and training or identify other health specialists to provide it. Depending on the program's needs, separate or joint workshops can be conducted for staff and parents. In addition, the health consultant might help plan health education for the children on topics such as hand washing, tooth brushing, eating healthy foods, and medical and dental check-ups. Health education for staff, parents, and children is most effective when it is desired by and builds on the experiences of participants, uses audiovisual aids, and allows for active participation. Traditional medical slide presentations are less effective than interactive and hands-on learning.

Reviewing Illness and Injury Logs

Health consultants should recommend that child care providers keep records of illnesses and injuries that children and staff experience in their program.[2,5,8] This documentation can be helpful for health care follow-up and for legal review, if necessary. The form should describe the illness or injury and what action was taken.[5,8] The health consultant can help the program director and staff to periodically review illness and injury logs to identify patterns, such as outbreaks of certain kinds of diseases or equipment frequently involved in injuries.[2] On the basis of the patterns of illnesses and injuries noted, the health consultant and child care staff can work together to develop plans to improve the prevention and management of illness and injury in the program.[11]

Providing Ongoing Child and Staff Health Consultation

Child care programs can benefit from having an ongoing relationship with a health consultant who is available to address whatever health issues may arise. When the consultant is familiar with the program's staff, families, routines, and facilities, the consultant's assessment and recommendations are better tailored to the program's particular needs. For example, a child care program might call the health consultant to explain that head lice has been a problem for children in the center for a month and to ask how they can stop the outbreak. If the consultant knows that "dress-up" play is very popular in the center, the consultant can quickly identify it as a potential contributor to the outbreak and advise the program to wash the play items, store them away for several weeks, and encourage other activities until the outbreak has passed. The health consultant can provide information and advice over the telephone or on-site or refer the program to resources, such as health care professionals or written or video materials. In addition, for sensitive issues, such as working with families whose children have chronic or recurring health problems, a trusting relationship with the health consultant is important. The health consultant can be instrumental in clarifying the issues and facilitating communication among child care providers, parents, and other service providers, when necessary.

LEGAL ISSUES

Health consultants must know the laws and regulations that apply to child care programs. These include their state child care licensing regulations, health and safety codes, medical and nurse practice acts; state and federal Early Intervention and Special Education laws; and the federal Americans With Disabilities Act,[9] Occupational Safety and Health Administration regulations,[10] and Head Start program performance standards. Consultants should know the child care program requirements for health consultation (eg, some states require monthly health visits to infant centers) and the health training requirements for caregivers (eg, some states require training in first aid and infection control). Consultants should also know the various state requirements for reporting incidents occurring in child care, such as communicable diseases and suspected child abuse and neglect—what is reportable and how and to whom to make reports.

To provide the highest standard of care and to limit liability, health consultants should follow the standards of practice for their profession and the most current recommendations from national health authorities, such as the AAP, APHA, and the Centers for Disease Control and Prevention.[2] Consultants should share a description of the child care responsibilities with their medical and nursing malpractice insurance carrier and ask for written confirmation of coverage for these activities, noting any restrictions or the need for additional coverage. Consultants should document their health consultation to maintain an ongoing health record for each program and for legal review, if necessary. At a minimum, written records should include the date, the client, the reason for consultation, and the information or advice provided.

If the child care program has requested that the health consultant provide direct services for individual children, such as health screening and mental health assessments, the consent of the child's parent or legal guardian is required. In addition, parental consent is required to contact a child's health care professional, if necessary. Confidentiality is an important issue. Child care providers must obtain parental consent for the consultant or anyone else to review their child's medical information. A consultant should discuss medical information about a child only with individuals who need to know to care for the child, and then only with the written consent of the parents or legal guardian. Consultants should never discuss the problems of one child care program with another program.

FUNDING SERVICES

Health consultants may or may not charge for their services. Having a contract and payment for services, however, can help clarify expectations and ensure accountability.[1] Health consultants may charge child care programs a fee for specific services or for consultation time. Consultants may have a fixed rate or a sliding scale depending on the needs and resources of the child care program. If the health consultant is a registered service provider for specific health plans, it might be possible to bill health insurance companies or Medicaid for some services, such as child health assessment. Governmental agencies (eg, Department of Health and Human Services, Department of Education), foundations, service organizations, and corporations may also provide grants for health consultation or research projects with child care programs.

Child care programs with limited funds may need health consultation free of charge. Public health departments might offer health consultation to child care programs as part of their community outreach and education on child health promotion and disease and injury prevention.[4] Health care professionals with another primary source of income, such as a private medical practice or hospital job, might consider providing free child care health consultation as part of their overall service to their community or patients. Some health care professionals may provide a certain number of hours per year of free services or offer free services to programs serving low-income children and families.

CONCLUSIONS AND RECOMMENDATIONS

Health care professionals should serve as child care health consultants to help promote the health and safety of children, families, and staff in child care settings. As with any other role, a health care professional must acquire the skills and knowledge to provide effective service as a health consultant.

REFERENCES

1. Aronson SS. Implementation: making it all happen. In: *Health and Safety in Child Care*. New York, NY: Harper Collins Publishers; 1991:194–211
2. American Academy of Pediatrics, American Public Health Association, and Maternal and Child Health Bureau. *Caring for Our Children. National Health and Safety Performance Standards: Guidelines for Out-of-Home Child Care Programs*. 2nd ed. Elk Grove Village, IL: American Academy of Pediatrics; 2002
3. Aronson S. Child care and the pediatrician. *Pediatr Rev*. 1989;10:277–286
4. Ulione M, Crowley AA. Nurses as child care health consultants. *Healthy Child Care America*. Elk Grove Village, IL: American Academy of Pediatrics. 1997;1:1

5. Aronson SS, eds. *Healthy Young Children: A Manual for Programs.* 4th ed. Washington, DC: National Association for the Education of Young Children; 2002

6. Dixon S. Talking to the child's physician: thoughts for the child care provider. *Young Child.* 1990;March:36-37

7. American Academy of Pediatrics, Pennsylvania Chapter Web site. Available at: http://www.paaap.org/mod.php?mod=userpage&menu=800&page_id=1. Accessed March 19, 2004

8. American Academy of Pediatrics, Pennsylvania Chapter. *Model Child Care Health Policies.* 4th ed. Rosemont, PA: American Academy of Pediatrics, Pennsylvania Chapter; 2002

9. Child Care Law Center. *Caring for Children With Special Needs: The Americans With Disabilities Act and Child Care.* San Francisco, CA: Child Care Law Center; 1995

10. US Department of Labor, Occupational Safety, and Health Administration. Occupational exposure to bloodborne pathogens. *Federal Register.* 1991;56:235

11. Ulione M, Dooling M. Preschool injuries in child care centers: nursing strategies for prevention. *J Pediatr Health Care.* 1997;1:111-116

ADDITIONAL RESOURCES

American Academy of Pediatrics and National Association for the Education of Young Children. *Caring for Our Children* (6 videos). Elk Grove Village, IL: American Academy of Pediatrics; 1995

California Department of Education. *Project Exceptional: A Guide for Training and Recruiting Child Care Providers to Serve Young Children with Disabilities, Volume 1.* Sacramento, CA: California Department of Education, Child Development Division; 1996

Child Care Law Center. *Caring for Children with Special Needs: The Americans with Disabilities Act and Child Care.* San Francisco, CA: Child Care Law Center; 1995

Dooling M, Ulione M. Health consultation in child care: a partnership that works. *Young Child.* 2000;55:23-26

Sokal-Gutierrez K. *Keeping Kids Healthy: Preventing and Managing Communicable Disease in Child Care* (manual and video). Sacramento, CA: California Department of Education; 1994

US Department of Health and Human Services. *Training Guides for the Head Start Learning Community* (8 guides). Washington, DC: US Department of Health and Human Services; 1994-1998

ORGANIZATIONS

American Academy of Pediatrics
141 Northwest Point Boulevard
Elk Grove Village, IL 60007
(Healthy Child Care America Campaign)
Phone: 888/227-5409
E-mail: childcare@aap.org
Web site: http://www.healthychildcare.org

American Public Health Association
800 I Street NW
Washington, DC 20001-3710
Phone: 202/789-5600
Web site: http://www.apha.org

Child Care Law Center
973 Market Street, Suite 550
San Francisco, CA 94103
Phone: 415/495-5498
Web site: http://www.childcarelaw.org

National Association of Child Care Resource and Referral Agencies
1319 F Street NW, Suite 810
Washington, DC 20004
Phone: 202/393-5501
Web site: http://www.naccrra.org

National Association for the Education of Young Children
1509 16th Street NW
Washington, DC 20036
Phone: 800/424-2460
Web site: http://www.naeyc.org

National Association of Pediatric Nurse Practitioners
1101 Kings Highway North, Suite 206
Cherry Hill, NJ 08034-1912
Phone: 609/667-1773
Web site: http://www.napnap.org

National Child Care Information Center
243 Church Street NW, 2nd Floor
Vienna, VA 22180
Phone: 800/616-2242
Fax: 800/716-2242
TTY: 800/516-2242
E-mail: info@nccic.org
Web site: http://www.nccic.org

National Resource Center for Health and Safety in Child Care
Campus Mail Stop F451
PO Box 6508
Aurora, CO 80045-0508
Phone: 800/598-KIDS (5437)
Web site: http://www.nrc.uchsc.edu

The Role of the Health Care Professional in Child Care: Education, Family Support, Community Involvement, and Child Advocacy

Angela A. Crowley, PhD, APRN, CS, PNP

LEARNING OBJECTIVES

- Define the role of the primary health care professional in parent education about child care.
- Describe effective communication patterns between health care professionals and child care providers that promote child health and family development.
- List community activities and advocacy efforts in which health care professionals can engage to improve children's health and the quality of child care.

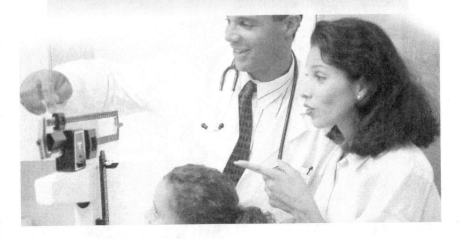

INTRODUCTION

During the past quarter century, social and economic forces have profoundly changed the definition of the American family and the roles parents play. Currently, more than 60% of mothers with children younger than 6 years are in the workforce.[1] Friedman et al[2(p376)] have described this change as a "watershed event...For the first time in history, the majority of infants living in the United States (are) receiving a significant amount of care from someone other than their mothers." Parents of young children are juggling multiple roles with few resources and some uncertainty about long-term outcomes. New brain research reveals that the quality of experiences during the first 3 years of life profoundly influence development.[3] Issues of quality, accessibility, and affordability of child care further compound the complexity of parenting in this decade. As the only professionals who most consistently interact with parents of young children, pediatric and family primary health care professionals are in a unique position to educate and support families about child care issues.

PARENT EDUCATION AND SUPPORT

The American Academy of Pediatrics (AAP) encourages parents to have a prenatal visit with a pediatrician and recommends 12 well-child visits during the first 5 years of life and yearly visits thereafter. These visits provide an opportunity to assess parents' child care needs, educate them about quality care, promote their access to community child care resources, and support the transition to care and the ongoing challenges related to combining working and parenting roles.

Before counseling parents, health care professionals must first examine their own knowledge and attitudes about out-of-home care for young children. In a survey initiated by the AAP Committee on Early Childhood, Adoption, and Dependent Care to explore pediatricians' attitudes and practices regarding child care issues, 59% of pediatricians said they discuss when a child can return to child care after an illness and 58% said they discuss returning to work after childbirth with mothers. Also, although 79% of pediatricians reported that they should be involved in a family's child care decisions, only 32% offer referrals to local child care resources or offer resources and information on child care to parents. Because working and substitute care are a necessity rather than an option for most families, it is imperative that health care professionals be well versed in criteria for and access to quality care as well as advantages and disadvantages of various forms of care. Ignoring the importance of child care decisions or conveying disapproval, such as negative comments about the association between illness rates and child care attendance, only discourages parents from sharing their concerns and need for education. At no time should a health care professional make a parent feel guilty about using child care.

Although the quality of child care is as vital to children's growth and development as are nutrition, safety, family environment, and other issues commonly reviewed at well-child visits, parents seldom initiate discussion of child care arrangements. However, they are eager to discuss this topic when health care professionals communicate the importance of quality care as it is related to children's health and family functioning and demonstrate knowledge and openness about this topic. Parents may not realize that many health care professionals are dealing with these same issues in their lives. They may appreciate learning how their health care professional successfully manages work and family issues.

Prenatally and during every well-child visit through the school-aged years, health care professionals should routinely inquire about mothers' anticipated return to work, including timing, the numbers of hours of work each week, and what child care arrangements, if any, have been planned. Discussion should include types of care options (family, in-home, or center-based), indicators of quality, how to find and assess child care, and parents' feelings about returning to work. Information about licensing, staff-child ratios, group size, staff turnover rates, philosophy, curriculum, access to a health consultant, and health and safety issues should be available to parents before they select care. Providing the name and contact information for the child care resource and referral agency in their locale or state would give parents access to information about each of these considerations (http://www.childcareaware.org).

Health care professionals should routinely inquire about mothers' anticipated return to work.

Parents frequently ask about the best time to return to work. If financial resources and job flexibility allow, mothers should be encouraged to take adequate leave time for recovery from delivery, for the infant to thrive and for developing a routine to establish breastfeeding, and for satisfying the mother's need to form an intimate, secure relationship with her infant. All of these variables will be unique for each family. In addition, parents should be encouraged to explore maternity or paternity leave benefits. Health care professionals can provide vital information to young mothers returning to work, such as how to access breast pumps and store their milk while working. Health care professionals may be able to assist families by filling out family leave forms, especially in the event of a premature or ill infant.

It is valuable to share with parents information about the normal development of separation anxiety and stranger fear between approximately 6 months and 1 year of age and its resurgence during the second year of life. Avoiding these times for returning to work or giving special attention to transitioning the child to a child care provider during these periods will facilitate the process. It is vital for parents to know that regardless of how well children adapt to child care, they will still exhibit some degree of separation anxiety at the appropriate stages similar to children who are reared at home.

Children and parents need time to feel comfortable with a child care provider and setting if it is outside of the home. A trial period in the child care setting with the parent at first present and then absent for brief intervals will afford the child time to develop trust with the provider and the parents an opportunity to develop confidence in the arrangement before the mother returns to work.

Once children enter child care, parents should be instructed to continuously monitor how the child is adapting. If a child develops symptoms of stress, such as poor eating and irritability or a change in sleep habits, closer attention to potentially precipitating factors in child care, such as change in staff, should be explored.

Child care providers and parents should be encouraged to communicate daily events during arrival and departure times to facilitate a child's transition from one environment to another. The loss of a pet at home or the illness of a friend at child care are important events that parents and child care providers need to communicate as they transfer care.

As children enter the preschool period, some parents may wish to reassess their child care arrangement to ensure a structured environment appropriate for the child's changing developmental needs. The educational component of child care becomes especially important in the preschool years. Again, the health care professional can offer advice about the various types of programs geared to this age group and suggestions about how to transition to a new program if this becomes necessary.

Although child care is usually associated with children younger than 6 years, supervision of school-aged children before and after school and during holidays and vacations is essential when parents are employed outside the home. Health care professionals should regularly inquire about parents' employment status and child care arrangements. Increasingly, school-aged child care programs are offered in schools or through community agencies. Health care professionals should discourage parents from allowing their children to be "latch-key" children and assist parents with finding supervision appropriate for this age group.

During the process of selecting child care, parents often fail to plan for the mild illnesses young children experience frequently. Although most minor childhood illnesses (such as colds and ear infections) do not require exclusion from child care, it is inevitable that at some point, a child will be excluded because of a specific contagious disease (such as strep throat or diarrhea) or because he or she is too ill for normal participation in the program. Without preparing an alternative care arrangement ahead of time, parents may feel they have no other option than to bring the sick child to his or her regular program. The presence of children who are contagious or unable to participate in normal program activities creates tension between child care providers, who are striving to maintain the health of the staff and other children, and parents. The health care professional can help avert these situations by counseling parents when they choose child care about the necessity for considering other arrangements that are more appropriate for mildly ill children, such as a parent taking family sick leave or flex time, care by a relative or friend, a developmentally appropriate child care program for mildly ill children, or in-home care through a home care agency. Health care professionals should also discourage inappropriate antibiotic use to allow the return of mildly ill children to child care. A recent study[5] revealed that many child care staff inappropriately exclude children and recommend antibiotics before the child is allowed to return.

To counsel parents about availability and options for regulated child care, the health care professional should be familiar with child care resources in the community. Many communities have child care resource and referral agencies that maintain a database of licensed child care providers and programs. These organizations may also offer counseling for selecting child care. Depending on the funding agent, these services may be provided free or at minimal cost. Other resources for finding child care include: child care associations or councils, family child care home associations, and the state or local chapter of the National Association for the Education of Young Children (NAEYC). Pamphlets with advice about selecting child care are available through the AAP, National Association of Pediatric Nurse Practitioners, and NAEYC and are useful for parents as an adjunct to counseling.

Health care professionals should also be familiar with the publication from the AAP, American Public Health Association (APHA), and Maternal and Child Health Bureau titled *Caring for our Children: National Health and Safety Standards: Guidelines for Out-of-Home Child Care Programs*[6] as well as their state's child care licensing regulations. This information is available through the National Resource Center for Health and Safety in Child Care Web site (see Resources). The standards in *Caring for Our Children* provide detailed recommendations for providing quality child care and are an excellent resource for all health care professionals and child care providers.

COMMUNICATION AND COLLABORATION WITH CHILD CARE PROVIDERS

Many health care professionals may have little to no contact with the child care providers of their patients, other than cursory notes written on yearly health forms. Yet, when one considers that many young children spend most of their waking hours with child care providers, it seems logical and necessary to facilitate communication via the parents for the health and well-being of the children.

In a study to determine communication patterns between child care providers and health care professionals, Rausch[7] compared child care health records with primary care charts. Although health care professionals usually reported acute illnesses to child care providers, in this sample there was no communication to child care providers about such chronic problems as developmental delay, chronic otitis media, hearing disorders, dental caries, or asthma. Needless to say, if child care providers are unaware of children's chronic health problems, they may misinterpret or even ignore important symptoms. In contrast, child care providers who are aware of children's health problems may often be the first to report untoward changes or to adapt programs to children's needs.

Health care professionals can foster communication with child care providers by providing comprehensive health assessment reports (see Appendix C), educating providers about children's health problems, and encouraging ongoing interaction. Parents should always be well informed of issues, and their permission for disclosure of information should be obtained. By encouraging communication, child care providers are more likely to collaborate with parents and health care professionals to foster the health and development of children.

THE HEALTH CARE PROFESSIONAL'S COMMUNITY INVOLVEMENT AND CHILD CARE ADVOCACY

Because of the variable quality, accessibility, and affordability of child care in every community, education and advocacy efforts are essential. In addition, pediatric health care professionals bring a unique perspective on children's health and family functioning to national and community organizations focused on child care issues. Some of the many organizations committed to improving the quality of child care include child care resource and referral agencies, such as the National Association of Child Care Resource and Referral Agencies, NAEYC, early childhood professional organizations, the AAP, and the National Association of Pediatric Nurse Practitioners. Furthermore, the Maternal Child Health Bureau, Community Integrated Service System/Health Systems Development Child Care grant initiatives exist in almost every state and in several territories. The purpose of these grants is to improve the health and safety of children in child care by linking health care professionals and organizations with the child care community. The AAP and the National Resource Center for Health and Safety in Child Care can provide state-specific information to interested health care professionals.

By offering to participate, health care professionals can broaden and strengthen the services of these organizations. For example, nurses, physicians, and physician assistants can develop health education programs for child care providers and parents, provide consultation to child care programs, write newsletter articles on child care health and safety, organize a local database of child care health consultants, and link child care providers with community health resources. They can also encourage local undergraduate and graduate schools that prepare health professionals to engage in these activities and integrate theory and experiences relevant to child care health into the curriculum.

The fluctuating condition of local, state, and national services for children and families requires that health care professionals provide ongoing testimony and advocacy for child care standards recommended by the APHA and AAP, educational training programs and resources, and monitoring of child care settings. Health care professionals can be a forceful voice in urging legislators and public officials to support children's issues and the family in the workplace.

CONCLUSIONS AND RECOMMENDATIONS

1. Discuss child care arrangements with parents prenatally and at each well-child visit from infancy through the school-aged years. Provide information about local resources.
2. Review characteristics of quality child care programs with parents.
3. Participate in active, ongoing communication with parents and child care providers to foster children's health and development.
4. Provide health consultation to child care programs.
5. Participate in national, state, or community child care organizations and advocate for accessible and affordable child care.

REFERENCES

1. US Department of Health and Human Services. *Child Health USA '99*. Washington, DC: Superintendent of Documents, Government Printing Office; 1999
2. National Institute of Child Health and Development, Early Childhood Network. In: Friedman SL, Haywood HC, eds. *Developmental Follow-up: Concepts, Domains, and Methods*. San Diego, CA: Academic Press; 1994:377–396
3. Shonkoff JP, Phillips DA, eds. *From Neurons to Neighborhoods: The Science of Early Childhood Development*. Washington, DC: National Academy Press; 2000
4. American Academy of Pediatrics. 1999 Periodic Survey of Pediatricians' Experiences With Child Care Health and Safety. Elk Grove Village, IL: American Academy of Pediatrics; 1999. Available at: http://www.healthychildcare.org/pdf/PedsSurvey.pdf. Accessed March 19, 2004
5. Skull SA, Ford-Jones EL, Kulin NA, Einarson TR, Wang EE. Child care center staff contribute to physicians visits and pressure for antibiotic prescription. *Arch Pediatr Adolesc Med*. 2000;154:180–183
6. American Academy of Pediatrics, American Public Health Association, and Maternal and Child Health Bureau. *Caring For Our Children. National Health and Safety Performance Standards: Guidelines for Out-of-Home Child Care Programs*. 2nd ed. Elk Grove Village, IL: American Academy of Pediatrics; 2002
7. Rausch KJ. Communication patterns between health care providers and child care workers. Unpublished master's thesis. New Haven, CT: Yale University School of Nursing; 1994

ADDITIONAL RESOURCES

American Academy of Pediatrics. *Choosing Child Care: What's Best for Your Family*. Elk Grove Village, IL: American Academy of Pediatrics

American Academy of Pediatrics. *The Pediatrician's Role in Promoting Health and Safety in Child Care*. Elk Grove Village, IL: American Academy of Pediatrics; 2001

Child Care Aware
1319 F Street NW, Suite 500
Washington, DC 20004
Phone: 800/424-2246
Web site: http://www.childcareaware.org

Healthy Child Care America
American Academy of Pediatrics
141 Northwest Point Boulevard
Elk Grove Village, IL 60007
Phone: 800/433-9016
Web site: http://www.healthychildcare.org

National Association for the Education of Young Children
1509 16th Street NW
Washington, DC 20036
Phone: 202/232-8777
Web site: http://www.naeyc.org

National Resource Centers for Health and Safety in Child Care
UCHSC at Fitzsimons
Campus Mail Stop F541
PO Box 6508
Aurora, CO 80045
Phone: 800/598-5437
Web site: http://nrc.uchsc.edu

Parent's Guide to Day Care
National Association of Pediatric Nurse Practitioners
1101 Kings Highway North, Suite 206
Cherry Hill, NJ 08034
http://www.napnap.org/catalog/catalog-nonmember.html

Sale JS, Kollenberg K, Melinkoff E. *The Working Parents Handbook*. New York, NY: A Fireside Book, Simon & Schuster; 1996

CHAPTER 16

Injury Prevention in Child Care, Preschool, and After-School Programs

James M. Poole, MD, and Donna J. Thompson, PhD

LEARNING OBJECTIVES

The reader of this chapter will gain an understanding of:

- The role of the pediatrician in injury prevention.
- Strategies for identifying and selecting high-quality care.
- Safety considerations unique to a child's age.

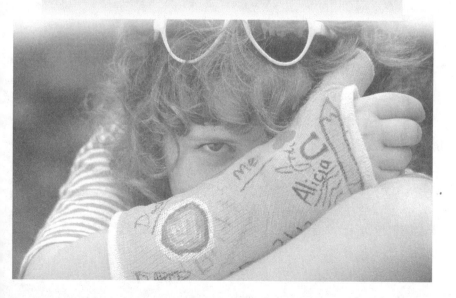

INTRODUCTION

The workplace has changed with the increase in the number of 2-wage-earner families. Coupled with this increase is the continual increase in the divorce rate and the number of single-parent families. In 2001, 61% of US children from birth through 6 years of age (not yet in kindergarten) were in some form of child care on a regular basis from persons other than their parents.[1] This translates to approximately 12 million children who attend some form of child care on a regular basis. The family and workforce are undergoing major changes. This change has been attributable to 1) the increased mobility of the workforce, with a resultant decrease in the extended family; 2) an increase in mothers entering the workforce; and 3) the increase in single parenting (by mother or father). More infants, toddlers, preschoolers, and school-aged children (before and after school) are spending their days in out-of-home child care programs. In 2002, 48 million (97%) children living with 2 parents had at least 1 parent in the workforce and 31 million (62%) were living in families with 2 parents in the workforce.[2] Of the 3.3 million children who lived only with their father, 2.9 million (89%) had fathers in the workforce. Among the 16 million children who only lived with their mother, 13 million (77%) had mothers in the labor force.[2] Compounding this problem is the fact that roughly 3% of children in kindergarten through third grade and 25% of children in fourth through eighth grade with working parents have no supervision after school.[1]

In 2002, the US Census Bureau reported that nearly 55% of mothers are returning to the workforce within a year of a child's birth and 72% of mothers with children older than 1 year are in the workforce.[3] The increases in the numbers of single parents and 2-wage-earner families have required the development of more child care centers and before- and after-school programs. The lack of availability of programs for the school-aged child in some communities has resulted in an increase in the number of "latch-key" children or children in "self-care." The demand for child care will result in a generation of children raised in such environments. According to predictions, the proportion of children needing care will continue to increase.[4] Associated with this increase in out-of-home care is the need to increase safety education and intervention strategies to prevent injury, a major cause of morbidity and mortality for children.

ROLE OF THE PEDIATRICIAN

Some pediatricians caring for the 13 million children in child care often focus on infectious diseases. There is also a great need and opportunity for pediatricians to instruct parents about injury prevention strategies in quality child care. This care extends from early childhood to before- and after-school programs. Pediatricians can make a major contribution to the health and safety of their young patients by educating themselves and parents about decreasing the risks of injuries to children in out-of-home child care. This will require that the pediatrician: 1) have knowledge of the child care environment and related health and safety issues;

2) be willing and able to spend time providing anticipatory guidance to parents; 3) understand effective community-based interventions; and 4) be able to offer specific suggestions and guidelines for the parent. No longer is this a role for only nonphysicians. The pediatric community must take the lead in ensuring that children receive safe, healthy, and developmentally appropriate child care.

It appears that a small number of children actually sustain the most injuries. This suggests that the risk is circumstantial or developmental. It is more important to identify individual, family, and environmental risk factors than to focus on the "incident-prone" child and also injuries most likely to occur at various ages.[5] Child care program directors are typically willing to develop lines of communication and assistance with a parent. This chapter will provide a brief overview of the problem for health care professionals as well as suggestions and reading materials for the parent. Pediatricians can bring needed expertise to the child care environment, assisting in the formation of new regulations, enforcing existing rules, and addressing safety issues in the community concerning places where young children spend their days.

To better understand child care structure, one must understand the various types of child care settings:

- Private centers: small (fewer than 25 children), medium (25–120 children), and large (120–300 children)
- Corporate centers: (50–300 children), subsidized totally or in part by a corporation
- Hospital based: (25–150 children), usually on-site
- Child care home: registered by state (6–25 children)
- Child care home, unregistered: the bulk of child care is provided in an unregistered child care home with 1 to 5 children

Inaccuracies in reporting make it difficult to determine the true scope of injuries in child care. Also, defining an actual injury, if handled by the caregiver at the center without health care professional intervention, is difficult.

One of the major variables with respect to child care-related injuries is the number of children allowed in a group setting and the staff-child ratio. For instance, a school-aged group may include as many as 25 children with only 1 staff member, whereas an infant group may be as small as 6 infants with 2 caregivers. State regulations and centers may vary substantially regarding group sizes, ages, and staff-child ratios. In general, the lower the staff-child ratio and quality of supervision, the lower the injury rate and the safer the environment becomes; therefore, pediatricians should work with state regulatory agencies to ensure appropriate ratios are maintained in the classroom and on the playground.

DEFINING QUALITY CARE

Because children are now spending more time at child care or before- and after-school programs than they are at home, it is important to examine the quality of these programs. Evidence suggests that the quality of programs and the provider-child relationship have a major influence on children's physical, emotional, social, and intellectual development. A 1995 study from the University of Colorado, University of North Carolina, Yale University, and University of California, Los Angeles found a direct link between quality of care and developmental outcomes in children. Children attending higher-quality programs scored higher in language ability and preacademic skills, had more positive attitudes toward their care, were more advanced socially, and had warmer, more open relationships with teachers.

High-quality child care combines nurturing care, developmentally appropriate activities for children, and trained staff members who interact with children to promote their social, emotional, and cognitive development. Quality centers manifest a safe and healthful physical environment that provides adequate stimulation, opportunities for a wide variety of learning experiences, and involvement with the child's family through clear and routine communication. Unfortunately, child care is expensive, approximately $4500 to $8000 per year for a preschool child, and the profit margin for child care centers was only 3.7%. Better-quality centers were generally more expensive or were heavily subsidized, usually by corporations. Child care is a relatively new frontier and is improving daily, but the bulk of child care occurs in centers that are small and financially vulnerable.

How to Quickly Evaluate for Quality

1. Look at toys and play equipment (in working order, no sharp edges or broken parts), safety items (shock stops, fire extinguisher, first aid kit), cleanliness, child-teacher interaction (respectful, pleasant), and upkeep (indoor and outdoor play environments maintained).
2. Listen to how the center sounds (happy teachers and children, noise level—excessively high or too quiet?).
3. Count group and class sizes, and ask about ratios (see Table 1.3).
4. Ask about the training and experience of the adults caring for your child and their ongoing professional development and training.
5. Be informed about how the center and the community are improving quality (accreditation in child care).
6. Evaluate activities to ensure they are safe, developmentally appropriate, and interesting and allow for a variety of motor, sensory, and cognitive experiences.
7. Monitor interaction between staff and children, other staff, and parents to ensure these interactions are positive, respectful, and conducive to an open, learning environment.

8. Verify that the curriculum is developmentally stimulating and incorporates new safety recommendations, such as the Back to Sleep campaign.

9. Watch for a safe play environment inside and outside.

MAKING SURE THE ENVIRONMENT IS SAFE AND HEALTHY

The increasing demand for child care and the large number of children in child care centers require an associated increase in child safety education and intervention to prevent injuries. Child care centers appear to be as safe as, or safer than, the home. In a study of 1000 injuries among 527 children in child care settings, there were 6 to 49 injuries per 1000 children every 8 hours, most being minor injuries with no fatalities or hospital admissions.[6] Safety precautions for child care require constant reassessment, improvement, and enforcement. Although currently there is not a nationally mandated standard, all states have regulations designed to protect the health and safety of children attending child care centers. Unfortunately, many family child care homes are unregulated, and many states do not have the staff or funding to adequately evaluate and monitor centers. Pediatricians are, therefore, an important link to help parents determine whether their child care setting is safe.

Factors influencing the risk of injuries in the child care setting include:

1. **SAFE** playgrounds including **S**upervision, **A**ge-appropriate Design, **F**all surfacing, and **E**quipment and surfacing maintenance[7] (see also Appendix B)
2. Age of children
3. Sex of children
4. Length of time in child care
5. Socioeconomic variables
6. Child-teacher ratio
7. Programs including swimming, field trips
8. Size of center
9. Quality of center and accreditation
10. Cost of care at the center
11. Time of day
12. Clothing (strangulation hazard)
13. Inappropriate surfaces, such as asphalt, cement, dirt, and grass

The most frequent safety hazards in licensed child care facilities include playground equipment without underlying impact absorbing surfaces, hot water ($\geq 130°$F), stairs without safety gates, and lack of prominently displayed emergency numbers.[8] Addressing these situations with the parent and the child care provider and making appropriate changes will lessen the rate of injuries at child care and at home. In a US study of public playgrounds by the National Program for Playground Safety, which included 1134 child care centers, less than 44% had enough absorbing surfaces on their playgrounds.[9] A large study in Sweden explored the location of injuries in child care centers (Table 16.1).

TABLE 16.1. Factors Contributing to Injuries in Child Care Centers[10]

Physical Characteristics	Injuries (%)
Playground equipment (climbing frames, slides, etc)	13.0%
Other child involved (pushing, collision, throwing)	12.8%
Furniture (chairs, bookshelves, etc)	11.5%
Part of building (doors, radiators)	10.7%
Vegetation (trees, berries)	8.4%
Toy	5.2%
Fixed equipment outdoors (fence, gate)	3.1%
Bicycle	2.5%
Sleds	2.5%
Stairs	1.7%
Outdoor surface (asphalt, cement)	1.5%
Other factors (including sporting equipment)	7.6%
Unspecified	19.7%

Children may have a lower incidence of injuries in child care, as Rivara reported. Emergency department-treated injuries in child care settings occur in 14.3 per 100 children, compared with 35 per 100 children in the community overall.[11] Briss also found child care centers to be relatively safe.[12] In contrast, the National Program for Playground Safety gave the child care center playgrounds assessed in its study (n=1163) an overall "C" grade and found that unacceptable. Children deserve "A" playgrounds.[9] Child care injuries may be overrepresented in emergency department reports, because child care injuries are more likely to be seen by a health care professional than are home injuries because of parental anxiety and costs of care being paid by insurance versus by the center.

A California study found child care center injuries to be 75% preventable, with 62% involving playground equipment, especially slides and swings.[13] Kotch found a similar rate of home and child care center injuries, 146 home injuries compared with 149 child care center injuries in 1 study.[4] The peak hours for child care center injuries in Atlanta were 11:00 am to 4:00 pm. This appears to be related to activity cycles and supervision. Warm months were associated with an increase in injuries, with the playground being the major site. Head injuries from falls were the most common, and 2-year-olds had the highest injury rates. Larger child care centers had higher rates of injuries than did smaller centers.[14]

Many child care providers are unaware of the temperature of the hot water in their centers.[8] This should be state regulated and enforced. The problem with hot water stems from the need to have hot water for kitchen cleaning and cooking, yet lower temperatures for the rest of the center. This requires separate hot water heaters, or safety valves for water temperatures.

Time of day and the nature of activities play a large part in when injuries occur. Injuries are more likely to occur when parents or substitute teachers who are not familiar with certain safety or center guidelines are present. The injury rate increases when children are tired (late afternoon or nap time), when the caregiver is distracted (when fixing lunch or changing activities), when another child is hurt or requires attention, and on field trips (supervision, unfamiliar environment, the environment is not child proofed).

Playground

One of the highest risk areas is the playground, accounting for more than 60% of child care center injuries. Problems include the surface material, safety gates, swings, and allowing mixed age groups onto the same playground at the same time (see Appendix B). These injuries also include falls from playground equipment and hanging injuries from entrapment on equipment. Safety training is important.

According to the Briss study,[15] only 61% of the child care centers surveyed have shock-absorbing surfaces on the playgrounds. The National Program for Playground Safety study indicated that 71% of child care centers surveyed had shock-absorbing surfacing. Further, they found that only 62% had the surfacing in the 6-foot use zone and that only 44% had the appropriate depth of surfacing proportionate to the height of the equipment.[9] Serious injury can occur from a 30-cm fall to asphalt or a 122-cm fall to packed surfaces.[16] Severe injuries occur above 2 meters (6.7 feet). Briss found that half of all fractures came from falls on the playground. Tinsworth[17] found that falls to the surface accounted for 48% of injuries to children younger than 2 years and 63% of injuries to children between 2 and 4 years of age. Tinsworth also noted that head and face injuries were most common for children ages younger than 5 years (49% of injuries), and arm and hand injuries occurred 30% of the time. Some states are now addressing this problem as an issue requiring more stringent regulations.

DECREASING THE RISK OF SUDDEN INFANT DEATH SYNDROME IN CHILD CARE

Two thirds of US infants spend at least some time in child care. These children spend an average of 22 hours per week in the care of someone other than their parent or primary caregiver. If you assume that sudden infant death syndrome (SIDS) occurs equally around the clock, you can calculate the following:

(67% of all infants are in child care) × (22 hours/week spent in child care)/ (168 total hours/week) = 8.8% of cases of SIDS will occur in child care.[18]

However, 20% of SIDS deaths occur in a child care setting. Approximately one third of SIDS cases in child care occur in the first week, and half of those occur on the first day. Most of these deaths are attributable to unaccustomed stomach sleeping or an infant who is used to sleeping on his or her back at home being put on the stomach by a secondary caregiver.

Child care providers can be proactive in decreasing the risk of SIDS in their home or center by implementing the *Caring for Our Children*[19] standards, being able to respond to and handle an infant medical emergency, being aware of bereavement resources, talking with a child care health consultant about SIDS risk reduction, discussing sleep position with families, and creating and using a safe sleep policy. The elements of a safe sleep policy include safe sleep practices and the creation of a safe sleep environment. General points it should include are:

- Healthy babies always sleep on their backs at nap time and night
- If a baby needs to sleep in a position other than on the back, a note from a child health professional that describes the medical condition that merits an exemption needs to be obtained by the child care center and kept on file and by the baby's crib to alert all staff
- Babies must always sleep in safety-approved cribs and firm mattresses and not on cushions, adult beds, water beds, sofas, or any other surface other than the infant's crib
- The crib should be free of toys, stuffed animals, excess bedding, crib bumpers, and wedges
- Practice the feet-to-feet rule (the baby should be placed at the foot of the crib; if a blanket is being used, it needs to be tucked under the baby's arm and tucked in to 3 sides of the crib)
- There should be only 1 baby per crib for naps and at night
- Room temperature should be 65°F to 75°F in the winter and 68°F to 72°F in the summer

Pediatricians can help by discussing safe sleep practices with their patients at prenatal visits and by encouraging them to talk to the secondary caregivers that will be taking care of their child about safe sleep. Everyone who cares for the baby needs to be informed about how the baby should sleep to keep him or her healthy and safe.

EVALUATING AN INJURY AS IT RELATES TO THE CHILD CARE PROVIDER

If a child comes into the health care professional's office with an injury, it is important not to focus on assigning blame. Identify the source of the problem, collect information concerning the incident, and ask about other children, supervision, and the environment. Could the injury have occurred at home? Was the injury unintended or inflicted? The parent feels some measure of guilt in most cases when their child is injured in the child care setting, and most children are very impulsive in their actions. Health care professionals must support the child care provider and the parent's decision to place their child in child care. At the same time, health care professionals must be concerned with the needs of the child and ensure that there has not been any measure of abuse or neglect.

If you feel that abuse or neglect is present, contact the local regulatory and investigating agency to file a report. Try to call the child care center director or provider and discuss in detail their perception of what took place. Pediatricians should support the family first, and that means supporting the entire situation without labeling child care as "bad."

Safety Items to Check (see also *Model Child Care Health Policies* from the Pennsylvania Chapter of the American Academy of Pediatrics [see resources]):

- Children are greeted on arrival and departure.
- Caregivers are trained in first response, cardiopulmonary resuscitation (CPR), and first aid.
- Outdoor area is fenced and has a variety of safe equipment. Caregivers can see the entire playground. Different age groups are separated (eg, 0-1, 2-3, 4-5).
- After-school children (5 to 12 years of age) are separated from younger children on the playground at the same time.
- Hot water is set to no more than 120°F.
- Toxic substances are eliminated.
- Monthly safety updates and meetings are held (see Resources for information on National Program for Playground Safety).
- Plastic bags are stored appropriately.
- CPR instructions are posted in rooms.
- Daily, weekly, or monthly playground safety checklist is completed (Table 16.2).
- Emergency phone numbers (ambulance, poison control, etc) are posted where all can find them.
- Reporting of injuries occurs without official reprimand, as this may decrease reporting (Fig 16.1).
- Daily log of all injuries, including those not requiring a health care professional visit, is maintained.
- On beach trips, swimming without lifeguard is not allowed (it is not appropriate to take a large group of children to an ocean, lake, or river).
- Swimming pool safety is strictly enforced: not allowing too many children, always having certified lifeguards, not allowing teachers to act as lifeguards, not allowing contract supervision of children (liability for center). The "10-20 rule" is always followed: because drowning may occur in 30 seconds, stay close enough to spot trouble within 10 seconds and rescue the endangered child within 20 seconds.[20] Recommended child-staff ratios should not be exceeded (infants and toddlers, 1:1; preschoolers, 4:1; school-age children, 6:1).

TABLE 16.2. Safety Checklist	
PARKING LOT	• Free of ice • Prevention from walking between cars • Ignition turned off when parent enters building • Children are hand held to car and not allowed to run free in front yard or parking lot
ENTRANCE	• All steps have handrails and are covered • Entrance and exit from ground level
HALLWAYS	• Kept clean • Spills cleaned up • No sharp corners (cover them) or head-height counters with sharp edges • Equipment not left in halls (both physical and fire hazard) • Safety glass for all door glass in building
KITCHEN	• Only authorized personnel allowed in kitchen • Grease should not be used • Fire extinguishers clear and tested for working condition • Shelves secured • Food and equipment stored safely • Food cans easily reached and not hazard to fall • Hand washing sink separate • Children not allowed in food preparation area
TOXIC CHEMICALS	• For kitchen and cleaning, chemicals should have their own locked storage unit • Cleaning solutions (ie, bleach solutions for mixing) for use in classrooms have a locked cabinet
CLASSROOMS	• Electrical sockets up high or covered • Locked cabinet or file box for medicine and diluted cleaning chemicals (never concentrated in classroom) • Cribs, tables, and bookcases have all screws and bolts checked monthly • No hot plates; appliances for warming bottles protected from being pulled off counter • No climbing on chairs or tables to hang items • No sharp corners on tables or equipment • Toys safe, no loose ornaments • Fire exit with one turn or pull down action from room • Hot surfaces, heaters, vents cannot be reached by children • Tap water 120°F or less • Good lighting in all rooms • Sleeping cots give clear walkway, and children arranged head to toe • Children are not left alone in high chairs or seats • No infant walkers, stationary "walkers" allowed • No pacifiers with strings longer than 6 inches
PLAYGROUND	• Check for 12 inches of loose-fill surfacing around stationary equipment • Bolts covered, soft swing seats • Soft impact-absorbing surfaces: sand, pea gravel may be used for children older than 3 years; wood or rubber products. Check state licensing requirements

TABLE 16.2. Safety Checklist, continued	
PLAYGROUND, continued	• Fenced with safety locks • Age appropriate, slides covered or with hand rails (only 1 child allowed at a time) • No space where child's neck could get stuck (<3.5 inches or >9 inches) • All areas supervised at all times by trained caregivers • Do not allow other adults to have a teacher conference on playground, because it is a distraction to caregiver watching others • Check for poisonous plants, trash, sharp objects surrounding yard • Do not allow children to play on playgrounds with strings in hoods • Remove helmets from children before allowing them to use playground equipment
COMPUTERS, ELECTRICAL EQUIPMENT	• Ensure children cannot get behind equipment (electrical hazard) • Serviced by authorized people only • No liquids allowed near equipment • Supervised at all times
VANS	• First aid kit • Car safety seats (use booster seats with shoulder harness for larger children) for children younger than 5 years. Booster seats required until child is approximately 8 years of age and at least 4 feet 9 inches in height • Seat belts working and used • Radio sound kept at minimum and appropriate for children • Monthly, check oil, tires, and brakes • Routine checks by service dealer • Driver with chauffeur license • Driver should be older than 21 years • Children not allowed in front seat • Check for sharp rusty metal on van
STAFF TRAINING	• Children taught safety, emergency procedures • Ongoing training hours required • CPR and first response training to a minimum of 3 on-site staff at all times
ART SUPPLIES	• Nontoxic, use natural materials such as dyes and water-based products • Avoid aerosol sprays and solvent-based glues
FIELD TRIPS	• Adequate supervision • Do not rely on the people at the location to be responsible for children • Some type of identification worn by each child • Children should hold hands in pairs or hold a rope when walking in a group
EQUIPMENT	• First aid kit well stocked • Sports equipment safe, soft
FIRE/SEVERE WEATHER DRILLS	• Children should be evacuated to safe area within 3 minutes • Monthly fire drills • Smoke detectors and alarm system

FIG 16.1. Injury Report Form		
CHILD'S NAME	DATE/TIME OF INJURY	INJURY DESCRIPTION
WHERE OCCURRED	HOW OCCURRED	PARENT NOTIFIED BY
WITNESSES	MEDICAL TREATMENT	
PREVENTIVE CHANGES	PARENT SIGNATURE DATE	STAFF SIGNATURE/DATE

- Sunscreen with a sun protection factor (SPF) of at least 15 is applied before outdoor activities, and hats and protective clothing are always worn when going out in heat of day 10:30 am to 3:30 pm.
- Sports: strenuous activities are not performed with high ambient temperature (risk of heat exhaustion or stroke), strenuous outdoor activities are decreased or eliminated when the heat index (a value that incorporates air temperature and relative humidity) is $\geq 90°F$.
- Barbecue: no open barbecue grills, dangers from hot dogs and choking are prevented.
- Fireworks are never allowed.
- Safety equipment (helmets, pads) always used with in-line skates, scooters, and bicycles. Children using scooters are closely supervised.

- On field trips, children are always checked for ticks, scented perfumes are not worn, long pants are worn if in woods or high grass, first aid for bee stings is available.
- Boating is never allowed.
- For visits to petting farms, including hay rides, caution is used in selecting the location, parent supervision is allowed and release forms are signed, and there is close supervision.
- For birthday parties, there is awareness of foods that a child may be allergic to (ie, peanut butter), caution is exercised in type and preparation of foods, parent involvement is encouraged, appropriate party favors are provided, no latex balloons are used.
- There are no unprotected accessible stairways.
- Screens cover all heat sources.
- High chairs have safety harnesses.
- Rice is considered instead of sand inside play bins.
- Sand boxes are covered.
- Cribs are inspected for loose bolts, mattresses are at lowest level, there is no soft bedding, and infants are placed on their backs to sleep (ie, Back-to-Sleep campaign).
- Changing tables have sides to prevent children from rolling off.
- Sports equipment needs to be soft (soft balls, no hard sticks or clubs).
- Poisonous plants are not in or around the center.

Injuries Most Commonly Seen by Child Care Providers

- Bee stings
- Broken arms
- Bumps on heads from falling
- Lip lacerations
- Choking on food
- Fingers pinched in doors
- Forehead lacerations and abrasions
- Lacerations elsewhere
- Nose bleeds
- Contusions from such activities as running into each other
- Scraped knees, arms, and hands
- Scratches from falling outside
- Human bites involving another child
- Injury to tongue from child's own teeth
- Tooth injuries
- Ankle, leg, head, and back injuries from tripping over toys and furniture

CHILDHOOD SAFETY

Each month and year that a child grows and develops brings his or her own set of increased abilities and from a safety standpoint, his or her own set of problems. The following list is by ages. In a child care setting, the staff ratios (trained supervisors should be the same outside as inside), group sizes, and teacher training and experience are all factors that may influence the rate of injuries. Some individuals consider the child's sex to be an important risk factor. However, impulsive, aggressive, risk taking behaviors are not exclusively found in males. Each of the following carries over year to year in this brief list.

Major Areas of Emphasis for Injury Prevention by Age

Birth to 3 Months of Age
- Car safety seats (see Fig 16.2)
- Protect against falls—crib rails up, diaper changing table with sides
- Avoid offering supplemental water to the healthy young breastfed or formula-fed infant unless recommended by the infant's pediatrician. In most circumstances, infants have their fluid needs met by breast milk or formula alone until the introduction of solid foods.
- Put to sleep on back
- Never leave unattended, do not mix different age groups
- Never shake infant's head or body vigorously
- No necklaces or pacifiers on a string (to prevent strangulation)
- Water temperature 120°F or less
- Never hold an infant while drinking something hot
- Do not suspend or rest an infant carrier above the floor; always secure the restraints on a child in the infant carrier
- Avoid direct sun exposure of a young infant

3 to 6 Months of Age
- Car safety seats (see Fig 16.2)
- Prevention from falling, sunburn, choking, poisoning (have poison control number in clear view)
- Stationary "walkers" only
- Toys should not have sharp edges or detachable parts
- Purses need to be up and out of way of crawling infants, as they may contain dangerous items
- Prepare electrical outlets and extension cords, making them inaccessible by children
- Beware of expanding gates; "v" shaped openings in top have been associated with infant and toddler strangulation

Fig 16.2. Car safety seats: selecting the most appropriate type[21]

The safest place in a vehicle for all children is the rear seat. Never place a rear-facing infant seat in the front seat of a vehicle with an activated passenger-side air bag.

5 lb	10 lb	20 lb Ages 5–15 mo*	30 lb	40 lb	50 lb	60 lb Age 8 y*	70 lb	80 lb

Infant-only seat, rear facing, never in front seat with passenger-side air bag. Car bed if medically indicated.

Convertible safety seat, rear facing until child is at least 1 year of age and at least 20 lb, then forward facing to the maximum weight and height allowed by seat.[†]

Combination seat with internal harness that transitions to a belt-positioning booster seat; forward facing only; weight varies.

Forward facing seat with internal harness; weight varies.

Integrated child seat: toddler seat with harness (20–40 lb) or some as belt-positioning booster seat with lap/shoulder belt (more than 35–40 lb), as long as child fits.[‡]

Belt-positioning booster seat[§] with lap/shoulder belt as long as child fits[‡]

The lap/shoulder belt fits when:
- Shoulder belt fits across mid chest and shoulder
- Lap belt low and snug across thighs
- Child can sit all the way back against vehicle seat and knees bend at edge of vehicle seat

Additional considerations:

Lap/shoulder belt is more protective than a lap only belt.
Restrained is safer than unrestrained.
Lap/shoulder belts can be retrofit in some vehicles.

Source: American Academy of Pediatrics, 2002

Weight limits on specific products vary, and this is indicated by dashed lines at the ends of bars. Always read and follow manufacturer's and vehicle instructions. Use of safety belts varies with vehicle belt system and height of child. For additional information on the use of car beds, see the AAP policy statement "Safe Transportation of Premature and Low Birth Weight Infants." For more information, or to locate a local child passenger safety technician, visit www.nhtsa.dot.gov/people/injury/childps

* Usual age range for this weight; individual children's ages will vary widely.
† If car safety seat accommodates children rear facing to higher weights, for optimal protection, the child should remain rear facing to the maximum weight for the seat as long as the head is below the top of the seat back.[3]
‡ Very tall children may require a combination seat or belt-positioning booster seat before 40 lb.
§ Crash injury data for children in this age group indicate that child safety seats provide more protection than seat belts.[8]

- No plastic bags or latex balloons near children
- **DO NOT USE A MICROWAVE** to heat food or milk (burn, explosive heat, heats unevenly)
- Exercise crib safety
- Place child on back to sleep
- No soft items (eg, pillows) in crib
- No corner post extensions or cut-outs on head boards
- Slats no more than 2½ inches apart
- Mattress fits snugly; no more than 2 fingers can fit between mattress and crib side
- 36 inches between mattress and top of crib rail
- Sheet fits tightly over a thin, firm mattress

6 to 12 Months of Age
- As the child becomes mobile, the risk of unintentional trauma increases
- Watch for sharp corners and edges (falls)
- Locks on all cabinets containing chemicals or medications, keep purses out of reach (infants may get into a purse with dangerous items)
- Do not serve food that could cause choking (peanuts, popcorn, hot dogs, carrots, celery sticks, grapes, etc)
- Car safety seats (face backward in back seat until 20 lb in body weight *and* 1 year of age); see Fig 16.2
- Water safety includes buckets, toilets, bathtubs, and pools
- Children require constant trained supervision
- Playpens are for sleeping, not for free play, because this limits the adult-child interaction
- Clean the carpet regularly
- **DO NOT USE A MICROWAVE** to heat food or milk

1 to 2 Years of Age
- Car safety seats (see Fig 16.2)
- Walking makes hazardous substances and situations even more accessible to the child
- Do not use collapsible gates within a classroom
- Tap water temperature 120°F or less
- Poison prevention
- Aspiration prevention
- Burn prevention
- Climbing and falling precautions, including shock-absorbing surfaces under play equipment whether outside or inside (mats are unacceptable[22])
- Street and parking lot safety (always hold or carry a small child)

- Dangerous food (jelly beans, peanuts, popcorn, chewing gum) should not be offered (if hot dogs are offered, they should be cut lengthwise and crosswise into small pieces)

2 to 4 Years of Age
- Car safety seats (see Fig 16.2)
- Water safety
- Prevention of ingestion of harmful substances
- Street safety
- Aspiration safety
- Fall prevention
- Burn prevention
- Shock safety
- Alter mini-blind loop cords to prevent strangulation (these cords are not appropriate in child care settings); use protective devices for rolling up cords
- The center should not allow pets because of such concerns as bites, scratches, and infections (turtles and reptiles may transmit *Salmonella* infection)
- Do not let children go unattended from the playground into the indoor setting (eg, to use the bathroom)
- Never leave a child unattended for any reason
- Supervise a child who is given time out
- Water play requires that each child has his or her own water bucket
- Empty small wading pools daily
- Use extreme caution when taking children to a swimming pool, using a staff-child ratio of 1 to 4

4 to 6 Years of Age
- Pay special attention to car and van safety (see Fig 16.2)
- Bicycle safety with use of helmets; take helmets off and store them before allowing children to use playground equipment
- Street safety
- Stranger safety (only leave by way of the front door with a designated adult)
- Climbing safety; age-appropriate equipment
- Equipment on the playground needs to be age appropriate (eg, 2–5 years with spaces for separation of children ages 0–1, 2–3, and 4–5 years)
- Teach children their home phone number and address
- No mechanical equipment or yard equipment where the children are
- Do not mow grass with children outside

CONCLUSIONS AND RECOMMENDATIONS

The increasing demand for child care and the large number of children in child care centers demand an associated increase in child safety education and intervention to prevent injuries. Pediatricians and other health care professionals should work with state regulatory agencies to ensure appropriate ratios are maintained in the classroom and on the playground and to ensure that recommended safety procedures are in place and should help parents to choose a child care program that is safe and developmentally appropriate for their child.

REFERENCES

1. Federal Interagency Forum on Child and Family Statistics. *America's Children: Key National Indicators of Well-Being, 2002.* Washington, DC: US Government Printing Office; 2002
2. US Census Bureau. *Children's Living Arrangements and Characteristics: March 2002.* Washington, DC: US Census Bureau; 2003. Available at: http://www.census.gov/prod/2003pubs/p20-547.pdf. Accessed March 19, 2004
3. US Census Bureau. Fertility of American Women: June 2002. Washington, DC: US Census Bureau; 2003. Available at: http://www.census.gov/prod/2003pubs/p20-548.pdf. Accessed March 19, 2004
4. Kotch JB, Loda F. Parents' reports of home and out-of-home injuries among children attending child care centers. *Early Child Dev Care.* 1993;96:183–193
5. Boyce WT, Sobolenski S. Recurrent injuries in school children. *Am J Dis Child.* 1989;143:338–342
6. Leland NL. Injuries to preschool-age children in daycare centers, a retrospective record review. *Am J Dis Child.* 1993;147:826–831
7. Thompson D, Hudson, SD. *The National Action Plan for the Prevention of Playground Injuries.* Cedar Falls, IA: National Program for Playground Safety; 1996
8. O'Conner MA. Self-reported safety practices in child care facilities. *Am J Prev Med.* 1992;8:14–18
9. Hudson SD, Mack MG, Thompson D. *How Safe Are America's Playgrounds?* Cedar Falls, IA: National Program for Playground Safety; 2000
10. Sellstrom E, Bremberg S, Chang A. Injuries in Swedish day-care centers. *Pediatrics.* 1994;94(6 Pt 2):1033–1036
11. Rivera FP. Injuries in day-care centers. *Am J Dis Child.* 1987;141:938
12. Briss PA. A nationwide study of the risk of injury associated with day care center attendance. *Pediatrics.* 1994;93:364–368
13. Chang A. Injuries among preschool children enrolled in day care centers. *Pediatrics.* 1989;83:272–277
14. Sacks JJ. The epidemiology of injuries in Atlanta day care centers. *JAMA.* 1989;262:1641–1646
15. Briss PA. A nationwide study of the risk of injury associated with day care center attendance. *Pediatrics.* 1994;93:364–368
16. Laforest S, Robitaille Y, Lesage D, Dorval D. Surface characteristics, equipment height, and the occurrence and severity of playground injuries. *Inj Prev.* 2001;7:35–40

17. Tinsworth DK, McDonald JE. *Special Study: Injuries and Deaths Associated With Children's Playground Equipment.* Washington, DC: US Consumer Product Safety Commission; 2001

18. Ehrle J, Adams G, Tout K. *Who's Caring for Our Youngest Children? Child Care Patterns of Infants and Toddlers.* Washington, DC: The Urban Institute; 2001

19. American Academy of Pediatrics, American Public Health Association, and Maternal and Child Health Bureau. *Caring for Our Children. National Health and Safety Performance Standards: Guidelines for Out-of-Home Child Care Programs.* 2nd ed. Elk Grove Village, IL: American Academy of Pediatrics; 2002

20. American Red Cross. *Stay Well.* Boston, MA: American Red Cross; 2001:24

21. American Academy of Pediatrics, Committee on Injury and Poison Prevention. Selecting and using the most appropriate car safety seats for growing children: guidelines for counseling parents. *Pediatrics.* 2002;109:550–553

22. Mack MG, Sacks JJ, Thompson D. Testing the impact attenuation of loose-fill playground surfaces. *Inj Prev.* 2000;6:141–144

ADDITIONAL RESOURCES

American Academy of Pediatrics. *Caring for Your Baby and Young Child: Birth to Age 5.* Shevlov SP, Hannemann RE, eds. Elk Grove Village, IL: American Academy of Pediatrics; 1998

American Academy of Pediatrics. *Choosing Child Care: What's Best for Your Family.* Elk Grove Village, IL: American Academy of Pediatrics; 2002

American Academy of Pediatrics. Moving Kids Safely Web resources. Available at: http://www.aap.org/family/cps.htm. Accessed March 19, 2004

American Academy of Pediatrics, American Public Health Association, and Maternal and Child Health Bureau. *Caring for Our Children. National Health and Safety Performance Standards: Guidelines for Out-of-Home Child Care Programs.* 2nd ed. Elk Grove Village, IL: American Academy of Pediatrics; 2002

American Academy of Pediatrics, Committee on Nutrition. *Pediatric Nutrition Handbook.* Kleinman RE, ed. 5th ed. Elk Grove Village, IL: American Academy of Pediatrics; 2003

American Academy of Pediatrics, Workgroup on Breastfeeding. Breastfeeding and the use of human milk. *Pediatrics.* 1997;100:1035–1039

Aronson SS, ed. *Healthy Young Children: A Manual for Programs.* 4th ed. Washington, DC: National Association for the Education of Young Children; 2002

Ashraf RN, Jalil F, Aperia A, et al. Additional water is not needed for healthy breast-fed babies in a hot climate. *Acta Paediatr Scand.* 1993;82:1007–1011

Centers for Disease Control and Prevention
National Center for Injury Prevention and Control
Mailstop K65
4770 Buford Highway NE
Atlanta, GA 30341-3724
Phone: 770/488-1506
Web site: http://www.cdc.gov/ncipc/

Child Care Aware
1319 F Street NW, Suite 500
Washington, DC 20004
Phone: 800/424-2246
Web site: http://www.childcareaware.org

Heining MJ, Nommensen LA, Peerson JM, et al. Intake and growth of breastfed and formula-fed infants in relation to the timing of introduction of complementary foods: the Darling study. *Acta Paediatr Scand.* 1993;82:999-1006

National Program for Playground Safety
University of Northern Iowa, School of HPELS, WRC 205
Cedar Falls, IA 50614-0618
Phone: 800/554-PLAY
Web site: http://www.uni.edu/playground

Pennsylvania Chapter, American Academy of Pediatrics. *Model Child Care Health Policies.* 4th ed. Rosemont, PA: American Academy of Pediatrics, Pennsylvania Chapter; 2002

National Resource Center for Health and Safety in Child Care
UCHSC at Fitzsimons
Campus Mail Stop F541
PO Box 6508
Aurora, CO 80048
Phone: 800/598-5437
Web site: http://nrc.uchsc.edu

National SIDS Resource Center
2070 Chain Bridge Road, Suite 450
Vienna, VA 22182
Phone: 866/866-7437
Web site: http://www.sidscenter.org

State resource and referral agencies and child care licensing agencies

US Consumer Product Safety Commission. *Handbook for Public Playground Safety.* Washington, DC: Consumer Product Safety Commission; 1997

CHAPTER 17

Prevention, Control, and Management of Infectious Diseases

Trudy V. Murphy, MD

LEARNING OBJECTIVES

This chapter will help the reader to:

- Understand the agents, routes of transmission, and morbidity from infection acquired in child care settings.

- Know how to provide a safe and healthy environment and prevent infection transmitted in child care settings.

- Recognize the infections that cause epidemic disease in child care settings and understand the principles and the resources for their management and control.

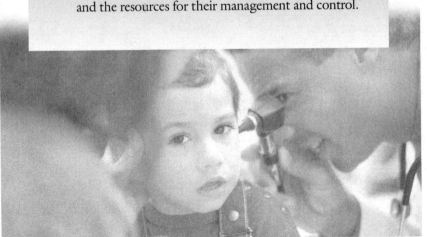

INTRODUCTION

Many infectious agents are transmitted in the child care environment. Young children are dependent on others to manage their body fluids, secretions, and excretions, and these are the primary vehicles for transmission of infectious agents. Hands and toys easily become contaminated with infectious agents, and children inoculate themselves by repeatedly placing their hands and toys to their nose and mouth. Spread of infection is efficient because of proximity. By virtue of their age, children are highly susceptible to infection. These illnesses are usually most contagious during early symptomatic periods of disease or even before the development of clinical symptoms. Copious respiratory secretions, coughing, and diarrhea facilitate transmission of agents that colonize the child's respiratory or gastrointestinal tract (shed asymptomatically) as well as agents that cause acute illness. Child care providers have many demands on their attention and, often, limited training and resources to carry out measures that promote a healthy environment. Health care professionals and parents can assist child care providers by sharing this heavy responsibility.

Some characteristics of infectious agents lead to especially efficient transmission by young children in child care settings (Tables 17.1 and 17.2). Agents that cause asymptomatic infection (eg, hepatitis A virus [HAV], cytomegalovirus [CMV], rotavirus) or that persist by establishing asymptomatic colonization (eg, group A β-hemolytic streptococci, *Giardia lamblia*) can be the reservoir of endemic infection, which persists for weeks or months. Agents that survive for relatively long periods (hours or days) on toys, handles, and other environmental surfaces are found widely in classes of toddlers. This contamination contributes to explosive outbreaks as well as endemic disease (eg, *Shigella* species, *Escherichia coli* O157:H7, *G lamblia*). Agents that have a low infective dose or are transmitted efficiently in aerosols are associated with epidemic disease (eg, *Shigella* species, respiratory syncytial and influenza viruses, and varicella zoster virus [VZV]).

Children who are younger than 3 years and who attend child care are at 2 to 3.5 times greater risk of infection than are children who receive care at home. This excessive risk is documented for upper respiratory and diarrheal illnesses, otitis media, hepatitis A virus infection, invasive bacterial infections (*Haemophilus influenzae* type b [Hib], *Streptococcus pneumoniae*), herpes simplex virus infection, VZV infection, and CMV infection. Children attending large child care facilities (centers) have the highest risk of infection, presumably because they are exposed to a large number of children. Some studies find children in family child care homes have a lower relative risk of infection than do children at centers. However, other recent studies by Cordell and Caulicer have documented more infection among children in family child care homes, possibly relating to differences in exclusion criteria between center-based and home-based child care. More hours attending child care also is associated with a higher risk of some infections.

The morbidity from infection acquired in child care settings ranges from minimal to life threatening. Even mild infections, such as upper respiratory illness or otitis

TABLE 17.1. Examples of Infections Caused by Agents Transmitted in Child Care Settings

Disease	Agents
Diarrhea	Rotavirus, astrovirus, calicivirus, enteric adenovirus, *Shigella* species, *Campylobacter* species, *Escherichia coli* O157:H7 and other *E coli* organisms, *Aeromonas* species, *Clostridium difficile, Giardia lamblia, Cryptosporidium* species, hepatitis A virus
Respiratory tract infection, upper and lower (laryngotracheal bronchitis, bronchiolitis, pneumonia)	Rhinovirus, respiratory syncytial virus, influenza and parainfluenza viruses, adenovirus, enterovirus, *Mycoplasma pneumoniae*
Otitis media	*Streptococcus pneumoniae*
Pharyngitis, stomatitis	Group A β-hemolytic streptococci, herpes simplex virus, enteroviruses
Serious or invasive bacterial infections including meningitis, pneumonia, bacteremia, cellulitis, arthritis, etc	*S pneumoniae, Haemophilus influenzae* type b, *Neisseria meningitidis,* group A β-hemolytic streptococci, *Staphylococcus aureus*
Aseptic meningitis	Enterovirus, echovirus 30, others
Hepatitis	Hepatitis A virus, hepatitis B virus
Skin and hair infection	Those causing pediculosis, ringworm, impetigo, scabies
Complicated or febrile infection	Varicella zoster virus, measles, influenza, *Bordetella pertussis, M pneumoniae, Mycobacterium tuberculosis**
Asymptomatic or mild illness	Many, including cytomegalovirus, parvovirus B19, rubella

* Transmission usually from child care provider.

media, often result in visits to health care professionals. Frequent illnesses result in more courses of antibiotics. A pattern of increased resistance to commonly prescribed antibiotics has been recognized for bacteria isolated from children attending child care settings. Most infectious agents spread efficiently in child care settings also are efficiently transmitted to household members and, thus, can be amplified in the community. The substantial role of child care settings as reservoirs of infection disseminated to family members is underappreciated and often unrecognized. Spread of infection to household members by symptomatic children younger than 3 years is best documented. It is common for 12% to 25% of susceptible household members to be infected by an ill child; symptomatic disease in household contacts occurs in as many as 50% to 60% of household contacts for *Shigella* species, enteroviral meningitis, and probably other infections. Spread of infection to household members by asymptomatic children is also well recognized, as with HAV infection. Susceptible mothers who are pregnant are at risk of VZV, CMV, and parvovirus B19

TABLE 17.2. Mode of Transmission of Infectious Agents Spread in Child Care Settings

Mode of Transmission	Example
Fecal to oral: contaminated hands or fomites contaminated with stool organisms (eg, toys, tables [rarely food]) to mouth; contamination of environmental surfaces common	Most agents causing diarrhea: bacteria (eg, *Escherichia coli* O157:H7, *Shigella* species, *Aeromonas* species, *Campylobacter* species), viruses (eg, rotavirus, astrovirus, calicivirus, enteric adenovirus, enteroviruses, hepatitis A virus), and parasites (eg, *Giardia lamblia, Cryptosporidium* species)
Respiratory to mucosal: aerosolized (cough, sneeze) or direct inoculation from hand or fomites contaminated with nasal, oral, or conjunctival secretions; survival on environmental surfaces common	Respiratory viruses (eg, respiratory syncytial virus, influenza, parainfluenza, adenovirus, measles, rubella, mumps, varicella zoster virus), bacteria (eg, group A β-hemolytic streptococci, *Streptococcus pneumoniae, Haemophilus influenzae, Neisseria meningitidis, Staphylococcus aureus, Mycobacterium tuberculosis, Bordetella pertussis*)
Oral to mucosal	Herpes viruses (eg, herpes simplex virus, cytomegalovirus, Epstein-Barr virus)
Oral or respiratory secretions and urine to mucosal: direct inoculation from contaminated hands, fomites	Cytomegalovirus, rubella
Blood or serous fluids to mucosa or broken skin: blood-containing drainage from nose, abrasion, dermatitis, human bite, bleeding gums	Hepatitis B, human immunodeficiency virus
Direct contact: inoculation from contact with skin or fomites	Varicella zoster virus, pediculosis (lice), tinea capitis, group A β-hemolytic streptococci, *S aureus*, scabies

infection acquired from their children; when transmitted to the fetus, severe disease or death occurs in an estimated 2% of VZV infections, 25% of CMV infections, and 4% to 10% of parvovirus B19 infections. Time lost from work or school, morbidity from illness, medical care, and antibiotic resistance result in substantial personal and societal cost.

PREVENTION OF INFECTION TRANSMITTED IN CHILD CARE

When selecting a child care environment, parents can be encouraged to assess the resilience of their child to illness and their own tolerance for infection. Care in a stable family child care home with few or no other children is a consideration for children with chronic health problems or immunodeficiency. Mothers who could become pregnant can be informed about the risk of CMV and parvovirus B19 infection; serologic screening for susceptibility to CMV may allay anxiety and encourage careful handling of respiratory secretions and urine. When family members, including the child, thoroughly wash their hands on return to their home, some studies report a relative decrease in illness in family members. Recognizing the modes of transmission (Table 17.2) and careful adherence to measures that prevent infection in child care settings (Table 17.3) are likely to provide a healthier environment for children, child care providers, and family members.

Parents can minimize their risk of infection through immunization; if the parent is susceptible, immunization against tetanus, diphtheria, measles, mumps, rubella, polio, VZV, HAV, and possibly hepatitis B should be considered. Annual immunization against influenza may decrease time lost from work when influenza is epidemic in the community; influenza is common in children attending child care.

Children attending child care should be immunized according to the most current recommendations of the Advisory Committee for Immunization Practices (ACIP) of the Centers for Disease Control and Prevention, the American Academy of Pediatrics, and the American Academy of Family Physicians (Fig 17.1 [updated annually]). Routine immunization with HAV vaccine currently is recommended for children in child care only during epidemics; when state, county, or community incidence of disease exceeds established levels; or for children at risk of severe infection because of underlying, chronic, or immunodeficiency disease. Hepatitis A infection generally is mild in young children. The purpose of immunizing children in child care is to prevent transmission of HAV to parents or to child care providers who can have debilitating disease. HAV vaccine is currently approved for children starting at 2 years of age, but studies are now being conducted to document safety and efficacy when the vaccine is given at 1 year of age.

Influenza immunization prevents some otitis media, generalized illness in the child, and transmission to other family members. Influenza vaccine can be given annually starting at 6 months of age. Infants and toddlers between 6 and 24 months of age are also at high risk of influenza-associated hospitalization; therefore, the American Academy of Pediatrics recommends influenza immunization for healthy children between 6 and 24 months of age. The American Academy of Pediatrics also recommends annual influenza immunization for all children with high-risk conditions who are 6 months and older. Parents, other family members, and child care providers having contact with children younger than 24 months are also recommended to be immunized to protect infants who are too young to be immunized. Immunization of contacts is particularly important. In addition, pregnant women in their second or third trimester during influenza season are also encouraged to be immunized.

Two pneumococcal vaccines are available for use in children, a protein conjugate pneumococcal vaccine and a purified polysaccharide vaccine. The pneumococcal conjugate vaccine contains 7 pneumococcal types and provides potential protection against 85% to 90% of the serious invasive infection caused by this organism. A 4-dose series (2, 4, 6, and 12–15 months of age) of the conjugate vaccine is

TABLE 17.3. Measures to Decrease Transmission of Infection in Child Care Settings

1. Full immunization (children, parents, and child care providers) according to recommendations of the Advisory Committee on Immunization Practices of the Centers for Disease Control, the American Academy of Pediatrics, and the American Academy of Family Physicians (see Fig 17.1 and Appendix E). Special indications for immunization against:
   - Influenza
   - Hepatitis A virus

2. Small, stable care group, stable child care providers, limited or no time shared with other groups

3. Low turnover, no "drop-in" children, no episodic care or changes in group assignment

4. Facilities
   - Sinks and toilets located conveniently and operational
   - Adequate supplies of soap, towels, toilet paper, and facial tissue for individual use
   - Store toilet items (tooth brush, towels, etc) to prevent shared use

5. Staff trained in effective hand washing techniques for themselves and for children:
   - On arrival
   - Before preparation of food
   - Before eating
   - After toileting and after changing diapers
   - After cleaning faces and nasal secretions
   - After outdoor play
   - On return to the child's home

6. Staff trained in diapering techniques:
   - Disposing of diapers
   - Disinfecting changing surfaces and hands

7. Different staff to prepare food and to care for children

8. Scheduled cleaning of environment and toys:
   - After toys are placed in the mouth or contaminated by body fluids (nasal, blood, urine, stool, vomit)
   - Daily (or as needed) use of freshly prepared bleach solution (a quarter cup bleach to 1 gallon water)

9. Regular staff education and monitoring; training in first aid and cardiopulmonary resuscitation

10. Prompt isolation or exclusion of children for:
    - Illness (see Table 17.5)
    - Potentially infectious condition

11. Develop partnership with parents:
    - Parents can share with facility personnel information about infections diagnosed in child and family members
    - Staff can promptly inform parents of agents infecting children at facility and recommend preventive measures (see Appendix D)
    - Staff can encourage parents to wash hands (child and other family members) on return home

12. Regular medical and public health consultation to:
    - Assess potential health problems at the facility
    - Develop and coordinate intervention

FIG 17.1. Recommended childhood immunization schedule, 2004*

Recommended childhood and adolescent immunization schedule[1] — United States, July-December 2004

Vaccine ▼ / Age ►	Birth	1 mo	2 mo	4 mo	6 mo	12 mo	15 mo	18 mo	24 mo	4-6 y	11-12 y	13-18 y
Hepatitis B[2]	HepB #1	only if mother HBsAg (-) HepB #2	HepB #2		HepB #3						HepB series	
Diphtheria, Tetanus, Pertussis[3]			DTaP	DTaP	DTaP		DTaP			DTaP	Td	Td
Haemophilus Influenzae Type b[4]			Hib	Hib	Hib[4]	Hib						
Inactivated Poliovirus			IPV	IPV	IPV			IPV		IPV		
Measles, Mumps, Rubella[5]						MMR #1				MMR #2	MMR #2	MMR #2
Varicella[6]						Varicella				Varicella	Varicella	
Pneumococcal[7]			PCV	PCV	PCV	PCV	PCV		PCV	PCV	PPV	
Influenza[8]						Influenza (yearly)				Influenza (yearly)	Influenza (yearly)	
Hepatitis A[9]										Hepatitis A series		

Range of Recommended Ages
Catch-up Immunization
Preadolescent Assessment

----- Vaccines below this line are for selected populations

1. Indicates the recommended ages for routine administration of currently licensed childhood vaccines, as of April 1, 2004, for children through age 18 years. Any dose not given at the recommended age should be given at any subsequent visit when indicated and feasible. ▨ Indicates age groups that warrant special effort to administer those vaccines not given previously. Additional vaccines may be licensed and recommended during the year. Licensed combination vaccines may be used whenever any components of the combination are indicated and the vaccine's other components are not contraindicated. Providers should consult the manufacturers' package inserts for detailed recommendations. Clinically significant adverse events that follow vaccination should be reported to the Vaccine Adverse Event Reporting System (VAERS). Guidance about how to obtain and complete a VAERS form is available at http://www.vaers.org/ or by telephone, 1-800-822-7967.

ISS081

(For necessary footnotes and important information, see reverse side.)

* Updated annually (available at http://www.aap.org and http://www.pediatrics.org).

FIG 17.1. Recommended childhood immunization schedule, 2004, continued*

2. **Hepatitis B vaccine (HepB).** All infants should receive the first dose of HepB vaccine soon after birth and before hospital discharge; the first dose may also be given by age 2 months if the infant's mother is HBsAg-negative. Only monovalent HepB vaccine can be used for the birth dose. Monovalent or combination vaccine containing HepB may be used to complete the series; 4 doses of vaccine may be administered when a birth dose is given. The second dose should be given at least 4 weeks after the first dose except for combination vaccines, which cannot be administered before age 6 weeks. The third dose should be given at least 16 weeks after the first dose and at least 8 weeks after the second dose. The last dose in the vaccination series (third or fourth dose) should not be administered before age 24 weeks. Infants born to HBsAg-positive mothers should receive HepB vaccine and 0.5 mL hepatitis B immune globulin (HBIG) within 12 hours of birth at separate sites. The second dose is recommended at age 1-2 months. The last dose in the vaccination series should not be administered before age 24 weeks. These infants should be tested for HBsAg and anti-HBs at 9-15 months of age. Infants born to mothers whose HBsAg status is unknown should receive the first dose of the HepB vaccine series within 12 hours of birth. Maternal blood should be drawn as soon as possible to determine the mother's HBsAg status; if the HBsAg test is positive, the infant should receive HBIG as soon as possible (no later than age 1 week). The second dose is recommended at age 1-2 months. The last dose in the vaccination series should not be administered before age 24 weeks.

3. **Diphtheria and tetanus toxoids and acellular pertussis vaccine (DTaP).** The fourth dose of DTaP may be administered as early as age 12 months provided that 6 months have elapsed since the third dose and the child is unlikely to return at age 15-18 months. The final dose in the series should be given at age ≥4 years. **Tetanus and diphtheria toxoids (Td)** is recommended at age 11-12 years if at least 5 years have elapsed since the last dose of tetanus and diphtheria toxoid-containing vaccine. Subsequent routine Td boosters are recommended every 10 years.

4. **Haemophilus influenzae type b (Hib) conjugate vaccine.** Three Hib conjugate vaccines are licensed for infant use. If PRP-OMP (PedvaxHIB® or ComVax® [Merck]) is administered at ages 2 and 4 months, a dose at age 6 months is not required. DTaP/Hib combination products should not be used for primary vaccination in infants at ages 2, 4, or 6 months but can be used as boosters after any Hib vaccine. The final dose in the series should be given at age ≥12 months.

5. **Measles, mumps, and rubella vaccine (MMR).** The second dose of MMR is recommended routinely at age 4-6 years but may be administered during any visit, provided at least 4 weeks have elapsed since the first dose and both doses are administered beginning at or after age 12 months. Those who have not received the second dose previously should complete the schedule by the visit at age 11-12 years.

6. **Varicella vaccine (VAR).** Varicella vaccine is recommended at any visit at or after age 12 months for susceptible children (i.e., those who lack a reliable history of chickenpox). Susceptible persons aged ≥13 years should receive 2 doses given at least 4 weeks apart.

7. **Pneumococcal vaccine.** The heptavalent pneumococcal conjugate vaccine (PCV) is recommended for all children aged 2-23 months. It is also recommended for certain children aged 24-59 months. The final dose in the series should be given at age ≥12 months. **Pneumococcal polysaccharide vaccine (PPV)** is recommended in addition to PCV for certain high-risk groups. See *MMWR* 2000;49(No. RR-9):1-35.

8. **Influenza vaccine.** Influenza vaccine is recommended annually for children aged ≥6 months with certain risk factors (including but not limited to asthma, cardiac disease, sickle cell disease, HIV, and diabetes), health care workers, and other persons (including household members) in close contact with persons in groups at high-risk (see *MMWR* 2004;53[No. RRE 430]:1-40) and can be administered to all others wishing to obtain immunity. In addition, healthy children aged 6-23 months and close contacts of healthy children aged 0-23 months are recommended to receive influenza vaccine, because children in this age group are at substantially increased risk of influenza-related hospitalizations. For healthy persons aged 5-49 years, the intranasally administered live, attenuated influenza vaccine (LAIV) is an acceptable alternative to the intramuscular trivalent inactivated influenza vaccine (TIV). See *MMWR* 2003;52(No. RR-13):1-8. Children receiving TIV should be administered an age-appropriate dosage (0.25 mL if 6-35 months or 0.5 mL if ≥3 years). Children aged ≤8 years who are receiving influenza vaccine for the first time should receive 2 doses (separated by at least 4 weeks for TIV and at least 6 weeks for LAIV).

9. **Hepatitis A vaccine.** Hepatitis A vaccine is recommended for children and adolescents in selected states and regions and for certain high-risk groups. Consult your local public health authority and *MMWR* 1999; 48(No.RR-12):1-37. Children and adolescents in these states, regions, and high-risk groups who have not been immunized against hepatitis A can begin the hepatitis A vaccination series during any visit. The two doses in the series should be administered at least 6 months apart.

Additional information about vaccines, including precautions and contraindications for vaccination and vaccine shortages is available at http://www.cdc.gov/nip or from the National Immunization Information Hotline, 800-232-2522 (English) or 800-232-0233 (Spanish). Approved by the **Advisory Committee on Immunization Practices** (http://www.cdc.gov/nip/acip), the **American Academy of Pediatrics** (http://www.aap.org), and the **American Academy of Family Physicians** (http://www.aafp.org).

Immunization Protects Children

Regular checkups at your pediatrician's office or local health clinic are an important way to keep children healthy.

By making sure that your child gets immunized on time, you can provide the best available defense against many dangerous childhood diseases. Immunizations protect against: hepatitis B, polio, measles, mumps, rubella (German measles), pertussis (whooping cough), diphtheria, tetanus (lockjaw), *Haemophilus influenzae* type b, pneumococcal infections, and chickenpox. All of these immunizations need to be given before children are 2 years old in order for them to be protected during their most vulnerable period. Are your child's immunizations up-to-date?

The chart on the other side of this fact sheet includes immunization recommendations from the American Academy of Pediatrics. Remember to keep track of your child's immunizations—it's the only way you can be sure your child is up-to-date. Also, check with your pediatrician or health clinic at each visit to find out if your child needs any booster shots or if any new vaccines have been recommended since this schedule was prepared.

If you don't have a pediatrician, call your local health department. Public health clinics usually have supplies of vaccine and may give shots free.

* Updated annually (available at http://www.aap.org and http://www.pediatrics.org).

recommended for all children (Table 17.4). Additional doses of one of the two 23-type pneumococcal polysaccharide vaccines are recommended for children who have underlying health problems increasing the risk of severe or life-threatening pneumococcal infection, particularly children with sickle cell disease or other functional or anatomic asplenia, or children who are members of populations with a higher incidence of severe pneumococcal infections, including American Indian/Alaska Native and black children. The pneumococcal polysaccharide vaccine is given as a single dose only in children at or older than 2 years of age; a booster dose may be repeated 3 to 5 years after the first dose. Children in group child care centers who are 24 to 59 months of age and all healthy children who are 24 to 35 months of age are also at higher risk of serious pneumococcal infection and should receive a single dose of pneumococcal conjugate vaccine if they have not previously been immunized as infants. As part of the routine infant immunization series, the pneumococcal conjugate vaccine is expected to have a significant effect on the incidence of otitis media, pneumonia, meningitis, and bacteremia in children younger than 5 years. The FDA has recently approved the pneumococcal conjugate vaccine to be considered in children with severe or recurrent otitis media. Also, by decreasing the use of antibiotics, it is hoped that the pneumococcal conjugate vaccine will diminish the incidence of antibiotic-resistant pneumococci among children in child care.

A polyvalent meningococcal conjugate vaccine is not yet available. However, a polysaccharide protein conjugate vaccine for group C meningococcal disease has been licensed in Europe, and research is ongoing to produce an effective vaccine to control meningococcal disease in all age groups.

Although few investigations have examined the efficacy of criteria to exclude children from child care, practical considerations and the usual duration of time children are contagious provide a basis for making these decisions (Table 17.5). Children should not attend child care if they are too ill to participate fully in the scheduled activities unless special resources are available for their care and isolation (see Chapter 18, Care of the Mildly Ill Child). Children with treatable agents causing infection can return when they are no longer infectious, as indicated in the *2003 Red Book,* and their ongoing care can be managed in their child care setting (some children with noncontagious diarrhea require too many diaper changes for child care staff to manage).

Parents who have difficulty leaving work for the duration of their child's illnesses may wish to identify temporary alternative care suitable for a child recovering from illness. During outbreaks of infection in child care, parents can be cautioned to follow the specific plan for control. If their child remains infectious despite feeling well, they should return to the usual facility rather than to alternative child care. Children who are taken to other child care centers can spread the infectious agent to a new group of children and amplify the epidemic.

TABLE 17.4. Summary of Recommendations for Use of 7-Valent Pneumococcal Conjugate Vaccine (PCV7) Among Infants and Children

Children for Whom PCV7 Is Recommended

All children younger than 23 months
Children 24–59 months of age with the following conditions:
- Sickle cell disease and other sickle cell hemoglobinopathies, congenital or acquired asplenia, or splenic dysfunction
- Infection with human immunodeficiency virus
- Immunocompromising conditions, including
  - ~ Congenital immunodeficiencies: B- (humoral) or T-lymphocyte deficiency; complement deficiencies, particularly c1, c2, c3, and c4 deficiency; and phagocytic disorders, excluding chronic granulomatous disease
  - ~ Renal failure and nephrotic syndrome
  - ~ Diseases associated with immunosuppressive therapy or radiation therapy, including malignant neoplasms, leukemias, lymphomas, and Hodgkin's disease; or solid organ transplantation
- Chronic illness, including
  - ~ Chronic cardiac disease, particularly cyanotic congenital heart disease and cardiac failure
  - ~ Chronic pulmonary disease, excluding asthma unless on high-dose corticosteroid therapy
  - ~ Cerebrospinal fluid leaks
  - ~ Diabetes mellitus
- Cochlear implants

Children for Whom PCV7 Should Be Considered

All children 24–59 months of age, with priority given to
- Children 24–35 months of age
- Children of Alaska Native or American Indian descent
- Children of African American descent
- Children who attend group child care centers*

*Defined as a setting outside the home in which a child regularly spends 4 or more hours per week with 2 or more unrelated children under adult supervision.

Adapted from Centers for Disease Control and Prevention. Preventing pneumococcal disease among infants and young children. *MMWR Morb Mortal Wkly Rep.* 2000;49(RR-9):1–38

ANTIBIOTIC USE AND ANTIMICROBIAL RESISTANCE

The National Center for Health Statistics of the CDC National Ambulatory Medical Care Surveys found more than a 25% increase in the use of antibiotics in children during the last decade. The largest portion of the antibiotics were prescribed for viral upper respiratory tract infections and otitis media. Antibiotics also were used to treat diarrheal illness, most of which is viral. Unnecessary use of broad, rather than narrow-spectrum, antibiotics has been observed as part of this trend. The most important factor predicting isolation of antibiotic resistant bacteria is use of an antibiotic within the previous 1 to 3 months. Bacteria isolated from children attending child care have coincidentally shown increasing resistance to commonly

TABLE 17.5. Criteria for Excluding Children From Child Care Settings

- Illness that prevents the child from participating comfortably in program activities.

- Illness that results in a need for care that is greater than the staff can provide without compromising the health and safety of other children.

- Any of the following conditions suggesting possible severe illness: fever, lethargy, irritability, persistent crying, difficult breathing, or other manifestations of possible severe illness.

- Diarrhea or stools that contain blood or mucus.

- Shiga toxin-producing *Escherichia coli,* including *E coli* O157:H7, or *Shigella* infection, until diarrhea resolves and results of 2 stool cultures are negative for these organisms.

- Vomiting 2 or more times during the previous 24 hours, unless the vomiting is determined to be caused by a noncommunicable condition and the child is not in danger of dehydration.

- Mouth sores associated with drooling, unless the child's physician or local health department authority states that the child is noninfectious.

- Rash with fever or behavioral change, until a physician has determined the illness is not a communicable disease.

- Purulent conjunctivitis (defined as pink or red conjunctiva with white or yellow eye discharge, often with matted eyelids after sleep and eye pain or redness of the eyelids or skin surrounding the eye), until examined by a physician and approved for readmission.

- Tuberculosis, until the child's physician or local health department authority states that the child is noninfectious.

- Impetigo, until 24 hours after treatment has been initiated.

- Streptococcal pharyngitis, until 24 hours after treatment has been initiated.

- Head lice (pediculosis), until after the first treatment.

- Scabies, until after treatment has been given.

- Varicella, until all lesions have dried and crusted (usually 6 days after onset of rash).

- Pertussis, until 5 days of appropriate antimicrobial therapy (which is to be given for a total of 14 days) have been completed.

- Mumps, until 9 days after onset of parotid gland swelling.

- Measles, until 4 days after onset of rash.

- Hepatitis A virus (HAV) infection, until 1 week after onset of illness or jaundice (if symptoms are mild).

*See Chapter 18.

†See Fig 17.1.

‡Criteria for specific agents are listed in American Academy of Pediatrics. *Red Book: 2003 Report of the Committee on Infectious Diseases.* Pickering LK, ed. 26th ed. Elk Grove Village, IL: American Academy of Pediatrics; 2003 or with medical clearance.

See Pennsylvania Chapter, American Academy of Pediatrics. *Preparing for Illness.* Available at: http://www.paaap.org/mod.php?mod=userpage&page_id=11&menu=. Accessed April 16, 2002 used antibiotics. Children in child care are now recognized as personal and institutional reservoirs for an array of bacteria that are resistant to commonly used antibiotics (Table 17.6).

Health care professionals treating children in child care face the triple challenge of adequately treating infection, minimizing the use of antibiotics, and educating families to the benefits of more judicious use of antibiotics. Antibiotics rarely benefit patients with common respiratory and diarrheal infections, which are viral. For otitis media, narrower-spectrum antibiotics (eg, amoxicillin) frequently have similar or better rates of cure than broad-spectrum and more costly alternatives (reviewed by Rosenfeld). For example, for otitis media, use of a cephalosporin or macrolide in preference to amoxicillin provides little clinical advantage in treating *S pneumoniae* with low-level resistance and no benefit in high-level resistance. In a publication from a CDC working group on drug-resistant *S pneumoniae,* amoxicillin was recommended as the drug of choice for treating otitis media. However, children at high risk of infection with drug-resistant organisms (younger than 2 years, recent antibiotic use, child care attendance) should have high-dose amoxicillin (80–90 mg/kg per day) as first-line therapy. Children at low risk of infection with drug-resistant organisms can continue to receive 40 to 45 mg/kg per day of amoxicillin. In the event of treatment failure, this report recommends the use of amoxicillin-clavulanate, cefuroxime axetil, or intramuscular ceftriaxone. Many factors unrelated to antibiotic resistance may contribute to treatment failures, including failure to comply with treatment regimen, poor absorption from the gastrointestinal tract, inadequate penetration of the antibiotic to the site of infection (eg, middle ear), unfavorable anatomy, or new infection. Otitis media with effusion is an asymptomatic condition, which is part of the natural history of resolving acute otitis media. It routinely persists for up to 3 months and does not respond to additional courses of antibiotics.

TABLE 17.6. Agents With Increased Prevalence of Antibiotic Resistance in Children Attending Child Care

Agent With Decreased Susceptibility	Antibiotic
Shigella species	Amoxicillin, trimethoprim-sulfamethoxazole
Escherichia coli O157:H7	Trimethoprim-sulfamethoxazole
Streptococcus pneumoniae	Penicillin, cephalosporins, trimethoprim-sulfamethoxazole, macrolides (erythromycin)
Group A β-hemolytic streptococci	Erythromycin (especially in Europe, Asia)
Haemophilus influenzae type b	Amoxicillin
Methicillin-resistant *Staphylococcus aureus*	Semisynthetic penicillins (eg, oxacillin, methicillin), cephalosporins, macrolides

Pharyngitis also is common with viral respiratory infections, including influenza. Treatment of pharyngitis with antibiotics benefits patients with laboratory-confirmed group A β-hemolytic streptococcal infection or, rarely, other bacteria (eg, diphtheria, *Arcanobacterium haemolyticum*). An important factor in decreasing parents' expectation for antibiotics is recovery from a previous viral respiratory illness without the health care professional prescribing antibiotics. Judicious use of antibiotics decreases selection of resistant strains of bacteria and the necessity for broad-spectrum antibiotics. Parents and child care providers may benefit from educational materials explaining the advantages of judicious use of antibiotics for their children.

CONTROL AND MANAGEMENT OF INFECTION TRANSMITTED IN CHILD CARE SETTINGS

Information from parents, child care providers, and health care professionals may make it possible to connect seemingly isolated cases of illness in family members with endemic or epidemic disease at a child care facility. Once information about illness is conveyed to the director or operator of the facility and to public health officials, a plan for control of infection can be developed. Parents and health care professionals in the community are more likely to comply with recommendations for intervention if informed promptly and fully about the infection and measures for control.

Hepatitis A

Recognizing epidemic HAV infection in child care settings requires a high degree of awareness. Hepatitis A infection typically is asymptomatic in infants; symptomatic illness occurs sporadically in older children and adult contacts. Transmission by the fecal-oral route is efficient in groups of infants who are in diapers. Epidemic HAV infection in a child care setting should be suspected when the infection is diagnosed in 1 or more parent, sibling, or care provider of an infant attending the facility (Table 17.7). Without intervention, transmission can continue for more than a year and account for a large number of cases in the community. Health care professionals caring for patients with HAV infection should determine whether the patient had exposure to an infant or toddler attending child care and report to public health officials the name of the contact child and the child care facility.

Comprehensive use of intramuscular immune globulin (IG) is effective in stopping epidemic disease in child care settings and decreases the incidence of HAV infections in the community (Table 17.7). Failures occur when IG is refused or when new children are enrolled at the facility without receiving IG prophylaxis or HAV vaccine. Active immunization with HAV vaccine can be given in addition to IG, although experience using this strategy is limited. Even 1 dose of HAV vaccine can be effective in preventing disease if administered early after exposure. Hepatitis A vaccine can be given to children whose risk of HAV infection is continuing. The

TABLE 17.7. Management of Hepatitis A Virus Infection in Child Care Facilities

1. Notify public health officials for assistance

2. Confirm diagnosis of recent infection: presence of immunoglobulin M antibody to hepatitis A virus in:
   - Patient
   - (Ideally) contact child or employee at the facility, even if asymptomatic

3. Review measures to decrease fecal-oral transmission:
   - Hand washing by staff and children
   - Procedures for changing diapers and preparing food
   - Exclusion policy for children with uncontained stool (diarrhea)
   - Use of bleach solution for environmental cleaning

4. Identify additional cases in household contacts of children at the facility

5. Close facility to new attendees until protected or for 6 weeks after the last case*

6. Allow patient to return to the facility when well, if more than 1 week from onset of illness

7. Administer immune globulin (IG [0.2 mL/kg of body weight, maximum 3 mL, once intramuscularly]) and hepatitis A vaccine[†] as follows:

Number of Cases	Patient's Relationship to Child Care Facility	IG[‡]
1	Child or employee, or parent of diapered child at the facility	Classroom contacts (children and employees)
2 or more	Contact of unrelated children attending the facility	All children and child care providers at the facility, household contacts of diapered children, and any new children enrolling at the facility for 6 weeks after the last case[†]

* Alternative: exclude newly enrolling children for 2 (to 4) weeks after administrating hepatitis A vaccine.

[†] Hepatitis A vaccine is approved for children 24 months or older and adults (see Fig 17.1). Experience using hepatitis A vaccine to control epidemic disease in child care is limited. Hepatitis A vaccine can be given with (but not as a substitute for) IG if administered at different sites. During vaccine trials, most patients who were given vaccine seroconverted 2 to 4 weeks after a single dose; initial serum concentrations of antibody were lower when vaccine was administered with IG than without but were similar after a booster dose. Administration of vaccine modified or prevented hepatitis A infection and decreased shedding of virus when administered early in the incubation period. Hepatitis A vaccine can be given widely if a continuing risk of hepatitis A infection is anticipated. Serologic screening for immunity to hepatitis A infection before immunization may be cost effective in adults and older children in populations at increased risk of hepatitis A. Serum must be obtained before administering IG.

[‡] Persons without documented history of hepatitis A infection.

vaccine is approved for use in adults and in children as young as 24 months. Studies are currently underway to determine safety and efficacy of this vaccine given at 1 year of age. Several states with high rates of hepatitis A have implemented mandates for routine HAV immunization before entry into school or child care. The ACIP currently recommends routine immunization for children 2 to 18 years of age who live in states, counties, or communities with high rates of hepatitis A infection (more than 20 cases per 100 000 population). In locales with intermediate rates of hepatitis A infection (more than 10 cases per 100 000 population), routine immunization against hepatitis A should be considered.

E coli O157:H7 Infection

Outbreaks of severe and complicated *E coli* O157:H7 infection are well described in child care settings. *E coli* O157:H7 belongs to a group of *E coli* that produce shigella-like toxin (verotoxins). Infection often results in hemorrhagic colitis, which can be followed by hemolytic-uremic syndrome in children (hemolytic anemia, thrombocytopenia, renal failure), or by thrombotic thrombocytopenia in adults. *E coli* O157:H7 is efficiently spread by fecal-oral transmission in child care settings and from infected children to household members. The highest symptomatic attack rate is in preschool-aged children. Diarrhea is the most common sign of the illness; fever is variable. Diarrhea commonly progresses from nonbloody to hemorrhagic and is accompanied by abdominal cramping. Hemolytic-uremic syndrome complicates *E coli* O157:H7 infection in 2% to 7% of children; fatality rates are 3% to 9%.

Most diarrheal illness caused by *E coli* O157:H7 resolves in 6 to 8 days in children. However, Manicle et al found that *E coli* O157:H7 continues to be shed in stool for a mean of 29 days and may be present for as long as 62 days. The duration of shedding is similar for children with hemorrhagic and nonbloody diarrhea. A small proportion of children shed this agent intermittently. Currently, there is no specific therapy (other than careful attention to fluid and electrolyte intake and renal and hematologic profiles) recommended for the treatment of *E coli* O157:H7 hemorrhagic colitis. Antimicrobial treatment does not appear to alter the course of the disease and may increase the risk of hemolytic-uremic syndrome. For this reason, antibiotics should usually be reserved for children in whom systemic infection is suspected. Infected children should not return to the facility until diarrhea has ceased and 2 consecutive stool samples spaced at least 48 hours apart are negative on bacteriologic culture.

Unlike the management of other epidemic diarrheal disease in child care, most experts recommend temporarily closing child care facilities to new admissions affected by *E coli* O157:H7 (Table 17.8). Exclusion of infected children increases the possibility that parents will enroll their child in another child care facility, thereby amplifying the outbreak. It is crucial that parents understand the serious implications of spread to other children. When reopened, child care personnel can be cautioned to scrupulously adhere to measures that decrease transmission (Table 17.3).

Other Diarrheal Illness

The management of other diarrheal agents affecting children in child care settings is similar to that for *E coli* O157:H7 (Table 17.9), except that the children generally are allowed to return to child care when they are asymptomatic. If the agent caus-

---

TABLE 17.8. Management of *Escherichia coli* O157:H7 Infection in Child Care Settings

1. Urgently report suspected or confirmed infection to public health officials and request assistance

2. Confirm diagnosis by culture of stool on selective medium (sorbitol)

3. Patients with diarrhea should remain at home until stools have returned to normal consistency, and 2 (or 3) consecutive stool specimen test results are negative for *Eschericha coli* O157:H7 using selective culture medium. Stool samples for culture are collected at least 48 hours apart when the child is not taking an antibiotic.

4. Enforce measures to decrease fecal-oral transmission:
   - Hand washing
   - Diaper changing techniques and disposal
   - Environmental cleaning with bleach solution

5. Close facility to new enrollees until:
   - All culture test results are negative
   - There are no new cases for at least 2 weeks after the last illness

6. Educate parents about:
   - Potential seriousness of infection
   - How to prevent spread of the agent
   - Not taking their child to another facility (and, thus, transmitting agent to other children)
   - Criteria for return to center (above)

7. No known benefit from use of antibiotic:
   - Does not modify course of disease
   - Does not prevent, and may increase the occurrence of, hemolytic-uremic syndrome

---

ing diarrhea is easily transmitted, infected children can be cohorted until a stool sample reveals that it is negative. Some agents, such as *G lamblia,* have become endemic in child care settings and are not eliminated from environmental surfaces with standard bleach solutions or other simple measures. Compliance with measures to control infections transmitted in child care (Table 17.3) is the hallmark of prevention and control of these agents.

Group A β-hemolytic Streptococci

Streptococcus pyogenes, or group A β-hemolytic streptococci (GABHS), infection is endemic in children attending child care. GABHS regularly colonizes the pharynx of about 25% of children, with the highest rates in older preschool-aged children. Colonization has been documented in up to 80% of children during the peak season of disease. Several strains of GABHS usually are present. Most infections are asymptomatic. Colonization persists for 3 months or more in at least one fifth of children. When the prevalence of colonization is high, GABHS is found widely on environmental surfaces. Toys and other items, which come in contact with nasal or oral secretions (eg, pillow, toothbrush), have the highest rates of contamination. Efficient transmission occurs through person-to-person spread and from environmental contact. About one quarter of parents, one third of siblings, and 10% to 25%

TABLE 17.9. Management of Diarrheal Disease in Child Care Settings*

1. Promptly report to public health officials and request assistance

2. Confirm specific diagnosis

3. Notify parents about:
   - Specific agent, symptoms, mode of transmission
   - Plan for controlling infection
   - When to seek medical attention
   - Informing child care staff of new cases
   - Criteria for return to the facility
   - Not taking child to another child care facility

4. Strictly enforce measures to decrease infection in child care, including hand washing, diaper changing techniques, and use of bleach solution[†] (Table 17.3)

5. Exclude symptomatic children with diarrhea until stools return to normal consistency

6. Mass screening to identify asymptomatic, infected children using bacteriologic culture; tests for ova and parasites or antigens are generally helpful only if the outbreak persists

Control Measure*	Agent
Enforce measures to decrease transmission: essential to stop epidemic	All agents: rotavirus, calicivirus, *Shigella* species, *Giardia lamblia, Cryptosporidium* species, *Escherichia coli* including *E coli* O157:H7,[‡] *Salmonella* species, *Campylobacter* species, *Clostridium difficile, Aeromonas* species, hepatitis A,[‡] etc
Close facility to new admissions during outbreak	*Shigella* species, *Cryptosporidium* species, *Salmonella* species, *E coli* O157:H7, others
Diagnosis and treatment of symptomatic children	*Shigella* species, *Campylobacter* species, *G lamblia, C difficile,* others
Treat asymptomatic, infected children	*Shigella* species
Mass treatment not effective in eradicating agent	*G lamblia, Salmonella* species, most other agents
Cohort infected, recovering children on return to the facility; assign dedicated child care providers	*Shigella* species, *Campylobacter* species, *Salmonella* species
Negative stool cultures (at least 2 cultures obtained 48 hours apart) before cohorted children return to regular group at the facility	*Shigella* species, *Salmonella* species (consider)

* No studies have determined optimal management of epidemic disease for many agents.

† Cysts of *G lamblia* and *Cryptosporidium* species are not killed by bleach solution or environmental disinfectants. Scrupulous hand washing is most effective in controlling epidemics. Symptomatic children with *G lamblia* infection should receive specific therapy.

‡ See Table 17.7 and Table 17.8 for management of hepatitis A and *E coli* O157:H7.

of child care providers become infected. In a Swedish study in which erythromycin resistance served as a marker, centers with high rates of infection served as a reservoir for continuing to spread GABHS to the community at large.

Symptomatic GABHS infection in child care occurs most commonly as pharyngitis in children older than 3 years and as purulent nasal discharge in younger children. Up to 25% of new infections can be symptomatic. Whether children attending child care have higher rates of symptomatic infection than do children who are not in child care has not been determined. Children suspected of having symptomatic GABHS infection should be tested via bacteriologic culture and treated if results are positive (Table 17.10). Ill children are most infectious early in the disease process and should be excluded from child care during the first 24 hours of antibiotic treatment. Return to the facility is contingent on recovering sufficiently to participate fully in activities while completing the course of antibiotics.

Invasive GABHS infection in children most often complicates VZV infection. Despite the high prevalence of GABHS colonization and efficient transmission of VZV in child care, severe or fatal invasive GABHS infection is rare. Subsequent cases of severe invasive GABHS infection are described in household contacts, usually in the elderly. More than one case of invasive GABHS infection has been described in child care classmates who also had VZV infection.

In some circumstances, bacteriologic culture and prophylactic administration of antibiotics are recommended for asymptomatic household contacts of patients with GABHS infection and have been given to child care classmates of a child with GABHS infection, regardless of the results of bacteriologic culture. However, no intervention is routinely recommended for asymptomatic child care contacts of

---

TABLE 17.10. Management of Invasive Group A β-Hemolytic Streptococci Infection in Child Care Settings

1. Encourage routine varicella immunization
   - Varicella infection is the most common predisposing illness in children with invasive group A β-hemolytic streptococci disease

2. Notify public health officials and request assistance

3. No consensus regarding the use of antibiotic prophylaxis for children attending child care with invasive group A β-hemolytic streptococcal disease

4. Consider:
   - Asymptomatic colonization with group A β-hemolytic streptococci is common in child care settings
   - Household contacts of children attending child care are a reservoir of group A β-hemolytic streptococci
   - Efficacy of prophylactic antibiotic regimens for eradicating asymptomatic colonization in children is low—50% to 70% 2 weeks after treatment
   - Benefit of extensive culture surveys (child care attendees, staff, household members) to determine who is colonized and might be treated is not defined
   - Children with local or systemic infection should complete 24 hours of antibiotic therapy before returning to the facility

patients with local or systemic GABHS infection. Suspected outbreaks and severe GABHS disease at a facility should be reported promptly to public health officials. Parents should be notified of sufficient details to allow full evaluation by the child's health care professional (see Appendix D). Attempts to eradicate colonization through comprehensive bacteriologic culture and administration of antibiotics have had limited success. Antibiotic regimens effective in treating symptomatic infection are less effective in eradicating colonization and are more effective in adults than in children. In the Swedish experience with an erythromycin-resistant strain, all children and child care providers and all of their household members were monitored with bacteriologic culture until negative for GABHS. Persons with positive cultures were treated with 2 or more courses of antibiotics. The rates of eradication were 97% for adults and 84% for children.

Head Lice

Head lice *(Pediculosis capitis)* is a common cause of infestation for children younger than 12 years, affecting approximately 6 to 12 million children annually. Although infestation is commonly associated with an intense emotional response on the part of parents and teachers, lice are principally a nuisance. They do not spread disease.

The adult louse is 2 to 3 mm long (about the size of a sesame seed). The adult female may lay 200 to 300 eggs during a 3- to 4-week life span. The eggs attach to the hair shaft close to the scalp by a strong chitin secreted by the louse. The eggs hatch in 7 to 10 days, and the emerging nymphs develop into mature adults within 9 to 12 days, at which time they begin reproducing. The empty egg casings remain attached to the hair shaft and move further from the scalp as the hair grows. In general, because body heat is required for incubation, any nits found more than a quarter inch from the scalp are probably empty egg casings and, therefore, not capable of infestation. The louse requires a blood meal from the host every 4 to 6 hours and cannot survive for more than approximately 48 hours away from the human host.

Lice crawl. They do not hop, jump, or fly, and they require close contact for transmission to occur. Head lice infestations occur with short and long hair, irrespective of good hygiene by the host.

Diagnosis requires finding live lice or viable nits. Nits must be within a quarter inch of the scalp to be viable and are best seen at the nape of the neck or behind the ears. Unlike dandruff, dry skin, or dirt, nits are firmly cemented to the hair shaft and are not easily removed. Because only a small proportion of children with nits within a quarter inch of the scalp (22%–33%) will actually become infested, some experts recommend making the diagnosis only when a living louse is found. Children with head lice usually scratch their head to relieve the itching and may develop secondary bacterial infections of the scalp and enlarged lymph nodes, especially at the back of the neck.

Treatment

A variety of potential treatments are available. When recommending a treatment modality, it is important to keep in mind the fact that head lice cause no known disease, and infestation is more a nuisance than a health threat. The following factors should be considered: safety, efficacy, expense, tolerability, and labor intensiveness of treatment. Topical insecticides, oral agents, rigorous wet combing, and numerous alternative therapies have been suggested.

Pediculicides are generally topical agents with activity against live lice and, to a variable degree, nits. Resistance has been reported to most pediculicides, but the extent of this problem is unclear.

Permethrin (1%), an over-the-counter synthetic pyrethroid, is currently the treatment of choice for head lice. It kills live lice and is ovicidal for 70% to 80% of eggs. Nix (Warner-Lambert Consumer Healthcare, Morris Plains, NJ), the commercially available product, is a creme rinse that is applied after shampooing and towel drying the hair, left on the hair for 10 minutes, then rinsed off. Permethrin 1% leaves a pesticidal residue that persists for up to 14 days to kill any emerging nymphs and prevent reinfestation. Treatment may be repeated in 7 to 10 days if live lice are seen or may be routinely recommended by some physicians.

Pyrethrins with piperonyl butoxide (eg, Rid [Bayer, Pittsburgh, PA]) are available over-the-counter as shampoos that are applied to dry hair and left on the hair for 10 minutes before rinsing. Retreatment 7 to 10 days later is recommended. Lindane 1% is a prescription organochloride shampoo with relatively low ovicidal activity, documented resistance, and potential neurotoxicity if used inappropriately. It is not currently recommended for the treatment of head lice.

Malathion 0.5% (Ovide [Medicis Pharmaceutical Corporation, Scottsdale, AZ]) is an organophosphate prescription lotion that is left on the hair for 8 to 12 hours before rinsing. It is highly effective against head lice and nits but is flammable because of its high alcohol content. For this reason, malathion lotion should be used with extreme caution and reserved as a second-line treatment if resistance is suspected. In addition, Ovide is contraindicated in neonates and infants because of the possibility of increased absorption. Package labeling also indicates that safety and efficacy has not been established through controlled trials for children younger than 6 years.

Oral medications, including the antibiotic trimethoprim-sulfamethoxazole and ivermectin, an anti-helminth, have been the topic of anecdotal reports and small studies that have suggested efficacy against lice. These products are not approved by the Food and Drug Administration as pediculicides and have not been rigorously studied for this purpose. Experience with ivermectin in children is limited, and this product may pose a risk of neurotoxicity, particularly in children weighing less than 15 kg.

Rigorous wet combing has been proposed as an alternative to pediculicides. Although limited efficacy data are available, one study found that only 38% of children were "cured" by wet combing alone. If performed to treat a head lice infestation, combing of wet hair (usually treated with a cream rinse to make combing easier) should be done frequently (daily to once every 3 days) for a period of approximately 2 weeks and then once or twice weekly for another several weeks. Each session should continue until no further lice are found on the comb, usually 15 to 30 minutes. Special fine-toothed combs should be used to wet comb the child's hair, and the comb should be inspected for live lice and rinsed after each stroke. The use of electrically charged combs is discouraged because of the risk of electrical shock.

Alternative agents, primarily occlusive agents, such as petrolatum, hair pomades, mayonnaise, and olive oil, are purported to work by obstruction of the respiratory apparatus of lice. Again, only anecdotal information is available regarding the effectiveness of these products, and some are so viscous that repeated shampooing is necessary to remove the residue.

After treatment with a pediculicide, manual removal of nits is probably not important in decreasing transmission. However, nit removal decreases the occurrence of misdiagnosis and overtreatment. Special, fine-toothed metal nit combs may facilitate the nit removal process and should be used on wet hair after shampooing.

"No-nit" policies are discouraged by the American Academy of Pediatrics and the National Association of School Nurses for school-aged populations. Less is known about head lice control in the child care environment, but it is likely that closer contact among children in this setting may increase transmission and, in some circumstances, may warrant stricter guidelines.

If children are discovered to have a head lice infestation while in child care, reasonable care to minimize head-to-head contact should be taken, and parents should be notified of the infestation by phone or privately when they arrive to pick up the child. Written guidelines regarding the diagnosis and treatment of head lice should be given to all parents, and parents of all children in the child care environment should be instructed to check their children for head lice at home. Children should not routinely be sent home from child care because of head lice.

Pediatricians should assist child care programs in developing appropriate guidelines and policies for the management of head lice infestations and accurate informational material for parents.

Meningitis and Other Invasive Bacterial Infections

Attending group child care increases the risk of severe infection caused by Hib, *S pneumoniae,* and probably *Neisseria meningitidis.* Strains of these bacteria are classified by the type of polysaccharide capsule elaborated by the bacteria. *H influenzae* strains are classified as nontypable (no capsule) or capsular types a to f. Nonencapsulated (nontypable) strains are common inhabitants of the respiratory tract and in otitis media; almost all serious infections in children are caused by encapsulated type b strains. Similarly, many of the more than 80 types of *S pneumoniae* colonize the respiratory tract during life and are isolated from middle ear and respiratory infections; only about 9 capsular types account for most cases of invasive disease in children. Among the capsular types of *N meningitidis*, serogroups A, B, C, W-135, and Y cause invasive disease. Serogroups B and C are most common in children in the United States.

The highest rates of serious infection caused by these bacteria are in children younger than 2 years, in the elderly, and in persons with immunodeficiency. Serious infection occurs infrequently in healthy older children and adults. The usual portal of entry is the upper respiratory tract. Spread from one asymptomatic child to another occurs in respiratory secretions, especially from the nose. Healthy children remain colonized for brief periods or for weeks or months. There is no defined incubation period. Invasion leading to severe infection is thought to be facilitated by coinfection with respiratory viruses. The immature antibody response to capsular polysaccharides in infants is likely to be a major factor responsible for the higher rates of disease in young children.

Meningitis, bacteremia, pneumonia, cellulitis, and arthritis are the most common diagnoses associated with these organisms. Serious infection, regardless of the diagnosis, has the same implications for management of contacts in child care. "Primary disease" in a child who attends child care is defined as a serious infection unrelated to contact with a previous case at the facility. The risk of primary disease caused by Hib and *S pneumoniae* is increased for susceptible children who attend child care. Wide use of Hib protein-conjugate vaccines has prevented most serious Hib disease in children in the United States. The risk of primary disease caused by *S pneumoniae* in children younger than 2 years is estimated about 2.5 times higher for children who attend child care than for children who receive care at home. No estimates are available for *N meningitidis*. It is anticipated that widespread use of the *S pneumoniae* conjugate vaccine will significantly decrease the incidence of invasive disease caused by this organism.

"Subsequent disease" in a child who attends child care is defined as serious infection that occurs soon after another case at the facility. It is assumed the patient with subsequent disease acquired the infection from a child with asymptomatic colonization or possibly from the previous patient. This concept differs from "secondary disease," which is defined by transmission from an index patient within a defined incubation period. Before universal immunization in the United States, the risk of subsequent disease caused by Hib was increased in some studies for child care classmates younger than 2 years. The risk of subsequent disease is not defined for *S pneumoniae* and *N meningitidis*; however, clusters of cases in child care settings have been reported uncommonly for both agents. Prophylactic antibiotics are recommended for contacts in child care after serious Hib and *N meningitidis* infection (Table 17.11).

TABLE 17.11. Management of Children in Child Care Exposed to a Patient With Invasive Bacterial Disease*

Background and Recommendation	Haemophilus influenzae type b	Streptococcus pneumoniae	Neisseria meningitidis
Increased risk of primary disease in child care	Yes; greater risk in center than in home care	Yes; greater in center care than in home care	Unknown
Increased risk of subsequent disease	Controversial, child younger than 2 y	Unknown, clusters of cases reported	Unknown, clusters of cases reported
Period of highest risk of subsequent disease	0–60 d	Unknown	Unknown; probably 30 d
Indications for intervention	Second case in classmate, within 60 d, and other classmates younger than 2 y not immunized	Undetermined	Primary case is child care attendee or employee
Notify parents and public health officials	1 case	1 case	1 case
Antibiotic prophylaxis indicated for all classmates and care providers[†]	2 cases: rifampin[‡] 20 mg/kg of body weight, once daily, orally for 4 d (maximum daily dose, 600 mg)	None	1 case: rifampin[‡] 10 mg/kg, twice daily, orally for 2 d (maximum daily dose, 600 mg) or ceftriaxone 125 mg (adults 250 mg), once intramuscularly
Immunization	Recommended for all children 2 to 60 mo; ensure up-to-date for age	See Fig 17.1	2 cases N meningitidis type A or C disease: all eligible children and adults

* Meningitis, bacteremia, pneumonia, arthritis, cellulitis, epiglottitis, etc.

† Supervised and simultaneous administration decreases, failures and recolonization. Indicated for all classmates and child care providers when any child is not immunized.

‡ Contraindicated in pregnancy, allergy, liver disease. Interacts with protein-bound drugs. Medication stains urine, tears, saliva, and soft contact lenses red-orange color. Birth control pills may be ineffective during use.

Agents Transmitted in Blood: Hepatitis B Virus and Human Immunodeficiency Virus

Transmission of hepatitis B virus and human immunodeficiency virus (HIV) occurs after virus in blood or blood-containing fluids reaches mucus membranes or broken skin. Nonsexual transmission among members of a household is well documented for hepatitis B infection. For both agents, anecdotal accounts suggest transmission is most likely to occur between siblings or to individuals providing medical care. Accounts of transmission after a human bite are anecdotal.

Transmission of hepatitis B has rarely been documented in child care settings; transmission of HIV infection has not been reported in a child care setting. The highest risk of transmission for hepatitis B infection is from asymptomatic, chronically infected children who are carriers of hepatitis B e antigen or from someone with acute hepatitis B infection. Because most young children in the United States are immunized against hepatitis B infection, the risk of acquiring hepatitis B infection in a child care setting is exceedingly low. The risk of acquiring HIV infection in the child care setting has not been estimated, because no transmission has been documented. With both infections, affected children or adults are likely to be asymptomatic or undiagnosed at the time they participate in child care. The basis for preventing acquisition of either agent is careful adherence to precautions for handling blood and blood-containing serous fluids.

Child care providers benefit from having written procedures for handling blood and serous fluids (eg, abrasion, epistaxis) and from having training in use of these protocols (Table 17.12). All children can be considered potentially infectious. It is important not to exaggerate or to minimize the risk of transmission. Persons cleaning spills of blood or serous fluids should wear gloves and use a bleach solution on environmental surfaces and toys (Table 17.13). Draining, actively bleeding, or oozing wounds should be covered, and the child should be removed from contact with other children until the potentially infectious body fluid is contained. Children who have aggressive or biting behavior place themselves and other children at increased risk of infection and can be excluded until the behavior is modified.

An important consideration for children with HIV infection is whether repeated infections place them at greater risk of progression of their disease or of more severe disease. Close medical supervision is recommended. Children with chronic infections, for example, with *Cryptosporidium* species, require evaluation for potential spread to other children. Infection with *Mycobacterium tuberculosis* requires particularly careful evaluation before allowing a child with HIV infection to attend child care. Some experts advise that one person at the child care center be informed when a child has hepatitis B or HIV infection so that potential exposures are managed appropriately. This information should remain confidential unless consent is given by the parent or guardian and is accompanied by education of other parents and child care providers.

TABLE 17.12. Prevention of Transmission of Bloodborne Diseases in Child Care

Characteristic	Hepatitis B	HIV
Transmission in child care	Rare	Not reported
Nonsexual transmission in households	Occurs	Rare
Transmission from bite	Reported, rare	Reported, rare
Specific measures to prevent transmission	Immunize children and child care providers	Strict compliance with procedures to manage blood and body fluids
Engage medical consultant if suspected or known exposure	Yes; public health officials	Yes; health care professional caring for child and exposed person
Postexposure prophylaxis	Obtain serum to determine immune status of source child and exposed person; administer hepatitis B immune globulin and vaccine. Complete vaccine series if exposed person is not immune	Obtain serum to determine HIV status of source child and exposed person. Start antivirals in exposed person if infection suspected in source child

General Measures

1. Standard precautions. Assume all children are potentially infected.

2. Have written procedures and protocols. Train child care providers in managing body fluids or stool with visible blood, on clothing or environmental surfaces.

3. Use gloves to decontaminate surfaces, touch oral mucosal surfaces, cover oozing lesions or manage body sites or fluids with bleeding, and change diapers with visible blood. Practice careful hand washing.

4. Decontaminate fomites and environmental surfaces contaminated with blood and body fluids with bleach solution (a quarter cup bleach to 1 gallon water).

5. Screen children who are immunodeficient for transmissible infections (eg, *Cryptosporidium* species infection) when indicated.

6. Exclude children with aggressive behavior (biting or frequent scratching) or difficult-to-manage body fluids containing blood (eg, generalized dermatitis or bleeding problem) until the problem or condition is resolved.

It is important to remember that transmission of tuberculosis in a child care setting is most likely to occur from an adult to a child rather than from child to adult or child to child. Preemployment screening of child care providers should include a Mantoux test and this should be repeated every 2 years.

TABLE 17.13. Housekeeping Procedures for Blood and Body Fluids.*

In general, routine housekeeping procedures using a commercially available cleaner (detergent, disinfectant-detergent, or chemical germicide) compatible with most surfaces is satisfactory for cleaning spills of vomitus, urine, and feces. Nasal secretions can be removed with tissues and discarded in routine waste containers. For spills involving blood or other body fluids, organic material should be removed, and the surface should be disinfected with freshly diluted bleach (1:10). Reusable rubber gloves should be used for cleaning large spills to avoid contamination of the hands of the person cleaning the spill, but gloves are not essential for cleaning small amounts of blood that can be contained easily by the material used for cleaning. People involved in cleaning contaminated surfaces should avoid exposure of open skin lesions or mucous membranes to blood or bloody fluids. Whenever possible, disposable towels or tissues should be used and properly discarded, and mops should be rinsed in disinfectant. After clean-up and after removal of gloves, hands should be washed thoroughly with soap and water. Gloves are not indicated for routine cleaning tasks that do not involve contact with body secretions, such as sweeping floors or dusting.

* Reprinted from American Academy of Pediatrics. Human immunodeficiency virus. In: Pickering LK, ed. *Red Book: 2003 Report of the Committee on Infectious Diseases*. 26th ed. Elk Grove Village, IL: American Academy of Pediatrics; 2003:360–382

CONCLUSIONS AND RECOMMENDATIONS

Health care professionals should work with child care providers to ensure that they understand the agents, routes of transmission, and health effects of infections acquired in child care settings. Child care providers should know how to provide a safe and healthy environment and prevent or decrease infections transmitted in child care settings. Health care professionals should recognize the infections that cause epidemic disease in child care settings and understand the principles and the resources for their management and control. Child care providers and the children in their care should be fully immunized according to current recommendations of the American Academy of Pediatrics, the Centers for Disease Control and Prevention, and the American Academy of Family Physicians.

RESOURCES

American Academy of Pediatrics. *2003 Red Book: Report of the Committee on Infectious Diseases.* Pickering LK, ed. 26th ed. Elk Grove Village, IL: American Academy of Pediatrics; 2003

American Academy of Pediatrics, American Public Health Association, and Maternal and Child Health Bureau. *Caring for Our Children. National Health and Safety Performance Standards: Guidelines for Out-of-Home Child Care Programs.* 2nd ed. Elk Grove Village, IL: American Academy of Pediatrics; 2002

Carabin H, Gyorkos TW, Soto JC, Penrod J, Joseph L, Collet JP. Estimation of direct and indirect costs because of common infections in toddlers attending day care centers. *Pediatrics.* 1999;103:556–564

Churchill RB, Pickering LK. Infection control challenges in child-care centers. *Infect Dis Clin North Am.* 1997;11:347–365

Cordell RL, MacDonald JK, Solomon SL, Jackson LA, Boase J. Illnesses and absence due to illness among children attending child care facilities in Seattle-King County, Washington. *Pediatrics.* 1997;100:850-855

Donowitz LG. At-a-glance guide to infection control in day care. *Contemp Pediatr.* 1999;11: 127-129

Holmes SJ, Morrow AL, Pickering LK. Child-care practices: effects of social change on the epidemiology of infectious disease and antibiotic resistance. *Epidemiol Rev.* 1996;18:10-28

Pennsylvania Chapter, American Academy of Pediatrics. *Preparing for Illness.* Available at: http://www.paaap.org/mod.php?mod=userpage&page_id=11&menu=. Accessed April 16, 2002

Rafanello D, Murray D. Controlling the spread of infectious disease in child care programs. *Healthy Child Care America Newsletter.* 2001;Winter:1, 6

Robinson J. Infectious diseases in schools and child care facilities. *Pediatr Rev.* 2001;22:39-46

Uhari M, Mottonen M. An open randomized controlled trial of infection prevention in child day-care centers. *Pediatr Infect Dis J.* 1999;18:672-677

Wald ER, Guerra N, Byers C. Frequency and severity of infections in day care: three-year follow-up. *J Pediatr.* 1991;118:509-514

Antibiotic Use and Antimicrobial Resistance

Adcock PM, Pastor P, Medley F, Patterson JE, Murphy TV. Methicillin resistant *Staphylococcus aureus* in two child care centers. *J Infect Dis.* 1998;178:577-580

Dowell SF, Butler JC, Giebink GS, et al. Acute otitis media: management and surveillance in an era of pneumococcal resistance—a report from the Drug-resistant Streptococcus pneumoniae Therapeutic Working Group. *Pediatr Infect Dis J.* 1999;18:1-9

Dowell SF, Marcy SM, Phillips WR, Gerber MA, Schwartz B. Principles of judicious use of antimicrobial agents for pediatric upper respiratory tract infections. *Pediatrics.* 1998;101: 163-165

Eliasson I, Holst E, Molstad S, Kamme C. Emergence and persistence of beta-lactamase-producing bacteria in upper respiratory tract in children treated with beta-lactam antibiotics. *Am J Med.* 1990;88(Suppl 5A):51S-55S

Hamm RM, Hicks RJ, Bemben DA. Antibiotics and respiratory infections: are patients more satisfied when expectations are met? *J Fam Pract.* 1996;43:56-62

McCraig LF, Hughes JM. Trends in antimicrobial drug prescribing among office-based physicians in the United States. *JAMA.* 1995;273:214-219

Reves RR, Jones JA. Antibiotic use and resistance patterns in child care centers. *Semin Pediatr Infect Dis.* 1990;1:212-221

Rosenfeld RA. An evidence-based approach to treating otitis media. *Pediatr Clin North Am.* 1996;43:1165-1181

Bloodborne Agents

American Academy of Pediatrics, Committee on Pediatric AIDS and Committee on Infectious Diseases. Issues related to human immunodeficiency virus transmission in schools, child care, medical settings, the home, and community. *Pediatrics.* 1999;104:318-324

Deseda CC, Shapiro CN, Carrol K, et al. Hepatitis B virus transmission between a child and staff member at a day-care center. *Pediatr Infect Dis J.* 1994;13:828-830

Renaud A, Ryan B, Cloutier D, Urbanek A, Haley A. Knowledge and attitude assessment of Quebec daycare workers and parents regarding HIV/AIDS and hepatitis B. *Can J Public Health.* 1997;88:23-26

Shapiro CN, McCaig LF, Gensheimer KF, et al. Hepatitis B virus transmission between children in day care. *Pediatr Infect Dis J.* 1989;8:870-875

Simonds RJ, Chanock S. medical issues related to caring for human immunodeficiency virus-infected children in and out of the home. *Pediatr Infect Dis J.* 1993;12:845-852

Diarrheal Agents

Bartlett AV, Moore M, Gary GW, et al. Diarrheal illness among infants and toddlers in day care centers. I. Epidemiology and pathogens. *J Pediatr.* 1985;107:495-502

Chorba TL, Meriwether RA, Jenkins BR, Gunn RA, MacCormack N. Control of a non-foodborne outbreak of salmonellosis: day care in isolation. *Am J Public Health.* 1987;77:979-981

Heijbel H, Slaine, Seigel B, et al. Outbreak of diarrhea in a day care center with spread of household members: the role of *Cryptosporidium. Pediatr Infect Dis J.* 1987;6:532-535

Hoffman RE, Shillam PJ. The use of hygiene, cohorting and antimicrobial therapy to control an outbreak of shigellosis. *Am J Dis Child.* 1990;144:219-221

Lemp GF, Woodward WE, Pickering LK, Sullivan PS, Dupont HL. The relationship of staff to the incidence of diarrhea in day-care centers. *Am J Epidemiol.* 1984;120:750-758

Mohle-Boetani JC, Stapleton M, Finger R, et al. Communitywide shigellosis: control of an outbreak and risk factors in child day-care centers. *Am J Public Health.* 1995;85:812-816

Roberts L, Jorm L, Patel M, Smith W, Douglas RM, McGilchrist C. Effect of infection control measures on the frequency of diarrheal episodes in child care: a randomized, controlled trial. *Pediatrics.* 2000;105:743-746

Steketee RW, Reid S, Cheng T, Stoebig JS, Harrington RG, Davis JP. Recurrent outbreaks of giardiasis in a child day care center, Wisconsin. *Am J Public Health.* 1989;79:485-490

Van R, Morrow AL, Reves RR, Pickering LK. Environmental contamination in child day-care centers. *Am J Epidemiol.* 1991;133:460-470

Van RV, Wun CC, Morrow AL, Pickering LK. The effect of diaper type and over clothing on fecal contamination in day care centers. *JAMA.* 1991;265:1840-1844

E coli O157:H7

Belongia EA, Osterholm MT, Soler JT, Ammend DA, Braun JE, MacDonald KL. Transmission of *Escherichia coli* O157:H7 infection in Minnesota child day-care facilities. *JAMA.* 1993;269:883–888

Pickering LK, Obrig TG, Stapleton FB. Hemolytic-uremic syndrome and enterohemorrhagic *Escherichia coli. Pediatr Infect Dis J.* 1994;13:459–476

Spika JS, Parsons JE, Nordenberg D, Wells JG, Gunn RA, Blake PA. Hemolytic uremic syndrome diarrhea associated with *Escherichia coli* O157:H7 in a child care center. *J Pediatr.* 1986;109:287–291

Swerdlow DL, Griffin PM. Duration of faecal shedding of *Escherichia coli* O157:H7 among children in day care centres. *Lancet.* 1997;349:745–746

Wong CS, Jelacic S, Habeeb RL, Watkins SL, Tarr PI. The risk of the hemolytic-uremic syndrome after antibiotic treatment of *Escherichia coli* O157:H7 infections. *N Engl J Med.* 2000;342:1930–1936

Head Lice

American Academy of Pediatrics, Committee on School Health and Committee on Infectious Diseases. Head lice. *Pediatrics.* 2002;110:638–643

Burkhart CN, Burkhart CG. Another look at ivermectin in the treatment of scabies and head lice [letter]. *Int J Dermatol.* 1999;38:235

Chesney PJ, Burgess IF. Lice: resistance and treatment. *Contemp Pediatr.* 1998;11:181–183

Roberts RJ. Clinical practice. Head lice. *N Engl J Med.* 2002;346:1645–1650

Roberts RJ, Casey D, Morgan DA, Petrovic M. Comparison of wet combing with malathion for treatment of head lice in the UK: a pragmatic randomized controlled trial. *Lancet.* 2000;356:540–544

Williams LK, Reichert A, MacKenzie WR, Hightower AW, Blake PA. Lice, nits, and school policy. *Pediatrics.* 2001;107:1011–1015

Hepatitis A

Hadler SC, Erben JJ, Matthews D, Starko K, Francis DP, Maylard JE. Effect of immunoglobulin on hepatitis A in day-care centers. *JAMA.* 1983;249:48–53

Shapiro CN, Hadler SC. Hepatitis A and hepatitis B virus infections in day-care settings. *Pediatr Ann.* 1991;20:435–441

Venczel LV, Desai MM, Vertz PD, et al. The role of child care in a community-wide outbreak of hepatitis A. *Pediatrics.* 2001;108(5). Available at: http://www.pediatrics.org/cgi/content/full/108/5/e78

Invasive Bacterial Infections

Black S, Shinefield H, Elvin L, et al. Pneumococcal epidemiology in childhood in a large HMO population. *Pediatr Res.* 1994;35:174A

Leggiadro RJ, Baddour LM, Frasch CE, et al. Invasive meningococcal disease: secondary spread in a day-care center. *South Med J.* 1989;38:511–513

Osterholm MT. Invasive bacterial diseases and child day care. *Semin Pediatr Infect Dis.* 1990; 1:222–333

Takala AK, Jero J, Kela E, et al. Risk factors for primary invasive pneumococcal disease among children in Finland. *JAMA.* 1995;273:859–864

Meningococcal Infections

Jodar L, Feavers IM, Salisbury D, Granoff DM. Development of vaccines against meningococcal disease. *Lancet.* 2002;359:1499–1508

Pneumococcal Infections

Centers for Disease Control and Prevention. Preventing pneumococcal disease among infants and young children. *MMWR Morb Mortal Wkly Rep.* 2000;49(RR-9):1–38

Respiratory Infections

American Academy of Pediatrics, Committee on Infectious Diseases. Recommendations for influenza immunization of children. *Pediatrics.* 2004;113:1441–1447.

Bridges CB, Fukuda K, Uyeki TM, Cox NJ, Singleton JA. Prevention and control of influenza: recommendations of the Advisory Committee on Immunization Practices (ACIP). *MMWR Morb Mortal Wkly Rep.* 2002;51(RR-3):1–31

Streptococcus pyogenes: Group A β-Hemolytic Streptococcus

Centers for Disease Control and Prevention. Outbreak of invasive group A Streptococcus associated with varicella in a child care center—Boston, MA, 1997. *MMWR Morb Mortal Wkly Rep.* 1997;46:944–948

Davies HD, Low DE, Schwarz B, et al. Evaluation of short-course therapy with cefixime or rifampin for eradication of pharyngeally carried group A streptococci. *Clin Infect Dis.* 1995;21:1294–1296

Engelgau MM, Woernie GH, Schwartz B, Vance NJ, Horan JM. Invasive group A streptococcus carriage in a child care centre after a fatal case. *Arch Dis Child.* 1994;71:318–322

Falck G, Kjellander J. Outbreak of Group A streptococcal infection in a day-care center. *Pediatr Infect Dis J.* 1992;11:914–919

Holmstrom L, Nyman B, Rosengren M, Wallander S, Ripa T. Outbreak of infections with erythromycin-resistant Group A streptococci in child day care centers. *Scand J Infect Dis.* 1990;22:179–185

Smith TD, Wilkinson V, Kaplan EL. Group A *Streptococcus*-associated upper respiratory tract infections in a day-care center. *Pediatrics.* 1989;83:380–386

CHAPTER 18

Care of the Mildly Ill Child

Angela A. Crowley, PhD, APRN, CS, PNP

LEARNING OBJECTIVES

This chapter will help the reader:

- Be able to define exclusion criteria for mildly ill children.
- Understand the developmental and emotional needs of mildly ill children.
- Be prepared to discuss alternative care arrangements for mildly ill children.
- Learn essential health guidelines for operating special facilities for mildly ill children.
- Understand the importance of family sick leave policies.

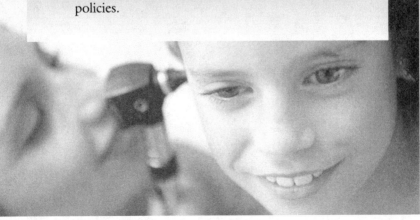

Although health care professionals are well aware of the frequency of mild illnesses among young children, particularly those enrolled in child care,[1] parents working outside the home are often unprepared for these illnesses and the ensuing disruption in family life and child care arrangements. In addition, confusion about appropriate exclusion criteria and differing needs or expectations may lead to tension and misunderstandings between child care providers and parents.

To adequately address this dilemma, health care professionals must consider several issues: the importance of clear, reasonable exclusion guidelines; the necessity for parent and child care provider education and communication; the emotional and developmental needs of ill children; the availability of alternate child care arrangements; and the value and importance of workplace family leave policies.

EXCLUSION OF ILL CHILDREN

One of the most common causes of tension between child care providers and parents is the issue of exclusion for illness. Understandably, child care providers and parents have different perspectives. Early childhood care providers are primarily concerned with maintaining the health of all the children and staff and minimizing the spread of communicable diseases. They also recognize that an ill child may not be able to participate in the regular program and may require more staff attention than can be provided.[2] In contrast, parents are typically unprepared when a child develops a mild illness and they are caught between job responsibilities and caring for their child.

Further compounding this dilemma is the wide variation in child care exclusion policies, which range from detailed to superficial to, most commonly, unwritten. Comparing exclusion recommendations among child care providers, parents, and pediatricians, child care providers are more likely than are parents to exclude for specific symptoms, and pediatricians are least likely to support exclusion.[2] Shapiro[3] and Landis and Chang[1] have challenged the common practice of excluding children with low-grade fevers and mild upper respiratory illnesses. Previous reports of respiratory and diarrheal illness have suggested a higher incidence of such illness among children attending child care centers (programs that provide care and education for 13 or more children), compared with children in small and large family child care homes (facilities that provide care and education for 7 or fewer children).[4-6] A recent report suggests that the incidence of illness may actually be greater among children in child care homes and that the increased absence attributable to illness among children in centers may reflect differences in exclusion policies and practices. The authors suggest that much of the absenteeism was attributable to mild respiratory illness that probably did not warrant exclusion.[7]

Through education and anticipatory guidance, pediatric primary health care professionals can clarify the confusion and modify the tension between parents and child care providers relevant to this issue. First, pediatricians and nurses can assist child care providers in developing exclusion policies as outlined by the American Public Health Association (APHA), Maternal and Child Health Bureau (MCHB), and American Academy of Pediatrics (AAP)[8,9] (see Chapter 17). Second, during well-child visits, pediatric primary health care professionals should counsel parents about the frequency of mild illnesses in young children, stress the importance of alternate care arrangements when children are infectious or unable to participate physically and encourage parents to plan in advance for those times. As consultants to child care programs, health care professionals can also recommend that child care providers understand the parents' dilemma, educate parents about the importance of exclusion policies, provide copies of the program's exclusion policy to all parents on enrollment and yearly, and encourage parents to develop alternative plans during illness.

DEVELOPMENTAL AND EMOTIONAL NEEDS OF ILL CHILDREN

To determine the appropriateness of alternate child care arrangements, it is essential to understand children's developmental and emotional needs, the impact of separation at various ages, and how children interpret illness. By considering these factors, health care professionals can appropriately counsel parents about selecting child care arrangements for ill children.

During infancy, the central developmental task is the formation of a relationship with a primary caregiver, usually a parent. Erikson[10] postulated that in the first stage of development—trust versus mistrust—a foundation for all later development is established. Infants acquire trust in others and themselves if their physical and emotional needs are consistently met with sameness and continuity by their caregiver. This process promotes a sense of hope. However, if these needs are unmet, infants develop mistrust and are apprehensive about future relationships.[10-12]

Between 18 months and 3 years of age, children progress to Erikson's[10] second stage, autonomy versus shame and doubt. They discover that their behavior is self-directed. Asserting oneself creates conflict between the joy of autonomy and the doubt and shame associated with parental disapproval.[11]

Mahler, Pine, and Berman[13] contend that children develop a sense of identity during the first 3 years of life through a process of separation-individuation. Newborns exist in a normal autistic state in which they are fused with their mother or primary caregiver. At approximately 4 to 5 months of age, they begin to emerge from this symbiosis.

During the second half of the first year of life, infants begin to develop object constancy, the ability to maintain constant relations with significant others ("object") regardless of their state of need.[14] By distinguishing and preferring constant caregivers, infants relinquish immediate gratification. Therefore, separation from their caregiver creates significant anxiety. This fear is often more acute in 15-month-olds as representational intelligence replaces sensorimotor intelligence.

At this age, children are more fully aware of their separateness and more clearly realize their relative helplessness. Parents play a prominent role as catalyst and anchor, encouraging initiative and providing security, while children attempt separation. As individuation proceeds, children develop the ability to maintain attachment to the caregiver while tolerating absences of increasing length.[11]

During the preschool years, children enter Erikson's[10] third phase of development—initiative versus guilt. Language, motor, and social skills flourish, and they are eager to undertake new tasks. Their world widens. Peers and socialization assume greater importance. Symbolic play provides the opportunity to explore various roles and behavior. Naturally egocentric at this stage, children experience guilt for real and imagined transgressions.[11]

School-aged children demonstrate significant maturation in language, fine and gross motor skills, and cognitive learning. Peers and the world of school take on increasing significance. Children derive a sense of capability and self-esteem from accomplishing tasks independently. Erikson[10] defines this period as industry versus inferiority.[11]

To comprehend the impact of sick child care arrangements on young children, it is necessary to understand how children interpret illness at various stages. The meaning of illness for young children varies with their developmental level, their individual capacities, and the context of the situation. Solnit[15] asserts that children's interpretation of illness cannot be fully understood without considering psychologic and emotional reactions.[11]

The meaning of illness for young children varies with their developmental level, their individual capacities, and the context of the situation.

During infancy, any tension, need, or frustration is probably felt as pain.[15] Very young children are unable to distinguish between diffuse discomfort and sharper, localized pain. Limited in expressive and receptive language, children cannot distinguish suffering caused by the physical illness from diagnostic and curative measures. In addition, the physical experience of pain is charged with psychic meaning. Anxiety is provoked by the specific vulnerabilities of each developmental struggle.[16] For example, reaction to physical discomfort for older infants and toddlers is heightened by fears of abandonment in the face of potentially overwhelming pain. Consistent with their developmental stage, preschool children may interpret illness and separation as punishment. Similar to adults, who lose bodily functions and independence in self-care during illness, children are also frustrated by their loss of control.[11]

Solnit[15] describes the parents' role during illness as irreplaceable. For young children who have not achieved object constancy, typically children younger than 3 years, the absence of parents during illness creates dual anxiety. Physical pain is amplified by the loss of the love object. Parents or caregivers who intimately and uniquely understand children's needs are absent in a time of stress when those needs are most acute. As children mature and are able to verbalize and interpret illness, they are capable of asserting their need for attention and actively participate in their own care. Older children, most often school-aged children and to some degree, preschoolers, feel the presence of their parents even in their absence. Still, parents play a primary role in helping children work through their fears and concerns about body intactness.[11]

ALTERNATIVE CARE ARRANGEMENTS

When children are ill and excluded from their usual out-of-home child care program, 3 options exist: in-home care, sick care in a special room at the child's regular program, or care in a separate facility exclusively for mildly ill children. Each of these options has inherent advantages and disadvantages, as measured by convenience, cost, and the emotional impact on the child (See Table 18.1).[1,11,17]

Care in the home takes 2 forms: care by a parent, relative, or friend or care by a trained provider. In a survey of mothers regarding sick child care preferences,[18] 84% of the respondents preferred in-home care, preferably by the parent. Care by the parent or significant other offers the ideal of a familiar caregiver in a familiar setting. Trained providers range from experienced nurses to individuals with limited short-term preparation specific to caring for mildly ill children. Although usually not known to the child, trained providers maintain the continuity of setting and, therefore, lessen the stress of separation.[11]

Most parents do not have the option of caring for their ill children without jeopardizing their jobs or losing wages. Relatives and friends are often unavailable. The trained in-home provider is the most expensive form of care and, consequently, is an option for only a small segment of the population. It is worth noting, though statistics are unavailable, that many preschool or school-aged children are left alone at home or with young, inexperienced siblings during times of illness when no other viable options exist.[11]

Care at the child's regular program refers to the integration of mildly ill children into the usual group or a separate but adjacent "get-well room." Family child care homes are more likely to offer the integrated option, as opposed to centers in which the integrated option has occurred primarily in research settings with an on-site health care professional.[1] This alternative again provides a familiar setting and often a familiar provider, because caregivers from the regular center usually manage the ill children exclusively. Because of seasonal fluctuations in illness, it is difficult to staff this type of center for fewer than 100 children, and most centers do not have readily available space for this purpose.[11]

Separate programs for ill children take 3 forms: a family child care home that is a satellite for 1 or more child care centers or is open to the larger community, a

TABLE 18.1. Advantages and Disadvantages of Sick Child Care Models[5]

TYPE OF CARE	ADVANTAGES	DISADVANTAGES
1. In home		
a. By parent, relative, or friend	Familiar provider and setting; most convenient	Work days lost if family sick leave unavailable; threat to job security
b. By trained provider in child's home	Familiar setting; very convenient	Unfamiliar provider; most expensive of all options May not be available in all locations
2. Child's regular child care program		
a. Child care center "get-well room"	Familiar provider and setting; very convenient	Not cost-effective for small to mid-sized programs Potential for cross-infection
b. Family child care home		
3. Separate facility		
a. Family child care home satellite of regular program that accepts sick children	Convenient; setting and provider may be familiar if orientation provided	Provider and setting may be unfamiliar May not be available in all locations
b. Center exclusively for mildly ill children	Convenient	Setting and provider unfamiliar
c. Center at parent's workplace	Very convenient; parents can visit during the workday	Unfamiliar setting and provider May require preregistration

center exclusively for ill children, or a center at the parents' workplace, which is most often hospital based.[19] Other than the satellite family child care home, these settings and caregivers are usually unfamiliar to the young child. The workplace option allows parents to visit, which may be comforting for the preschool or school-aged child but not sufficient to offset the fears of an infant or toddler. Unless subsidized, each of these programs requires additional costs for the parents who must simultaneously pay for the regular child care program.[11]

The emotional impact on young children of unfamiliar ill child care programs and providers has not been studied, and the literature on separation effects is of only limited value because of the length and circumstances of the separation experiences studied as well as methodologic issues. Although the stage theories of development and attachment are not without question, there remains serious concern about placing very young children, especially infants and toddlers, in these situations. Without having achieved adequate autonomy, object constancy, and cognitive ability, strange situations provoke undue anxiety. The short- and long-term impact of these experiences on development remain unknown. Hospitalized children unquestionably require close parental contact, and it can be argued that very young children cannot distinguish mild from serious illness and require that same level of attention. Further, children who are enrolled in less-than-adequate child care may be placed at even greater emotional risk by exposure to additional unstable arrangements.[11]

Preschool and school-aged children theoretically may be capable of adapting to unfamiliar environments and caregivers during illness. However, each child should be assessed individually, keeping in mind the normal regression associated with illness. At a minimum, these age groups should have the opportunity to visit, explore, and discuss this option well in advance of an illness.[11]

HEALTH GUIDELINES FOR OPERATING CHILD CARE FACILITIES FOR MILDLY ILL CHILDREN

Facilities for mildly ill children should provide the opportunity for healthy, safe, and developmentally appropriate care with special consideration for the unique needs of mildly ill children. Therefore, in addition to meeting the AAP, APHA, and MCHB standards[8] for child care programs for well children, it is essential that facilities adhere to the specific requirements determined by licensing agencies. The information presented here highlights the recommendations of the second edition of *Caring for Our Children*.[8] The reader is referred to that document for a full description of standards and rationale.

Child care providers who offer this service need to develop a plan of care for ill children that addresses the following areas: levels of severity, space, staffing, child-staff ratio, training, and policies and procedures.[8] It is imperative that health consultants actively participate in the development and ongoing management of such programs. The health consultant should be a health care professional with training and expertise in child care health consultation. In addition to providing consultation about the management of ill children, the health consultant should assist in the development and review of written policies and procedures, specifically admission, inclusion, and exclusion criteria; health evaluation procedures to determine appropriateness of attendance and need for additional health care; and plans for caring for children with communicable diseases, surveillance of illnesses managed, staff training, injury prevention, emergency care, and communication with parents and health care professionals.

Levels of Severity

Facilities for mildly ill children can potentially manage children with 3 levels of illness severity. Severity level 1 includes children who are primarily contagious, such as those with bacterial conjunctivitis or varicella infection but whose activity is otherwise unaffected. Severity level 2 comprises those children who have a medium activity level as a result of their illness, and severity level 3 includes children who, because of their symptoms, have a low activity level and, therefore, are primarily engaged in rest, sleep, or passive activities. Each facility should define in their procedure manual which levels of illness severity they can accommodate.

Space

All child care programs must attend to healthy practices that decrease the incidence of contagious diseases, and principles of infection control are of special importance within a facility serving ill children. Table 18.2 lists the environmental requirements necessary to limit the spread of infectious diseases within and outside the facility.

Staffing

In addition to the general qualifications listed in the guidelines from the AAP, APHA, and MCHB, the staff in facilities serving ill children should meet additional requirements because of the unique needs of this population. In addition to holding an undergraduate degree as defined in the standards, the director should have at least 12 credit hours of college-level training in child development or early childhood education, a minimum of 2 previous years' successful experience as a director of a regular facility, and at least 40 hours in prevention and control of communicable disease and care of ill children. Staff members should have a minimum of 2 years' successful work experience as a caregiver in a regular child care facility.

TABLE 18.2. Space Requirements in Special Facilities for Ill Children

- If in same location as regular program—no sharing of furniture or equipment

- No sharing of indoor space with the exception of a cook who has no other responsibilities

- Separation of children with:
  - ~ infections of the gastrointestinal tract (such as diarrheal diseases) and liver diseases
  - ~ varicella (space must be externally ventilated)

- No commingling of space, staff, or toys and equipment among children in different rooms

- Hand washing sink in each child care room

- Diaper changing area adjacent to hand washing sink in each room with nontoilet-trained children

- Minimum of 1 toilet with privacy for every 10 children

- Minimum of 35 square feet of useable indoor floor space per child

- Cups, plates, and utensils must be cleaned by (both of which meet local sanitation standards):
  - ~ using a mechanical dishwasher; or
  - ~ 3-compartment sink

- Disposable eating utensils can be substituted

- Mechanical washing machine and dryer on-site, or contract with a laundry service

- Children have access to rest and nap areas without disturbance from other children

Training

All staff members in facilities that care for children meeting the criteria for severity levels 2 and 3 must attend 20 hours of preservice orientation training. The training should address the following topics:

- Orientation to the facility and its policies
- Pediatric first aid, including management of a blocked airway, rescue breathing, and first aid for choking
- General infection control (Table 18.3)
- Care of children with common mild childhood illnesses (Table 18.3)
- Child development activities appropriate for sick children

In addition, the director and staff must have a minimum of 6 clock hours of continuing education annually related to the care of ill children and the prevention and control of communicable diseases in addition to continued training in general aspects of infection control. On being hired, employees should begin orientation to the facility and its policies, and documentation of the orientation should be kept in each employee's file.

TABLE 18.3. Training in Special Facilities for Mildly Ill Children	
General Infection Control Procedures	Care of Children With Common Mild Childhood Illnesses
• Understanding of disease transmission principles • Hand washing • Proper handling of contaminated items • Use of sanitizing chemicals • Safe food handling • Washing and sanitizing toys	• Recognition and documentation of illness signs and symptoms • Temperature taking • Administration and recording of medications (see Appendix F) • Knowledge of nutrition for ill children • Communication with parents of ill children • Knowledge of immunization requirements • Knowledge of when and how to call for medical assistance or notify the local public department of communicable diseases • Emergency procedures

Child-Staff Ratio

Ill children require more attention than well children. Therefore, the APHA/AAP standards reflect closer supervision in the child-staff ratio for all age groups (Table 18.4). These ratios are the maximum allowable in facilities for ill children. When there are mixed age groups in the same room, the child-staff ratio should be consistent with the age of the youngest child.

Procedures

Daily communication with the parent on the child's progress is essential. In addition, caregivers require information about the child's diagnosis, status of the illness, and directions specific to the child's care for each day of care at the facility (Table 18.5). Although ill children who are excluded from their regular program can be safely cared for in special facilities for ill children, there are some conditions that necessitate exclusion from these settings (see Table 18.6).

TABLE 18.4. Child-Staff Ratio in Special Facilities for Mildly Ill Children	
Age of Children	Child–Staff Ratio
2–24 mo	3 children to 1 staff member
25–71 mo	4 children to 1 staff member
72 mo and older	6 children to 1 staff member

TABLE 18.5. Daily Documented Information Required in Special Facilities for Mildly Ill Children

- Child's diagnosis and the source of information

- Status of the illness: potential for contagion, diet, activity level, illness duration

- Health care information, including release form to obtain emergency care

- Diet

- Medication plan and authorization to administer medications (see Appendix F)

TABLE 18.6. Signs and Symptoms Requiring Exclusion From Facilities for Mildly Ill Children

- Fever with stiff neck, lethargy, irritability, or persistent crying

- Diarrhea (3 or more stools in an 8-hour period or an increased number of stools compared with the child's normal pattern and with increased stool water or decreased form), in addition to signs of dehydration or blood or mucus in the stools unless at least 1 stool culture demonstrates an absence of *Shigella* species, *Salmonella* species, *Campylobacter* species, and *Escherichia coli* O157:H7
  - ~ Child with diarrhea caused by *Camplyobacter* species or *Giardia lamblia* may be readmitted 24 hours after treatment is initiated and the child's health care professional gives clearance.
  - ~ Child with diarrhea attributable to *Shigella* species or *E coli* O157:H7 should be excluded until diarrhea resolves and 2 stool cultures 48 hours apart test negative.

- Vomiting 3 or more times or with signs of dehydration

- Contagious states of pertussis, measles, mumps, varicella, rubella, or diphtheria, unless the child is appropriately isolated from children with other illnesses or grouped exclusively with children with the same illness

- Untreated infestation (eg, scabies, head lice, etc)

- Untreated tuberculosis

- Undiagnosed rash

- Abdominal pain that is intermittent or persistent

- Difficulty breathing

- Undiagnosed jaundice (yellow skin and whites of eyes)

- Lethargy such that the child does not play

- Other conditions as determined by the director or health consultant

FAMILY SICK LEAVE POLICIES

Although it is essential to educate parents and child care providers about all the aforementioned topics related to caring for mildly ill children, health care professionals foremost must advocate for family sick leave policies in the workplace, which would alleviate much of the stress related to this issue. When surveyed, parents most often prefer the option of caring for their sick child,[18] and no doubt, children would prefer recovering from mild illnesses at home with their parents. As child advocates, pediatric primary health care professionals are a critical voice in promoting policies that support the best interests of families.

CONCLUSIONS AND RECOMMENDATIONS

1. Prepare parents who use out-of-home child care for the frequency of mild illnesses in young children and the need for prearranged alternative care.
2. Discuss with parents the emotional, developmental, and health needs of young children when considering sick child care alternatives.
3. Assist child care providers with developing health exclusion policies.
4. Offer health consultation to child care programs for mildly ill children.
5. Support family sick leave policies in the workplace.

REFERENCES

1. Landis SE, Chang A. Child care options for ill children. *Pediatrics.* 1991;88:705–718
2. Landis SE, Earp JA, Sharp M. Day-care center exclusion of sick children: comparison of opinions of day-care staff, working mothers, and pediatricians. *Pediatrics.* 1988;81: 662–667
3. Shapiro ED. Exclusion of ill children in day-care centers. Policy and practice in New Haven, CT. *Clin Pediatr (Phila).* 1984;23:689–691
4. Hurwitz ES, Gunn WJ, Pinsky PF, Schonberger LB. Risk of respiratory illness associated with day-care attendance: a nationwide study. *Pediatrics.* 1991;87:62–69
5. Reeves RR, Morrow AL, Bartlett AV III, et al. Child day care increases the risk of clinic visits for acute diarrhea and diarrhea due to rotavirus. *Am J Epidemiol.* 1993;137:97–107
6. Bartlett AV, Morrow M, Gary GW, Starko KM, Erben JJ, Meredith BA. Diarrheal illness among infants and toddlers in day care centers II. Comparison with day care homes and households. *J Pediatr.* 1985;107:503–509
7. Cordell RL, MacDonald JK, Salomon SL, Jackson LA, Boase J. Illnesses and absence due to illness among children attending child care facilities in Seattle-King County, Washington. *Pediatrics.* 1997;100:850–855
8. American Academy of Pediatrics, American Public Health Association, and Maternal and Child Health Bureau. *Caring for our Children. National Health and Safety Performance Standards: Guidelines for Out-of-Home Child Care Programs.* 2nd ed. Elk Grove Village, IL: American Academy of Pediatrics; 2002
9. American Academy of Pediatrics. Children in out-of-home child care. In: Pickering LK, ed. *2003 Red Book: Report of the Committee on Infectious Diseases.* 26th ed. Elk Grove Village, IL: American Academy of Pediatrics; 2003

10. Erikson EH. *Childhood and Society.* 2nd ed. New York, NY: Norton; 1963

11. Crowley AA. Sick child care: a developmental perspective. *J Pediatr Health Care.* 1994;8: 261–267

12. Freiberg KL. *Human Development: A Life Span Approach.* 3rd ed. Boston, MA: Jones and Bartlett Publishers; 1987

13. Mahler MS, Pine F, Bergman A. *The Psychological Birth of the Human Infant: Symbiosis and Individuation.* New York, NY: Basic Books Inc; 1975

14. Hartmann H. The mutual influences in the development of ego and id. *Psychoanal Study Child.* 1952;7:66–68

15. Solnit AJ. Foreword. In: Eissler RS, Freud A, Kris M, Solnit AJ, eds. *Physical Illness and Handicap in Childhood.* New Haven, CT: Yale University Press; 1977:vii–xii

16. Lewis M. *Clinical Aspects of Child Development: An Introductory Synthesis of Psychological Concepts and Clinical Problems.* Philadelphia, PA: Lea & Febiger; 1971

17. Fredericks B, Hardman R, Morgan G, Rodgers F. *A Little Bit Under the Weather: A Look at Care for Mildly Ill Children.* Boston, MA: Work/Family Directions Inc; 1986

18. Landis SE, Earp JA. Sick child care options: what do working mothers prefer? *Women Health.* 1987;12:61–77

19. Herman RE, Koppa D, Sullivan P. Sick-child day care promotes healing and staffing. *Nurs Manage.* 1999;30:46–47

ADDITIONAL RESOURCE

Freud A. The role of bodily illness in the mental life of children. In Eissler RS, Freud A, Kris M, Solnit AJ, eds. *Physical Illness and Handicap in Childhood.* New Haven, CT: Yale University Press; 1977:1-12

CHAPTER 19

Health Issues for the Child Care Provider

Rene R. Gratz, PhD, and Judith A. Calder, BSN, MS

LEARNING OBJECTIVES

The learning objectives for the reader of this chapter are:

- To become familiar with the common occupational health hazards in child care work and have a basic understanding of disease transmission and prevention practices (including immunization) that affect adult child care providers.
- To appreciate the special problems of pregnant child care staff, including infectious disease and physical stressors.
- To understand the ergonomic implications of an adult work environment that was designed for children, especially musculoskeletal injuries.
- To understand the importance of appropriate staff health policies and current laws and regulations with implications for staff health.

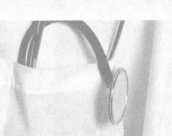

INTRODUCTION

The personal health and safety of the child care provider has a substantial impact on, and consequences for, child care programming. As stated in *Caring for Our Children,* the "quality and continuity of the caregiving workforce is the main determining factor of the quality of care."[1]

The child care workforce in group child care centers and family child care homes predominantly comprises women of childbearing age. In terms of number of providers in this country today, family child care home providers are a particularly important group. Although some studies have looked at the job stress of family child care providers, they have not been included in most epidemiologic studies of health in child care. Child care providers work in physically and emotionally demanding settings, receiving low pay and few, if any, benefits. In addition, family child care home providers working with smaller groups of children experience isolation, as they are usually the only adults with the children each day. Isolation is also, at times, a problem for the few men who work in child care.

The susceptibility to illness and injury of adults employed in child care is usually a secondary focus of studies of health in child care, if reported at all.[2,3] At the International Conference on Child Day Care Health held in Atlanta in June 1992, occupational health was highlighted as a major area of untapped information; it was also suggested that perhaps some of the undervaluing of child care providers is attributable to limitations in our knowledge of the health and health risks of those caregivers.[4]

Gratz and Claffey[3] surveyed child care center staff and directors and family child care home providers to document the health status, health behaviors, and concerns of child care providers. Among their findings was that most of the sample rated their current health as good or excellent, although approximately one third of the total group (but almost one half of center staff) reported being sick more often since beginning to work in child care; more than 80% of each group reported working when they were ill, often because of lack of substitutes or needing the income from that day's work.

The health of the program director, who may have less contact with the children, also is important. The director of a child care center provides leadership and is a role model for staff, parents, and children. He or she is in a position to influence policy and curricular changes; his or her interest in health and safety issues has the potential to modify or drastically alter current program conditions.

This chapter discusses health issues for the adult child care provider, including areas that currently are seen as of special concern: disease transmission and prevention practices; immunizations; special problems of pregnant staff; ergonomics, musculoskeletal injuries, and body mechanics; stress and burnout; staff health policies; and laws and regulations.

INFECTIOUS DISEASE

Many infectious diseases, including upper respiratory tract infections, influenza, diarrhea, and skin conditions, such as scabies and impetigo, affect adults as well as children in the child care environment. Other diseases may manifest primarily in children (eg, varicella and otitis media). Still, others may be transmitted readily from adults to children (eg, tuberculosis and pertussis from unrecognized adult carriers). Some infections, such as hepatitis A and giardiasis, may be inapparent in children but clinically symptomatic in adults. Some diseases (eg, cytomegalovirus [CMV], rubella, parvovirus B19, and varicella) may have particular significance because of the potential for severe consequences for pregnant women or for persons who are immunocompromised.

Factors That Increase Risk of Disease to Caregivers

The same factors that increase the risk of disease in children in child care settings also affect their caregivers, and some of these diseases can be serious enough to be considered occupational risks. The first factor to be considered is immune status. Just as children acquire immunity through experience with disease, there is anecdotal evidence that caregivers new to the field experience more illness than seasoned employees who have developed immunity from previous exposures. Caregivers who may not have developed antibody resistance to common childhood illness and adults with compromised immunity because of disease, disability, allergy, or medication may be more susceptible to child care-acquired diseases and their complications. In addition, caregivers not fully immunized are at risk of acquiring vaccine-preventable diseases, such as rubella and measles.

Environmental characteristics that increase adult exposure to infectious organisms are large facility size, large group size, age group mixing, and age of children in care. Child care providers who care for nontoilet-trained children with undeveloped hygiene habits have more opportunity to come into contact with infectious agents. For example, the seroconversion rate for CMV is higher among caregivers of children younger than 2 years.

Routine habits that increase adult exposure to disease are poor personal hygiene practices, poor environmental sanitation practices, lack of specific training about disease transmission and prevention, poor monitoring of health practices, and lack of equipment (eg, soap, disposable towels, sinks, and disposable gloves). It is important for the child care program director to provide employee health assessments (see Appendix G), benefits, good working conditions supportive of health, clear policies related to health and safety, continuing education programs, and guidelines for the exclusion of ill child care staff. The lack of any of these in the work setting can be detrimental to the health of child care providers.

Infectious Diseases That Are Potentially More Serious in Adults Than in Children

Varicella often produces more serious disease in nonimmune infected adults. All adults working with children should be assessed as part of a health history or by titer for immunity to varicella (chickenpox) and immunized if not immune (see Appendix E).

Cytomegalovirus is of particular concern for adults or children with certain immune deficiencies, because the deficiency puts them at high risk of severe disease if infected with CMV. Nonimmune pregnant caregivers are also at risk. Primary CMV infection during pregnancy usually results in asymptomatic infection for the mother. However, there is a 40% to 60% chance that the fetus will be infected, especially early in pregnancy. If infected, there is a 10% to 25% chance that the infant will have permanent neurologic sequelae that may include hearing or visual loss or impairment, mental retardation or developmental delay, cerebral palsy, or seizures. Rigorous personal hygiene is important to prevent transmission of the virus from children to adult providers. After infection, CMV may be excreted in the urine or saliva of asymptomatic children for weeks to months. Immunocompromised adults should consult their health care professionals for further information and recommendations. Information about CMV, including methods and risks of transmission, should be provided to susceptible women planning pregnancy or who are pregnant. Education should include hygienic measures to decrease exposure to CMV and the availability of medical counseling and testing for serum antibody to CMV to determine immune status. Pregnant women who are nonimmune should be counseled about the risks of working with preschoolers, especially children who are in diapers.

Hepatitis A virus is spread primarily by fecal-oral transmission. Young children show few if any symptoms, but adults become more ill with fever, jaundice, loss of appetite, nausea, weakness, and dark brown urine. If hepatitis A is diagnosed in a child attending out-of-home child care or in a staff member, the local health department will recommend specific measures that may include administration of immune globulin and immunization to prevent transmission. Routine hepatitis A immunization of children is recommended in some states and/or regions and for certain high-risk groups. Consult the local public health authority for recommendations.

Hepatitis B virus (HBV) is transmitted through blood, by sexual contact, and rarely through saliva. The Occupational Safety and Health Administration (OSHA) bloodborne pathogen standard (see "Prevention of Diseases Spread Through Blood" in this chapter) for employers requires that employers inform new employees of this occupational risk, prevention practices, and recommendations for HBV immunization. Employees who have any occupational exposure to blood and who are not immunized should receive HBV immunization within 24 hours of exposure to blood. In general, there is no reason to exclude HBV carriers. However, carriers with dermatologic conditions resulting in open weeping lesions or children with aggressive behavior (eg, biting or scratching) or bleeding problems may pose a risk to others and usually are excluded. Because recommendations may change, contact your health department for the latest information. Routine immunization of all children with HBV vaccine has decreased the risk of transmission.

Parvovirus B19 presents risks for infected adults who may develop a rash or more serious consequences, such as arthritis. Individuals with certain forms of anemia may experience a severe worsening of their condition with infection. Parvovirus B19 infection that occurs during pregnancy can cause fetal hydrops and death, especially if infection occurs during the first half of pregnancy (see Table 19.1).

Prevention Practices to Reduce Disease Transmission

Child care providers must understand that preventive health practices, such as hand washing, not only protect children in child care from infectious disease but also protect the child care provider and, secondarily, their household members and other close contacts. This critical information should be repeated and continually reinforced. Hopefully, this education will improve compliance with routine practices and decrease disease transmission to all members of the child care community. These practices include hand washing, standard precautions (previously called "universal precautions"), environmental cleaning and sanitation, health checks, and exclusion guidelines as described in Chapter 17.

Prevention of Diseases Spread Through Blood

The OSHA considers child care providers as a group of employees who could be "reasonably anticipated" to have contact with blood as a result of performing their job duties. Child care workers are covered by the bloodborne pathogen standard to limit occupational exposure to blood and other infectious material that could spread bloodborne disease. In a child care setting, this most always includes blood that is the result of an accident or that appears in nasal mucus, stool, or vomit.

All child care employers, including family child care home providers who hire assistants, must comply with the standard. One element of the standard is an exposure control plan that lists job classifications and tasks during which occupational exposure to blood may occur. This plan must be in writing and reviewed annually. It also requires "standard precautions" (formerly known as universal precautions), which emphasize hand washing and use of gloves when handling blood, as described in Chapter 17. Employers must provide protective equipment, such as gloves and cardiopulmonary resuscitation shields and disinfectants. Methods of cleaning and disinfecting surfaces and laundering items in contact with blood must be described and distributed as part of the control plan.

TABLE 19.1. Prevention and Possible Fetal Effects of Illness and Stress During Pregnancy

Illness and Risk	Effect	Prevention*
Rubella (German measles) (10%–20% of young adults lack immunity)	Depends on gestational age at time of exposure. Deafness, microcephaly, CNS disease, heart defects, cataracts.	Blood test if immunity uncertain. Avoid contact if not immune; immunize if not pregnant.
HBV (rarely transmitted in child care setting)	Newborn infection; up to 90% of infected neonates will develop chronic infection and be at lifelong risk of cirrhosis and liver cancer.	Avoid contact with blood or blood products; offer immunization if not pregnant; preemployment immunization recommended. If blood exposure occurs, contact public health officials for recommendations.
CMV (annual rate of infection of child care providers is 8%–20%)	If infected for first time during pregnancy, approximately 50% of fetuses will be infected and 10%–25% of infected infants will be damaged. Impaired hearing or vision, microcephaly, CNS disease including mental retardation, seizures, cerebral palsy.	Blood test for immunity, hand washing, consider use of gloves when handling urine and saliva; if pregnant and not immune, avoid contact with urine and saliva. Do not kiss children on hands, face, or mouth.
Varicella-zoster (chickenpox) (8% of adults lack immunity)	First and early second trimester: small size, limb atrophy, scarring of skin, CNS disease, cataracts, chorioretinitis. Perinatally: neonatal death.	Blood test if immunity uncertain; avoid contact if not immune; immunize if not pregnant.
Fifth disease (parvovirus B19; approximately 50% of adults lack immunity)	If infected first half of pregnancy rarely: fetal hydrops; anemia, jaundice, enlarged liver; stillbirths; miscarriage >10%.	Blood test for immunity; hand washing; avoid shared utensils; consult health care professional if not immune and exposed.
Toxoplasmosis (66% of adult women lack immunity)	Infection depends on stage of pregnancy; spectrum of abnormalities similar to CMV.	Eat only well-done meat, thorough hand washing after handling raw meat and vegetables, outdoor sandbox play, and gardening; pregnant women should not clean cat litter box.

TABLE 19.1. Prevention and Possible Fetal Effects of Illness and Stress During Pregnancy, continued

Illness and Risk	Effect	Prevention*
HIV infection and acquired immunodeficiency syndrome (no reports of child care transmission)	Fetal infection.	Appropriate precautions when handling blood and body fluids.
Herpes simplex virus (HSV) 2 – sexually transmitted (different from herpes simplex 1 virus, which is usually transmitted through oral secretions)	Fetal infection may involve skin, liver, lung, eyes, other organs, encephalitis with permanent CNS damage (mental retardation, seizures, microcephaly), visual impairment.	Hand washing, use of gloves when handling body fluids will decrease transmission of HSV from skin, mouth, or eye lesions. Sexual transmission of HSV does not occur in the child care setting in the absence of sexual abuse/sexual contact.
STRESS Physical and psychologic	Miscarriage, prematurity, toxemia, preeclampsia, nausea, prolonged labor.	Decrease sources of stress; relaxation techniques; good diet; exercise; rest when fatigued—elevate feet.

Adapted with permission from Gratz RR, Boulton P. Health considerations for pregnant child care staff. *J Pediatr Health Care.* 1994;8:18–26.

CNS indicates central nervous system; HBV, hepatitis B virus; CMV, cytomegalovirus.

*Standard precautions should be taught, monitored, and routinely reinforced (See Chapter 17).

Another component of the plan requires that HBV immunization must be made available to all employees who may have occupational exposure to blood within 10 days of assignment or within 24 hours of exposure at no cost to the employee. Employees must sign a form if they choose not to be immunized. Postexposure evaluation and follow-up procedures apply to all employees who have had an exposure incident. An exposure incident has occurred if an employee comes in direct contact with blood or blood-containing body fluids on the employee's eye, mouth, mucous membrane, nonintact skin (cut or chapped), or punctured skin (from a needle, bite, etc).

The child care program is required to train all employees at the time they start work. This training should cover an explanation of human immunodeficiency virus, HBV, and hepatitis C virus exposure risk; an explanation of standard precautions; the types of tasks that might involve exposure; a description of the exposure-reporting procedure; information on HBV vaccine; and an opportunity to ask questions. Record of this training must be kept on file.

A health consultant can be extremely valuable in helping programs develop this plan and keeping the risk in perspective. There have been no reports of HIV transmission in child care settings, and evidence indicates the risk of HBV transmission is low. However, standard precautions are reasonable and will contribute to preventing the spread of common illness as well. The local OSHA office will be helpful in providing the state regulations, and the California/OSHA handout from the Child Care Law Center (see Resources) can help in developing an implementation plan specific to a child care program.

Staff Exclusion Policies

Staff with infectious diseases may transmit them to young children. Additionally, adult staff with certain illnesses may require rest to recuperate. The following guidelines from *Caring for Our Children*[1] apply to caregivers who have contact with children (see Chapter 17 for exclusion guidelines for children; the *2003 Red Book*[5] also provides information on exclusion policies).

Standard 3.069: Staff Exclusion for Illness

A facility shall not deny admission to or send home a staff member or substitute with illness unless one or more of the following conditions exists. The staff member shall be excluded as follows:

a) Chickenpox: until all lesions have dried and crusted, which usually occurs by 6 days;

b) Shingles: only if the lesions cannot be covered by clothing or a dressing until the lesions have crusted;

c) Rash with fever or joint pain: until diagnosed not to be measles or rubella;

d) Measles: until 4 days after onset of the rash (if the employee is immuno-competent);

e) Rubella: until 6 days after onset of rash;

f) Diarrheal illness: 3 or more episodes of diarrhea during the previous 24 hours or blood in stools, until diarrhea resolves; if *Escherichia coli* 0157:H7 or *Shigella* species are isolated, until diarrhea resolves and 2 stool cultures test negative;

g) Vomiting illness: 2 or more episodes of vomiting during the previous 24 hours, until vomiting resolves or is determined to result from noncommunicable conditions, such as pregnancy or a digestive disorder;

h) Hepatitis A virus infection: until 1 week after onset or as directed by the health department when immune globulin has been given to appropriate children and staff in the facility;

i) Pertussis: until after 5 days of appropriate antibiotic therapy (which is to be given for a total of 14 days) and until disease preventive measures, including preventive antibiotics and vaccines for children and staff who have been in contact with children infected with pertussis, have been implemented;

j) Skin infection (such as impetigo): until 24 hours after treatment has been initiated;

k) Tuberculosis: until noninfectious and cleared by a health department official;

l) Strep throat or other streptococcal infection: until 24 hours after initial antibiotic treatment and end of fever;

m) Head lice: until after the first treatment; scabies: until after treatment has been completed;

n) Purulent conjunctivitis, defined as pink or red conjunctiva with white or yellow eye discharge, often with matted eyelids after sleep, and including eye pain or redness of the eyelids or skin surrounding the eye: until 24 hours after treatment has been initiated;

o) *Haemophilus influenzae* type b: prophylaxis (immunization); excluded until antibiotic treatment has been initiated;

p) Meningococcal infection: until all staff members for whom antibiotic prophylaxis has been recommended have been treated;

q) Respiratory illness: if the illness limits the staff member's ability to provide an acceptable level of child care and compromises the health and safety of the children.

Child care providers who have herpes cold sores shall not be excluded from the child care facility, but shall: 1) cover and not touch their lesions; 2) carefully observe hand washing policies; and 3) refrain from kissing or nuzzling infants or children, especially those with dermatitis.

ADULT IMMUNIZATIONS

Just as children in child care must be up-to-date on their immunization schedules, adults working in child care should be current as to their immunization status as well. Adult immunization recommendations include:

- Diphtheria, tetanus (Td): complete a primary series and boosters every 10 years
- Measles, mumps, rubella (MMR): 2 doses for those born after 1956
- HBV: 3 doses
- Varicella: 2 doses if nonimmune (no history of disease and seronegative)
- Hepatitis A: persons at increased risk, persons who have chronic liver disease
- Influenza: every year for persons 50 years of age and older and for those who care for infants and children 2 years or younger

Immunizations recommended for older adults and for people with chronic illness include:

- Pneumococcal vaccine: at age 65 or with chronic disease

SPECIAL CONCERNS FOR PREGNANT STAFF

Infectious Diseases

As a professional group that comprises predominantly women of childbearing age, pregnancy is a common occurrence among the child care workforce. It is a time that usually poses special concerns for women; employment as a child care provider presents additional considerations because of the close contact with infants and young children. Table 19.1 presents a summary of the currently known effects of illnesses and stress during pregnancy, known risk data, and suggested prevention practices.

Other Concerns for Pregnant Staff

Many women feel that pregnancy, emotionally and physically, is both the best and worst of times. Common problems for pregnant child care staff (Table 19.2) include fatigue, exposure to infectious diseases (see above), back problems, frequent urination, swollen feet, and varicose veins. Pregnant child care providers should consult their own health care professional with any specific questions or concerns.

ERGONOMICS AND MUSCULOSKELETAL INJURIES AND HAZARDS

The need to lift, carry, bend, and sit on small furniture and the floor is a basic part of the child care day. Daily routines provide many opportunities for muscle pulls, strains, and sprains, which research cites as the most common occupational injuries. According to the few studies conducted to date, most child-care related physical injuries occur to the lower back.[6,7] When these or any other work-related injuries do occur, they should be documented on a form similar to the children's injury report form (see Chapter 16).

TABLE 19.2. Common Problems and Recommendations for Pregnant Child Care Staff

Problem	Recommendation
Fatigue	• Always take scheduled breaks • Rest on left side or with feet elevated during breaks and lunch • Keep each workday to no more than 8 hours • Rest when fatigued
Exposure to infectious diseases	• Use frequent and proper hand washing techniques • Use gloves and *standard precautions** where appropriate • Establish informational network for parents and staff to communicate child's diagnosis by a physician • Alert health care professional of child care work and potential for this exposure
Back problems	• Use proper lifting and carrying techniques • Avoid heavy lifting • Maintain good standing and seated posture • Use adult-sized furniture; bring an adult-sized, easily movable, comfortable chair from home if necessary • Avoid floor sitting • To avoid constant bending, have children climb up to child care provider (if developmentally appropriate) • Trade strenuous chores of lifting and moving heavy objects with other staff
Frequent urination	• Have other staff available to cover room assignment to maintain staff-child ratios
Swollen feet, varicose veins	• Wear support hose • Exercise • Change position frequently • Rest with feet elevated

Reprinted with permission from Gratz R, Boulton P. Health considerations for pregnant child care staff. *J Pediatr Health Care.* 1994;8:18–26

* Standard precautions should be taught, monitored, and routinely reinforced (See Chapter 17).

Child care providers spend much of their workday sitting on the floor with children; they regularly move heavy equipment and furniture; and when they are not sitting on the floor, they are frequently sitting on small, child-sized chairs.[3,8] The workplace analysis by King et al[9] on the ergonomics of child care identified 8 problem areas creating physical demands on child care providers and suggests recommendations for prevention of musculoskeletal injuries (Table 19.3).

Professionals have spent much time and effort designing environments to facilitate optimum child development (see Chapter 4); early childhood environments also should be studied and designed with the adult child care worker's optimum ergonomic health as a priority.[9,10]

TABLE 19.3. Analysis of the Child Care Work Environment

Problem	Recommendations
1. Incorrect lifting of children, toys, supplies, equipment, etc	1. Education on proper lifting and carrying techniques (see Fig 19.1) 2. Promote job rotation where possible 3. Encourage independence in children whenever feasible
2. Inadequate work heights (eg, child-sized tables and chairs)	1. Create a chair that would allow the staff to slide their legs under the table 2. Use sit and kneel chairs 3. Educate staff on proper body mechanics 4. Provide the staff with adult-sized chairs for occasional use
3. Difficulty lowering and lifting infants into and out of cribs	1. Modify crib sides to enable them to slide down or modify the legs of the cribs to accommodate the staff 2. Educate staff on the proper use of body mechanics
4. Frequent sitting on the floor with back unsupported	1. When possible, have staff sit up against a wall or furniture for back support 2. Perform stretching exercises 3. Educate staff on proper body mechanics
5. Excessive reaching above shoulder height to obtain stored supplies	1. Redesign kitchen area, placing heaviest items at waist height 2. Reorganize snacks and supplies to simplify snack preparation procedures 3. Use step stools when retrieving items that are above cupboard height
6. Frequent lifting of infants and toddlers on and off diaper changing tables	1. Educate staff on proper body mechanics? 2. Have toddlers use steps to decrease distances staff members are lifting
7. Forceful motions combined with awkward posture required to open windows	1. Use step stool to allow for better leverage and decrease awkward posture 2. Have maintenance staff improve quality of window slide
8. Carrying garbage and diaper bags to dumpster	1. Provide staff with cart to transport garbage 2. Relocate garbage cart closer to work area 3. Decrease size and weight of loads

Reprinted with permission from King P, Gratz R, Scheuer G, Claffey A. The ergonomics of child care: conducting worksite analyses. *Work.* 1996;6:25–32

Back belts, also called "back supports" or "abdominal belts," increasingly are being used by workers in numerous industries, including child care, to prevent injury during lifting. The National Institute for Occupational Safety and Health[11] has reviewed the scientific literature and concluded the current evidence does not support their use as protective equipment against back injury. Rather than relying solely on back belts, child care programs should implement an ergonomics program.

This involves modifying the environment to decrease lifting and staff training in the use of safe lifting techniques.

Body Mechanics for Child Care Workers

Good posture and safe lifting can help prevent musculoskeletal injuries. According to ergonomics professionals, it's not how much you lift or carry, but how you do it. The main idea of proper body mechanics is to distribute the work over several sets of muscles and make use of the strongest one(s). Maintaining good posture at work, in movement, and at rest conserves energy, preserves muscle and joint mobility, and decreases the risk of injury.

Specialists in this area recommend always warming up with light stretching before starting any physical activity. They also recommend a sitting position with back straight in the chair and both feet on the floor, thighs parallel to the floor. When seated on the floor, use proper posture and always support the back against the wall or furniture.

Child care providers lift children and equipment frequently. Proper lifting techniques (see Fig 19.1) can prevent back and shoulder strain and serious injury when lifting children off the floor, in and out of high chairs and cribs etc, and on and off nap cots and changing tables. When using proper lifting techniques, you should: get a firm footing; bend your knees, do not bend at the waist; lift with your legs, using strong leg muscles rather than weaker back muscles; keep the child as close as possible to your body; and avoid twisting and jerking motions.[12]

To avoid injuries, Gratz et al[12] also recommend that child care providers squat rather than bend when working at low counters, tables, or sinks; if you have

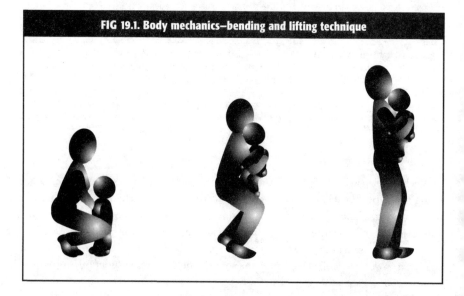

FIG 19.1. Body mechanics–bending and lifting technique

difficulty getting up from a squatting position, support yourself on a stable surface (such as a table or chair) and push up with your hands in addition to your legs; when reaching, use a sturdy step stool to get closer to the desired object; do not stretch with hands over head, stand on tip toes, or stretch your back; avoid leaning back too far when reaching for toys or food from high shelves; encourage independence in children whenever possible. For example, one could utilize stairs for children to climb onto changing tables); use a cart when transporting garbage to a dumpster; always push, do not pull, heavy objects.

STRESS AND BURNOUT

Caring For Our Children listed stress as 1 of 4 "major occupational health hazards" in child care work.[1(p410)] Those factors noted under stress include:

- Undervaluing of work (in both monetary compensation and status)
- Inadequate break time, sick leave, and personal days
- Working alone
- Responsibility for children's welfare
- Inadequate training
- Inadequate facilities
- Fear of liability

The major sources of stress in early childhood education also include aspects of the work environment, such as novelty and uncertainty, frustrations and barriers, pressures to achieve, and separation and loss. Child care settings are filled with examples of stressful situations each day. There are "…few other professions where the unexpected is so much to be expected."[13(p26)]

Sources of job stress in child care have been studied in greater detail for child care providers in group programs than for those who are family child care home providers. For family child care home providers, sources of stress have been suggested to be balancing multiple roles, maintaining positive relationships with parents, and maintaining a sense of accomplishment; "…the task of combining home and caregiving responsibilities may prove stressful—or even debilitating—if the caregiver does not plan carefully how to balance workloads and does not enlist the approval and support of others in the home environment."[14(p50)]

In group child care centers, sources of stress include similar factors experienced by family child care home providers (eg, long hours of continuous contact with children, little autonomy, role ambiguity, the physical demands of the job, income compared with other working parents, insufficient break time, unpaid overtime, and low salaries) and the additional potential stressor of relationships at work.[15] Additionally, communicating with parents; relationships between directors and staff and among staff; working in a predominantly female environment; and the children's behaviors and demands of the beginning and end of the workweek (ie, Mondays and Fridays) also have been noted as sources of stress in child care.[3,16]

Signs of emotional job stress can be psychologic, behavioral, or physiologic. They may manifest as various physical symptoms (eg, frequent headaches, difficulty sleeping, digestive problems, tenseness or irritability, fatigue, and feeling unmotivated or sad[17]) as well as lowered resistance to disease attributable to changes in immunocompetence.[13]

Stress can also lead to "burnout...a syndrome of emotional exhaustion and cynicism found in health and service personnel"[18(p6)] with which there is a loss of concern for the people one is working with.[19] Factors including personal characteristics, such as age, sex, marital status, educational experience, and ethnic background, are thought to influence burnout as well as external factors, such as the emotional intensity of involvement with people, a negative focus on problems, lack of positive feedback, and poor peer contact in the job setting.[20]

A number of early studies of burnout of workers in child care centers[18,19] found aspects of the work environment that were related to increased levels of burnout, ie, larger child-staff ratios; longer working hours on the floor with children; a less structured program; infrequent staff meetings; and fewer staff breaks. Burnout can also be traced to the nature of child care work as well as employment conditions. The focus of the work (the intensive child-adult relationship), staff personalities (idealistic, motivated to improve the lives of children), and employment conditions (wages, hours, benefits, responsibilities) lead to a description of many child care staff as "underpaid and overworked."[15,21]

Hyson[13] suggests 3 methods for coping with stress: seeking information; maintaining and regaining autonomy; and maintaining internal equilibrium. General information about growth and development and specific information regarding children in their care can make the "unfamiliar familiar."[13(p29)] A curriculum with structure that still enables flexibility is also beneficial to decreasing stress. Exploring ways to regain control in programming as well as of a staff member's emotional outlook are also stress decreasers.

Whitebook et al[15] recommend 1) an increase in staff involvement in decision making; 2) examining job title distinctions; and 3) improving break and substitute policies to decrease stress and increase levels of job satisfaction. Aronson[17] describes relaxation routines to decrease job stress (eg, exercise, talking things out, laughing, making lists, daydreaming, and relaxation exercises).

Dimidjian[14(p55)] suggests 4 strategies for family child care home providers to better cope with the stresses of in-home child care:

1. Acquiring additional knowledge and skills to deliver better caregiving
2. Forming affiliate support networks with other caregivers
3. Learning stress and time management techniques
4. Practicing monitoring one's own environmental demands, capabilities, and performance

PREVENTING OCCUPATIONAL INJURIES AND ILLNESSES

Preventing occupationally related illnesses and on-the-job injuries is the responsibility of not only the child care provider but also health care professionals concerned with the child care environment (see Chapter 15). The following guidelines can assist in providing an effective and ongoing prevention program.[22]

1. **Development of proper attitudes:** Positive attitudes toward health and safety can be encouraged through personal example of directors and health care professionals as well as by reinforcing these attitudes with child care providers.

2. **Knowledge of safe work procedures:** Keeping current with health and safety guidelines and research can assist in fostering a healthy work environment.

3. **Orientation and training of employees:** All formal training and education programs for child care providers should include an emphasis on health and safety issues and licensing regulations regarding health (see Chapter 2).

4. **Detection of employee personal difficulties:** Directors and other staff members can play an important role in areas such as stress and burnout to foster a healthy work setting.

5. **Enforcement of safe practices and regulations:** Maintaining proper staff-child ratios, hand washing, proper food preparation and storage, sanitation techniques, etc are essential to providing a safe and healthy child care program.

6. **Conducting planned observations:** Child care providers and program directors need to participate in ongoing opportunities to see that safe and healthy practices are being implemented.

7. **Prevention of unsafe conditions:** Unsafe conditions are a result of omission and commission. Worn-out equipment, peeling paint, etc should be removed or repaired quickly. Use of proper body mechanics for all activities should be taught and reinforced.

8. **Conducting planned safety inspections:** The program director and health care professionals can help prevent unsafe conditions with frequent and thorough inspections of the child care environment inside and outside the building.

9. **Conducting safety meetings:** Health and safety issues should be included as a permanent part of planned staff meetings as well as the focus of targeted meetings, brainstorming sessions, and in-service workshops.

10. **Correcting unsafe conditions:** When identified, unsafe conditions and activities should be remedied immediately.

11. **Investigating injuries and illness outbreaks:** An up-to-date log of injuries allows inquiry into the circumstances of the injury as soon as possible after it has occurred, and causes of the problem can be located and attended to. Record keeping of staff illnesses can provide documentation necessary to learn about how and when illnesses are spreading within a program.

STAFF HEALTH POLICIES

Staff Health Appraisal

Requiring employee health assessments identifies child care providers who are susceptible not only to infectious diseases but also to other occupational risks, such as back injuries, allergies, and stress. Ideally, assessments should be performed for new staff before contact with the children, after the job has been offered but before employment begins. Although state child care regulations regarding employee health assessments vary greatly, it is recommended that the staff members who have contact with children have a health appraisal within the first month of employment and every 2 years thereafter. Tuberculosis tests should be repeated every 2 years or as directed by local health departments. It is important to be informed of the legalities regarding employee health issues in accordance with the Americans With Disabilities Act; an example of such information is included in the Resources at the end of this chapter. Appendix G is a sample staff health assessment form. A thorough staff health assessment should include the following, at a minimum[1](Standard 1.045):

a) Health history;

b) Physical examination;

c) Dental examination;

d) Vision and hearing screening;

e) The results and appropriate follow-up of a tuberculosis screening using the Mantoux intradermal skin test, 1-step procedure (see Standard 6.014);

f) A review and certification of up-to-date immune status (measles, mumps, rubella, diphtheria, tetanus, poliovirus, varicella, influenza, pneumonia, hepatitis A, and hepatitis B) (see Standard 3.005 through Standard 3.007);

g) A review of occupational health concerns based on the performance of the essential functions of the job (see Standard 1.048);

h) Assessment of risk from exposure to common childhood infections, such as parvovirus, CMV, and chickenpox;

i) Assessment of orthopedic, psychological, neurologic, or sensory limitations or communicable diseases that require accommodations or modifications for the person to perform tasks that typical adults can do.

The national standards in *Caring for Our Children*[1] also address return to work and health limitations of staff in Standard 1.047: staff and volunteers must have a health care provider's release to return to work in the following situations:

a) When they have experienced conditions that may affect their ability to do their job or require an accommodation to prevent illness or injury in child care work related to their conditions (such as pregnancy, specific injuries, or infectious diseases);

b) After serious or prolonged illness;

c) When their condition or health could affect promotion or reassignment to another role;

d) Before return from a job-related injury;

e) If there are workers' compensation issues or if the facility is at risk of liability related to the employee's or volunteer's health problem;

f) When there is suspicion of a communicable disease.

If a staff member is found to be unable to perform the activities required for the job because of health limitations, the staff person's duties shall be limited or modified until the health condition resolves or employment is terminated because the facility can prove that it would be an undue hardship to accommodate the staff member with the disability.

Personnel Policies

The facility should have and follow written personnel policies. All written policies should be reviewed and signed by the employee affected by them on hiring and annually thereafter. Although the business plan of the child care program will determine the scope of benefits that can be offered, outlined below are the types of basic benefits that are recommended according to the staff benefit Standard 1.050, which applies to centers as well as large and small family child care homes[1]:

a) affordable health insurance;

b) sick leave;

c) vacation leave;

d) Social Security or other retirement plan;

e) workers' compensation;

f) holidays;

g) personal leave;

h) educational benefits;

i) family, parental, and medical leave.

The following measures recommended in Standard 1.049 should be offered to lessen stress for the staff and should be implemented to the maximum extent possible[1]:

a) Wages and benefits that fairly compensate the skills, knowledge, and performance required of caregivers, at the levels of wages and benefits paid for other jobs that require comparable skills, knowledge, and performance;

b) Job security;

c) Training to improve skills and hazard recognition;

d) Stress management and reduction training;

e) Regular work breaks;

f) Appropriate child-staff ratios;

g) Liability insurance for caregivers;

h) Staff lounge separate from child care area;

i) The use of sound-absorbing materials;

j) Regular performance reviews, which in addition to addressing any areas requiring improvement, provide constructive feedback, individualized encouragement, and appreciation for aspects of the job well performed;

k) Stated provisions for back-up staff, for example, to allow caregivers to take necessary time off when ill without compromising the function of the center or incurring personal negative consequences from the employer. This back-up should also include a stated plan to be implemented in the occasional event where a staff member needs to have a short, but relatively immediate break away from the children.

Employee Assistance Programs

Child care employees, like those of any organization, suffer the stresses and strains of daily life. Concerns such as marital and family and relationship problems; alcohol and drug abuse; legal troubles; emotional, psychologic, and financial problems; and job stress can affect employee health and performance. An employee assistance program provides confidential, professional assistance to employees and their families who are experiencing personal problems that could affect their well-being and job performance.

Many child care programs affiliated with large systems, such as school districts, government offices, colleges, and corporations, may have an employee assistance program. However, most community-based child care programs do not. In this case, a health consultant is well positioned to make referrals to resources in the community that may help resolve the personal problems of employees. A health consultant may also be called on to assist in starting an employee wellness program. Familiarity with community resources, such as health education centers and Head Start resources (see Resources at end of chapter) can provide some guidance.

OTHER LAWS AND REGULATIONS

Although the child care program director is responsible for all aspects of site administration, the child care health consultant should be aware that other statutes and regulations may provide guidelines or mandates that affect staff health and safety issues.

Child care regulations vary greatly among the states and may require staff health assessments, staffing ratios, staff training, and other health requirements. Head Start and child care systems under public auspices may have additional requirements.

Federal and state labor laws assert that employees of child care programs are entitled to the same legal rights as most other workers. Both federal and state laws protect employees with respect to minimum wage, overtime pay, and a variety of working conditions. When an area is covered by state and federal law, whichever offers the greatest protection prevails. The federal law is the Fair Labor Standards Act and is enforced by the US Department of Labor. Local contacts may be listed in a variety of ways in the government listing of the phone book, such as "Industrial Relations," or "Labor Standards Enforcement," or call the information number for your state government and ask what office enforces labor laws.

Workers' compensation for an illness or injury resulting from one's job is required by law in all states, although requirements vary among states. Its foundation depends on employees reporting job-related illnesses or injuries to their supervisor, who in turn files a report with the workers' compensation insurance carrier. Among the benefits an injured or ill employee may receive are medical care and treatment, short- or long-term disability benefits, and vocational counseling.

Federal and state OSHA requirements are designed to improve workplace health and safety. About half of the states administer their own programs. General requirements ask that employers inform employees of occupational risks and measures to decrease those risks, including training and the provision of protective equipment. Risks should be specific to the facility and may include infectious diseases, stress, noise, injuries, injuries from back strain and biting, skin injury from frequent hand washing, and environmental exposure to art supplies and cleaning and disinfecting materials.

All staff and volunteers are required to read and sign a statement that they have been informed of the risks, will abide by measures to decrease risks, and will inform their supervisor of any work-related illness or injury. Material safety data sheets on potentially hazardous materials should be kept on site. An OSHA poster must be placed where employees can see it, and some record keeping is involved. Samples of appropriate language are included in *Model Child Care Health Policies*.[23] For more information, call the local or regional OSHA offices.

The Americans With Disabilities Act applies to child care employee applicants and employees with disabilities to provide them with equal employment opportunity and to integrate them into the program's staff to the extent feasible, given the individual's limitations (see Resources).

The Family and Medical Leave Act of 1993 applies to companies that employ 50 or more workers; thus, it does not cover many programs for young children. It allows an employee to take up to 12 weeks of unpaid leave in any 12-month period for birth or adoption of a child; to take care of a child, spouse, or parent with a serious health condition; or for the employee's own health reasons.

The Pregnancy Discrimination Act of 1978 requires that pregnancy be treated no differently from other disability. Employers must permit physically able pregnant employees to work.

PROFESSIONAL ORGANIZATIONS

Professional organizations and associations can provide information and support regarding health and safety issues for the child care provider. The National Association for the Education of Young Children publishes a number of informative resource materials. The mission of the National Center for the Early Childhood

Workforce, formerly The Child Care Employee Project, is to ensure high-quality, affordable child care services by upgrading the training and compensation of teachers and providers. The mission is addressed through policy and program development, research and evaluation, and public education activities at the national, state, and local levels. Examples of some of the types of information and services they provide include:

- Surveys of early care and education programs, staff salaries, and working conditions
- Assessments of child care quality enhancement programs
- Conducting and publishing research on child care staffing issues
- Providing technical assistance for staff training and leadership development, grass roots organizing, and mentoring programs.

Local chapters of the American Academy of Pediatrics, community pediatricians, and many other professional organizations and associations can provide information and resources about health and safety issues. Information on national headquarters is included at the end of this chapter for selected organizations. Local chapters of these groups can also provide speakers and publications that child care centers may find useful for in-service meetings and workshops. Two- and 4-year college and university programs for training health care professionals as well as medical and dental schools are also excellent resources for providing health care personnel and information for child care providers.

CONCLUSIONS AND RECOMMENDATIONS

The child care health consultant may have the strongest impact in the area of staff health. Administrators and often child care providers themselves overlook their own needs. The health and safety of the child care provider is basic to providing quality care in group and family child care home settings. The partnership between the child care provider and the health care professional influences the health of the entire child care community: children, parents, and providers.

REFERENCES

1. American Academy of Pediatrics, American Public Health Association, and Maternal and Child Health Bureau. *Caring for Our Children. National Health and Safety Performance Standards: Guidelines for Out-of-Home Child Care Programs.* 2nd ed. Elk Grove Village, IL: American Academy of Pediatrics; 2002

2. Reves RR, Pickering LK. Infections in child day care centers as they relate to internal medicine. *Ann Rev Med.* 1990;41:383–391

3. Gratz R, Claffey A. Adult health in child care: health status, behaviors, and concerns of teachers, directors, and family child care providers. *Early Child Res Q.* 1996;11:243–267

4. Calder J. Occupational health and safety issues for child-care providers. *Pediatrics.* 1994; 94:1072–1074

5. American Academy of Pediatrics. *2003 Red Book: Report of the Committee on Infectious Diseases.* Pickering LK, ed. 26th ed. Elk Grove Village, IL: American Academy of Pediatrics; 2003

6. Whitebook M, et al. *Creating a Better Work Environment. Working for Quality Child Care. Vol 2.* Berkeley, CA: Child Care Employee Project; 1989

7. Brown MZ, Gerberich SG. Disabling injuries to childcare workers in Minnesota, 1985 to 1990. An analysis of potential risk factors. *J Occup Med.* 1993;35:1236-1243

8. Gratz R. *Wisconsin Early Childhood Professionals Occupational Health Survey: Preliminary Report and Recommendations From the Pilot Study.* Milwaukee, WI: Department of Health Sciences, University of Wisconsin-Milwaukee; 1994

9. King PM, Gratz R, Claffey A. The ergonomics of child care: conducting worksite analyses. *Work.* 1996;6:25-32

10. Markon P, LeBeau D. *Health and Safety at Work for Day-Care Educators.* Universite du Quebec: Chicoutimi, Quebec, Canada; 1994

11. National Institute for Occupational Safety and Health. *Back Belts. Do They Prevent Injury?* Washington, DC: US Department of Health and Human Services; 1994. DHHS Publication No. 94-127

12. Gratz R, Claffey A, Scheuer G. Taking care of yourself: the physical demands and ergonomics of working with young children. Paper presented at the Annual Conference of the National Association for the Education of Young Children; November 1996; Dallas, TX

13. Hyson MC. Playing with kids all day: job stress in early childhood education. *Young Child.* 1982;37:25-32

14. Dimidjian VJ. Understanding and combating stress in family day care. *J Child Care.* 1982; 1:47-58

15. Whitebook M, Howes C, Darrah R, Friedman J. Caring for the caregivers: staff burnout in child care. In: Katz LG, ed. *Current Topics in Education.* Vol 4. Norwood, NJ: Ablex Publishing; 1982:211-235

16. Gratz RR. *Violence in the Lives of Urban Children: Determining the Training and Support Needs of Teachers of Young Children.* Milwaukee, WI: Urban Research Center, University of Wisconsin-Milwaukee; 1995

17. Aronson S. Health concerns of caregivers. *Child Care Inf Exch.* 1987;54:33-37

18. Pines A, Maslach C. Combating staff burn-out in a day care center: a case study. *Child Care Quarterly.* 1980;9:5-16

19. Maslach C, Pines A. The burn-out syndrome in the day care setting. *Child Care Quarterly.* 1977;6:100-113

20. Maslach C. Burnout: *The Cost of Caring.* Engelwood Cliffs, NJ: Prentice Hall; 1982

21. Whitebook M, Howes C, Darrah R, Friedman J. Who's minding the child care workers? A look at staff burn-out. *Child Today.* 1981;10:15-20

22. Wisconsin Department of Administration. *Safety Fundamentals for Supervisors.* Madison, WI: Bureau of State Risk Management; 1994

23. Pennsylvania Chapter, American Academy of Pediatrics. *Model Child Care Health Policies.* 4th ed. Rosemont, PA: American Academy of Pediatrics, Pennsylvania Chapter; 2002

ADDITIONAL RESOURCES

Canadian Paediatric Society. *Well-beings: A Guide to Promote the Physical Health, Safety and Emotional Well-being of Children in Child Care Centres and Family Day Care Homes.* 2nd ed. Toronto, Canada: Creative Premises; 1999

Centers for Disease Control and Prevention. *The ABCs of Safe and Healthy Child Care: A Handbook for Child Care Providers.* Atlanta, GA: Centers for Disease Control and Prevention; 1996. Available at: http://www.cdc.gov/ncidod/hip/abc/contents.htm#top. Accessed March 19, 2004

Child Care Law Center. *HIV and AIDS: Employment Issues in Child Care.* San Francisco, CA: Child Care Law Center; 1995

Child Care Law Center. *The Americans With Disabilities Act: Employing People with Disabilities in Child Care.* San Francisco, CA: Child Care Law Center; 1996

Gratz RR, Boulton P. Health considerations for pregnant child care staff. *J Pediatr Health Care.* 1994;8:18–26

Head Start Information and Publication Center. *Enhancing Children's Growth and Development* and *Preventing and Managing Communicable Disease.* Available at: http://www.headstartinfo.org/cgi-bin/pubcatstore.cfm?CatID=52&do=detail. Accessed March 19, 2004

Reves RR, Pickering LK. Impact of child day care on infectious diseases in adults. *Infect Dis Clin North Am.* 1992;6:239–250

ORGANIZATIONS

American Association of Occupational Health Nurses
2920 Brandywine Road, Suite 100
Atlanta, GA 30341
Phone: 770/455-7757
Web site: http://www.aaohn.org

American Occupational Therapy Association
Work Programs Special Interest Section
PO Box 31220
Bethesda, MD 20824-1220
Phone: 301/652-2682
　　　　800/377-8555 (TDD)
Web site: http://www.aota.org

California Child Care Health Program
1322 Webster Street, Suite 402
Oakland, CA 94612-3218
Phone: 510/281-7917
Web site: http://www.childcarehealth.org

Child Care Law Center
973 Market Street, Suite 550
San Francisco, CA 94103
Phone: 415/495-5498
Fax: 415/495-6734
Website: http://www.childcarelaw.org

National Association for the Education of Young Children (NAEYC)
1509 16th Street NW
Washington, DC 20036-1426
Phone: 202/232-8777
        800/424-2460
Web site: http://www.naeyc.org

National Center for the Child Care Workforce (formerly The Child Care Employee Project)
733 15th Street NW, Suite 1037
Washington, DC 20005-2112
Phone: 202/737-7700
        800/896-7849
Fax: 202/737-0370
Web site: http://www.ericps.crc/wiuc.edu/nccic/org

National Institute of Occupational Safety and Health (NIOSH)
Humphrey Building, Room 715 H
MS P06
200 Independence Avenue SW
Washington, DC 20201
Phone: 800/356-4674
Fax: 513/533-8573 (Publications Office)
Web site: http://www.cdc.gov/niosh

National Safety Council
1121 Spring Lake Drive
Itasca, IL 60143-3201
Phone: 800/621-7615
Web site: http://www.msc.org

Occupational Safety and Health Administration (OSHA)
US Department of Labor
200 Constitution Avenue NW
Washington DC 20210
Phone: 202/219-8151 (Office of Public Affairs)
        202/219-8148 (General Information)
        202/219-4667 (Publications)
Web site: http://www.osha.gov *(lists local consultation offices)*

Office of Women's Health
US Department of Health and Human Services
US Public Health Service
200 Independence Avenue
Washington, DC 20201
Phone: 202/690-7650

CHAPTER 20

Families With Special Needs

Lois S. Sadler, PhD, RNCS, PNP, and Leslie Nield-Anderson, PhD, APRN-BC

LEARNING OBJECTIVES

This chapter discusses children living in families with the following characteristics: poverty, a single parent, substance abusing parents, depressed parents, adolescent parents, and parents with mental retardation. Often, several or possibly all of these conditions may coexist. The reader should:

- Understand the unique background, developmental, and behavioral characteristics of families with special needs and be able to clarify common myths about these family compositions.

- Identify areas of risks and strengths that require assessment by health care professionals and child care providers who interact with children of families with special needs.

- Learn about community resources, barriers faced by these families, and general and specific prevention and intervention strategies to foster positive coping in families with special needs who are raising young children.

INTRODUCTION

In assessing and understanding children and families with special needs, it is important for the health care professional to think about the many facets of the child and family that may contribute to the risk or the resiliency of the child and the family system in which the child lives. Bronfenbrenner[1] describes the child as unfolding within a series of nested systems that all influence the course of development. The individual child is at the center, surrounded by the family system, then the local community system, and finally the largest, societal or cultural system. Often, the child care center or child care providers intersect the child's family and community spheres and become influential sources of support for families and children. Conceptual frameworks that address family stress and adaptation for vulnerable parents, such as those who are poor, single, depressed, substance abusing, cognitively limited, or adolescents, are helpful to health care professionals and child care program planners.[2] Family stress and adaptation models depict the family's coping resources and include individual parents' resources such as self-esteem or mastery, the characteristics of the individual child, and family level resources including the way in which the family views the stressor, and resources in the environment which either assist or hinder the family's efforts to adapt or adjust to stressful situations.[2]

In each family situation described in this chapter, there are common areas, such as parental competence, parent-child relationships, parents' understanding of their children, children's development, the parenting role, parental behaviors, adequacy of child supervision for safety issues, and the potential for child neglect or abuse. Factors that contribute to strength and resiliency among family members living in harsh environments include personal resources (such as intelligence, self-efficacy, coping skills, or strategies), family environments that foster cohesion and promote competence in family members, and extended family and community supports that provide structure and aid to families.[3,4]

CHILDREN AND FAMILIES LIVING IN POVERTY

There are more than 12.1 million children living below the federal poverty level in this nation.[5] The number has increased for the second straight year. Nearly all of the increases occurred among black and Hispanic children. Children younger than 6 years and African American and Hispanic children experience disproportionately high rates of poverty, although the total number of young children living in poverty is highest for white children.[5-7] Of greatest concern are the 15% of children living in poor families in which poverty has lasted 10 years or more, because these children and families suffer the worst and longest-lasting effects of poverty.[5,8] Poor families are more likely to be headed by young female single parents, have low levels of parental education and earning potential, and have high levels of parental underemployment.[7,8]

Poverty affects children's health and well-being by acting directly and indirectly on their lives. Nutrition (undernutrition and excess empty calories), access to health care, home environments and stability, parental interactions with children, parental mental health, and neighborhood conditions are influenced by poverty. Toxic neighborhoods, including social hazards as well as environmental hazards, are especially worrisome in isolated urban pockets of severe poverty. These neighborhoods often have concentrations of hazardous environmental conditions, such as heavy industry, interstate highways, neighborhood violence, drug and alcohol abuse, and substandard public services, such as housing, schools, shopping areas, health care centers, and safe recreational facilities. Problems associated with families and children living in rural poverty often include geographic isolation and difficulty with transportation for access to social or community support services. Prevailing community attitudes concerning the family's acceptance of social service programs or assistance also vary from setting to setting and need to be understood and incorporated into any plan for outreach or support for poor families.

Poor families with young children (most often headed by a single mother) represent about 36% of the nations' homeless shelter population.[5,9] Beyond the reported figures, there are many more families with young children who experience "hidden homelessness," which occurs when families undergo multiple household changes over the course of a year or often double-up households with friends or family members. Either form of homelessness places enormous stressors on parents and children, including periods of living in crowded, unsafe environments, loss of privacy, disrupted schooling and health care, family separations, and lack of the basic necessities of life. Health problems experienced by these children are more serious than for poor children in general and include behavioral and developmental problems, nutritional and growth disorders, asthma, anemia, lead poisoning, upper respiratory illnesses, skin problems, ear and eye infections, and low levels of childhood immunizations.[9]

Poor families with young children (most often headed by a single mother) represent about 36% of the nations' homeless shelter population.

There are significant and long-term health and mental health problems affecting children who grow up in poor families. One in 6 children living in the United States has no health insurance.[7,10] Child health varies by parental income. Children living in the poorest families have the greatest incidence of health problems and receive the least amount of preventive pediatric care.[5,7] Available data suggest that the earlier in childhood that poverty occurs, the more serious the health and social consequences are.[8] When compared with children living in families above the poverty threshold, poor children are almost twice as likely to be born at low birth weight, are twice as likely to be reported to be in fair or poor health, and are less likely to be up-to-date in their immunizations. Poor children have higher rates of infant and childhood mortality, injuries, and chronic conditions, such as asthma and dental problems, and are more than 3 times as likely to be exposed to lead poisoning. They are more likely to suffer from malnutrition and short stature than are non-poor children.[8,11] Further, an association has been reported between the length and the depth of the family's poverty and greater decreases in children's IQ. Similar trends are seen in school achievement in that children who experience poverty before 5 years of age are more likely to experience school failure than are children who live in poverty that starts after 5 years of age.[5,8] Mental health effects are not as striking, but poor children are more likely to suffer from anxiety, depression, social withdrawal, aggression, and acting-out behavior.[5]

Parents raising children in poverty environments experience worse physical and mental health than do nonpoor parents. Economic stress and emotional stress undermine parenting efficacy, confidence, and adaptive parenting behaviors.[12] Although child abuse occurs in families from all economic levels, the additional burdens of poverty on parents, especially young single parents who may also be experiencing mental health or substance abuse problems, greatly increases the likelihood of harsh parental discipline and abuse.[13]

Assessing and Promoting Positive Family Coping

An assessment of families living in poverty environments begins with an assessment of how the family system is able to meet the basic needs of its members. The quantity and quality of social support are important to assess, including the levels of tangible support (help with basic needs), advice and coaching support, emotional support, any recent significant losses in the support network, and the degree of satisfaction versus intrusiveness that the family feels about the support. Family support networks commonly include extended family members, friends, neighbors, coworkers, and health or social service professionals. Especially when gaps are identified within the support network, it is necessary to assess the need for referrals to local community-based or state or federal programs providing essential services for young families such as housing, food, utilities, transportation, health insurance, and income support. The family assessment should examine how the family perceives and copes with stress, whether family members work together in cooperative modes or competitive modes, and the family's developmental stage. In some cases, the stage of family development may contribute additional developmental stressors to the already economically stressed family system.[2] For example, there are several life cycle stages that most families find expensive and emotionally demanding, and these include the early stages of the transition to parenthood and the stage of raising adolescents. When family stages overlap (as in the case of adolescent parenthood) the stressors are often compounded. The family assessment should also include a history of major life events (moves, deaths in family, previous unresolved losses, etc) as well as how the parents cope with the more mundane but persistent daily hassles (car trouble, arguments with neighbors, etc) and parenting hassles (child whining for toys or candy while shopping, etc).

Family cohesiveness and unity are often buffers that may help families to withstand some of the adverse effects of poverty on family members. Individual and group interventions should help families focus on ways they can increase their sense of family cohesiveness, such as relying on family traditions and rituals (such as birthday or holiday celebrations), the role of spirituality in the family, finding tension-reducing strategies or activities (physical exercise, opportunities for recreation, etc), and reframing the cause of the poverty situation (if in fact it is attributable to larger shifts in the economy) to help decrease some of the individual shame and guilt felt by parents.[14] An important goal of clinical work with parents living in poverty is to help them restore their parenting confidence, which is often closely linked to maternal self-esteem.[9] Mentor programs and parental skill-modeling programs offered through the child care center with child care staff as role models or use of home visitors to help with parental behaviors and skills provide opportunities for valuable intervention.[15,16]

Assessment of health services, which includes issues of access and involvement with parental health and mental health services and substance abuse treatment, is essential. It may be necessary to educate parents about ways to find consistent health care professionals for their children and how to use the phone more effectively (if phone service is available) for obtaining phone advice about health questions and episodic illnesses or conditions and how to avoid unnecessary health care and emergency room visits. Health care professionals may need to be particularly resourceful in helping parents living in poverty obtain preventive dental care for their children; this is one of the most neglected areas of preventive health care in poor children. Health care professionals or child care staff may need to assume an advocacy and mentoring role while assisting parents to negotiate the many systems and bureaucracies necessary to obtain needed services (see http://www.medical-homeinfo.org). It may be useful to encourage families to use available community resources in a proactive way rather than waiting for a crisis (eg, applying for nutritional supplement programs rather than relying on food pantries or soup kitchens when there is no food in the house). As advocates for families, it is important for pediatric health care professionals and child care providers to be aware of and support programs that use collaborative community empowerment models to improve living conditions and services in the neighborhoods in which poor families and children live.

CHILDREN OF SINGLE-PARENT FAMILIES

There is much diversity in family structure among the approximately 32% of families in the United States that are single-parent family units.[7] Single-parent families include families in which parents have never married (51% mother-headed and 7% father-headed), families after divorce (37% mother-headed and 5% father-headed), and single-parent families resulting from widowhood (1%).[6] Additionally, families such as military families may have 2 parents, but 1 is often away from the family for extended periods of time, and the family suffers many of the same stressors as does a single-parent family. Adolescent parents constitute a particularly vulnerable category of single-parent families because of their combined developmental issues, single-parent status, and greater likelihood of living in poverty (see section on adolescent parents in this chapter).

Rates of single-parent families are increasing largely because of an increase in the number of single women having children across all age groups. The 2 groups with the greatest increase include highly educated professional women and undereducated younger women living in poverty.[17] In the United States, between 85% and 90% of single-parent families are headed by females, and this finding is associated with a greater likelihood that the family unit will experience the effects of poverty.[2,5] However, not all single-parent families are struggling or living in poverty. For example, single-parent status may be planned and desired, as with some professional women later in childbearing age with resources to help mediate the stresses of raising and supporting a child. Additionally, families exist in which single-parent status exists on paper only, as there are partners or household members who are actively involved and committed to helping raise the children in the family.[17] If this is the case, the children of these couples (either heterosexual or gay or lesbian) have similar outcomes regarding their adjustment and school performance as children who live within more traditional married couple family constellations.[17,18]

Risk Factors

The likelihood that many single-parent families will experience poverty is a significant stressor for these family units. Additional stressors for these families include the negative public perceptions that are perpetuated by descriptive terms such as "illegitimate children" and "unmarried mothers." Single-parent family status is still associated with a stigma.[2,17]

Within single-parent families, there may be couple relationships, partnerships, and household members that often change and contribute to confusion and instability within the family system or possibly provide additional sources of support. It is important that health care professionals and child care providers not hold universal assumptions about single-parent families, but rather always assess support systems and household or family members who may serve as parental figures or provide important assistance for the family and for the children.

Children whose mothers never married have not experienced the stresses of the divorce process, and they are commonly raised by their mothers and extended family members. Children born to single women are at greater risk of adverse birth outcomes related to less prenatal care, poor nutrition, less weight gain during pregnancy, smoking during pregnancy, and being more likely to live in poverty.[7] Health risks of children growing up in these single-parent families continue to be linked to issues of family stressors, finances, and availability of health insurance and accessible health care.[5] Mothers in these families work more hours and receive less social support and parenting support, especially when raising sons.[17]

Each parent's own developmental history contributes to parenting behaviors and styles they will use with their own children.[19] It is, therefore, important to also assess whether the single parent experienced abusive parenting behaviors as a child, because the stresses of being a single parent may contribute to feeling overwhelmed and in some cases may lead to harsh or abusive behavior toward their own children. These behaviors may be mediated by the presence of a supportive network of friends or family members.

Approximately 28% of all US families are divorced single-parent families, and it is estimated that approximately 40% to 50% of all children living in the United States will spend some time in a single-parent home.[20] During the process of separation and divorce, parents and children undergo tremendous periods of disruption and reorganization of household and family routines. Most children manifest some emotional and behavioral problems in the months before and after the divorce, and many researchers are finding that these problems may persist into adulthood.[21,22]

During this time, parents have to cope with a change in household, usually a changing economy of family resources involving less money initially if not permanently, custody issues while reworking their parenting roles and adult roles, and a potential change in residence after divorce.[2] As a result of divorce, a family's standard of living (including housing, food, clothing, and access to health care and insurance) often declines rapidly and is highly dependent on the reliability of child support payments.[17] Single-parent mothers who enter the workforce as a result of divorce often have to cope with low salaries, poor benefits, high child care costs, and significantly less time available to spend with children. Feeling the failure of the marriage often raises emotional issues in parents, including depression, anxiety, and loneliness. During the period of transition, there is an increased incidence of alcohol and drug use, depression, somatic complaints, and health problems in parents. These issues usually moderate during the 2 years after the divorce.

Single-parent families describe positive aspects of their families that helped them cope with single parenthood status, including a large and helpful social support network, the ability of family members to communicate with one another, and being involved in a religious organization.[23] Adaptive family coping patterns, commonly described in black families, include traditions of relying on geographically close domestic networks of family and friends for exchanging needed goods and services and shared child care or periods of child keeping as ways to relieve some of the stresses (financial and emotional) for single parents and their children.[24,25] In single-parent families for which there are few or no family supports, health care professionals may need to create or locate available support systems or groups within the community (such as parenting self-help groups, mentor programs, parent support groups within churches or synagogues). For especially high-risk single-parent families, home visitation programs in the early stages of parenting may be helpful.[15] Child care centers and child care providers often become a significant part of family support systems, especially in the case of single-parent families for which there are no other available extended family members. Because the parent's own store of personal resources (such as self-esteem, ability to solve problems, and sense of mastery) are so important in enacting the parenting role, it is important to assess and encourage single parents to try to schedule adult recreational and relaxation time for themselves, if possible, on a periodic basis to give themselves a respite and restore their energy and perspective.

DEPRESSED PARENTS AND THEIR CHILDREN

A major depressive disorder, also referred to as affective disorder, mood disorder, and unipolar depression, is a disturbance in mood. Its clinical characteristics are associated with a loss of interest or pleasure in activities (anhedonia) and a depressed mood most of the day, nearly every day, for 2 weeks. There is often a change in weight (increase or decrease) with accompanying changes in appetite; changes in sleeping patterns (increase or decrease); decreased energy with fatigue and tiredness; a diminished ability to concentrate; feelings of worthlessness, hopelessness, or excessive guilt; and possibly recurrent thoughts about death. A dysthymic disorder is a chronically depressed mood that occurs most of the day for more days than not for at least 2 years. For a complete description and discussion regarding classifications and diagnostic criteria for mood disorders, see the *Diagnostic and Statistical Manual of Mental Disorders, Fourth Edition (DSM-IV)*[26] or the *Diagnostic and Statistical Manual for Primary Care (DSM-PC)*[27] for primary care providers.

Depression has been identified as the most common psychiatric problem seen in primary care settings. It is estimated that one third to one half of individuals with depression are not accurately diagnosed, and treatment is therefore delayed or inadequate. Depressive disorders tend to be chronic and recurrent. Individuals with a major depression experience 5 to 6 episodes in a lifetime, with most episodes resolving in 6 to 9 months.[28] Depression occurs approximately 2 times more frequently in women than in men, with first onset typically developing before 20 years of age, across diverse cultures. Depression in women not only has an earlier onset than in men, but episodes tend to last longer and recur more often in women than in men. However, for men and women, the onset of depression usually occurs during the childbearing and child-rearing years. Depressive episodes are often preceded by an anxiety disorder. Depressive disorders impair work performance and attendance and family functioning and incur high health care expenses.[29]

Approximately 8% of mothers are clinically depressed at any given time. After childbirth, major depression occurs in 10% to 15% of new mothers, generally within the first 2 weeks after delivery. The cause of postpartum depression is not known. It has been postulated that changes in estrogen, progesterone, cortisol, and β-endorphin levels are responsible for mood changes, and treatment with estrogen has been effective in some cases.[29,30] Postpartum depression can begin within the first 3 postnatal months and extend beyond 12 months. Risk factors include psychosocial stressors, marital discord, and a history of depression. It is estimated that 20% to 30% of pregnant women with a history of depression will experience postpartum depression, and the risk of recurrence with subsequent pregnancies is 50% when there have been previous episodes of depression.[29-31] Depression in fathers after childbirth has not been widely studied. However, there seems to be a higher rate of postnatal depression in fathers when there has been a history of depression with a father and when a wife or partner experiences depression during pregnancy or soon after delivery.[31]

Research in the area of children of depressed parents has focused on prevalence rates of psychiatric disorders in offspring, underlying explanations involving genetic factors, and the influence of living with depressed parents on children's development and adjustment. Studies of twins and adoptions demonstrated that genetic factors only partially account for the problems of children with depressed parents. There is increasing evidence that marital distress, family stress, family interactional patterns, and the more intrinsic factors of depression, such as low self-esteem, contribute comparable effects.[28,32-34]

Studies investigating the impact of parental depression on children have primarily addressed the influence of mothers' depression, as primary caregivers, on children. A survey by Kessler et al[35] confirms the importance of continued research in this direction. Maternal depression was identified by female participants to be the greatest childhood adversity; male participants identified their mothers' depression to be the second greatest adversity and fathers' aggression to be their greatest adversity. It remains, however, a challenge to health care professionals and researchers to continue to unravel the complicated genetic factors and family dynamics for why some children from depressed families develop psychiatric disorders, others suffer from impaired social functioning, and still others develop adaptively.[36]

Parental Depression and Related Problems

Parental depression has been associated with increased rates of substance abuse, suicide, medical hospitalizations, outpatient primary care medical visits, marital and family problems, domestic violence, child abuse, and psychiatric, social, and academic problems in children. The presence of other medical and family difficulties can overshadow an accurate diagnosis of depression as an important contributing factor.[37]

Depressed individuals frequently suffer with the mental disorder of depression and a cooccurring substance-induced disorder, commonly referred to as a dual diagnosis. Thirty-two percent to 44% of individuals with a substance-related disorder suffer from a cooccurring major depression, with the first onset of depression and use of substances occurring during child-rearing and childbearing years.[38-41] Poverty, homelessness, unemployment, domestic violence, child abuse, marital and family turmoil, and legal difficulties have been consistently related to the cooc-currence of substance-related disorders and depressive disorders, placing children at higher risk of academic, social, and health problems as well as anxiety, depression, and conduct disorders.[35,37]

Depression can be a physiologic consequence to many medical illnesses and pharmacologic agents or a psychologic response to a medical condition.[42] Medical illnesses (multiple sclerosis, diabetes, sickle cell anemia, traumatic injuries, cardiac disease, arthritis, cancer) are associated with increased incidences of depression and mortality, placing greater demands on family life. A parent who is depressed and medically ill spends more days in bed, has increased somatic complaints with corresponding increased outpatient medical visits, has longer and more frequent hospitalizations, and experiences more physical pain and functional impairment than does a nondepressed parent with a medical illness.[34,42] Families with a depressed medically ill parent find themselves managing psychiatric and medical regimens as well as associated medical and psychiatric crises. Families must contend with trans-portation difficulties, often to several treatment sites, increased strains on family finances, overburdened family and social networks, and strained personal coping and adjustment skills. Family members struggle, along with their medically ill member, with fatigue, uncertainty, and helplessness.[43] Health care professionals them-selves can become overwhelmed when treating families with the complexities of cooccurring disorders. A problem for health care professionals and their patients occurs when depressive episodes are not identified as the family interacts with many professionals and agencies.

Depressed parents commonly experience other psychiatric difficulties. Anxiety disorders, personality disorders, and what is referred to as "double depression" often cooccurs with a major depression. Double depression refers to individuals who suffer from a major depression while suffering also from the more enduring depression, dysthymia. It is estimated that double depression develops in approxi-mately 40% of individuals with major depression.[28]

Depression in parents threatens a child's family life and physical safety. Family violence does not occur out of the blue. Children of depressed parents are more likely to lose a parent from suicide. Also, an estimated 60% of women who murdered their children indicated that they had sought assistance from a physician for a med-ical problem 4 to 6 weeks before the incident.[42] Mothers who are abusive with their children consistently report significantly greater depressive symptomatology with accompanying negative feelings of self-worth, a diminished sense of self-competence, lower social support networks, and family strife; these characteristics can significantly interfere with a child's developmental, intellectual, and social needs.

Parental Depression, Family Dynamics, and Assessment

When a parent is suffering from depression, it is difficult for him or her to function and participate in family life. Children living with parents with recurring depression are particularly vulnerable to parents' diminished ability to interact with them positively, to socialize them to the larger world, and to expose them to a variety of experiences needed for developmental independence and intellectual enrichment.

The Touch Research Institute at the University of Miami School of Medicine has ongoing investigations on the influences of interactional patterns between depressed parents and their infants.[44,45] Two predominant interactional patterns have been identified. In one interactional pattern, withdrawn and understimulating, there is a decrease in a depressed mother's positive facial expressions, vocalizations, tactile stimulation, and affectionate playful contacts. Mothers are disengaged and less responsive and respond primarily when their infants are distressed. In the other interactional pattern, mothers are intrusive and overstimulating; interactional behaviors are haphazard, abrupt, disconnected, and looming.[44,45] Infants' responses to their mothers' interactional style varies, ranging from less attentiveness, looking around, fewer contented expressions, and lower activity levels to attempting to avoid contact with their mothers, protesting, and being fussy. Interestingly, mothers with sustained depressions of 3 to 6 months after delivery seem to have right frontal activation on electroencephalograms (EEGs), low vagal tone, decreased serotonin, and elevated norepinephrine and cortisol levels. Similarly, their infants have a decreased responsivity to facial expressions, elevated norepinephrine and cortisol levels, right frontal activation on EEG, and a tendency to sleep excessively. Elevated norepinephrine and cortisol levels suggest interactional stress between depressed mothers and infants.[46,47] The significance of the EEG activation pattern is not known, but it has been hypothesized that it may be a biologic marker for infant vulnerability toward an anxious and fearful disposition and future difficulties with social withdrawal during preschool and adult depression.[45,47] Infants of chronically depressed mothers have lower scores on mental, motor, and growth percentiles (weight and length) at 1 year of age.[45] Importantly, if a mother's depression goes into remission during the first year of an infant's life, there appears to be no lasting effects, strongly supporting the necessity for early detection and intervention.[47]

The importance of early detection and intervention in parental depression was noted earlier by Billings and Moos.[48] They found, from a 1-year follow-up of depressed parents with children 18 years or younger, that children of chronically depressed parents had higher levels of depression, anxiety, physical health problems, and more difficulties academically and in peer interactions than did children who did not have a depressed parent. The children whose parents were not chronically depressed were able to function at higher levels than were children whose parents were chronically depressed, and both sets of children were more disabled than were children from homes in which there was not a depressed parent. Parents' functioning levels and self-esteem significantly improved when their depression went into remission, and their functioning capability and self-esteem were similar to nonde-pressed parents.[48] These results suggest that the effects of parental depression on offspring are associated with symptom duration and can be buffered with early assessment and intervention.

Many studies document an increased risk of major depression in children whose parents are depressed. Few studies of offspring of depressed parents, however, have followed offspring longitudinally into adulthood to document the nature and extent of risk. At the Yale University Depression Research Unit in New Haven, Connecticut, Weissman et al[49,50] conducted a 10-year follow-up study of children who initially were between 6 and 23 years of age when treated at the unit and who had 1 or both parents with diagnosed major depression. They reported that the children of depressed parents had fewer children and higher rates of major depression, phobias, panic disorder, and alcohol dependence than did children of nondepressed parents. Female children of depressed parents in the study had an onset of major depression that peaked between 15 and 20 years of age. Males had a gradual rise in the onset of major depression after puberty. After 20 years of age, the incidence rates were not only similar for males and females but also decreased. The peak incidence of anxiety for males and females was between 5 and 10 years of age. The onset of separation anxiety and phobias occurred at approximately 5 years and 6.5 years of age, respectively, with a decrease in

Children of depressed parents had fewer children and higher rates of major depression, phobias, panic disorder, and alcohol dependence than did children of nondepressed parents.

incidence rates after 12 years of age. The incidence of alcohol dependence, on the other hand, for males and females increased at 15 to 20 years of age and after 25 years of age. The most frequently reported feeling of the children was worth-lessness, and many experienced poor overall functioning in work, family, and mar-riage. Offspring were less likely to go for treatment when they needed it and less likely to receive treatment when they were depressed and frequently received no treatment at all. An early report of this study (2-year follow-up)[51] found first onset of suicide attempts, major depression, anxiety disorders, conduct disorders, and substance abuse higher among children of depressed parents. The recurring familial nature of major depression and comorbidity with other disorders found in this study concurs with other researchers' findings across settings, populations, and cultures and further supports the importance of early diagnosis and treatment for depressed parents and offspring.

Depressed parents have been observed to exhibit less affection and respond less positively and more negatively, with quickened anger, hostility, and irritability. Hostile transactions between depressed parents and their children are more pro-nounced in older school-aged children, who are more active and challenging to authority—shouting, slapping, and coercion are more apparent during exchanges rather than negotiation and offering choices. Interestingly, depressed mothers commonly describe angry, aggressive, destructive, and depressed behaviors in their children. It remains unclear whether these are negative and distorted maternal self-appraisals projected onto children, leading to children's future depression and common comorbid difficulties, such as conduct disorders and substance use, or are foretelling observations by mothers' about their children's vulnerabilities. Nevertheless, it emphasizes the need for health care professionals to examine parents' perceptions of their children's behavior and determine the need for a more extensive evaluation of parent and child for depression.[28,34,52,53]

Severity and duration of family stress influences children's ability to function interpersonally and academically. Depressed parents usually have several family stressors occurring simultaneously, and the relationship among stress factors and parental depression is not well understood. The stressors may be a consequence of a parent's depression, depression may be an additive effect of stressors, or a parent's depression may be a consequence of circumstances outside the family related to neighborhood and economic conditions.[28,48,54,55] Nevertheless, the stress of low socioeconomic conditions and inadequate partner and social supports are highly related to depression in mothers. Poor families are more likely to be headed by young female single parents who have never been married or are divorced, living in impoverished neighborhoods (see Children and Families Living in Poverty in this chapter). In addition, low self-esteem and low self-confidence are more prevalent in women than in men, as are beliefs about poor parenting competencies, higher unemployment rates, higher rates of childhood abuse, and less education. Health care professionals need to evaluate mothers routinely for depression when financial situations are strained and mothers are living alone with their children. Whether a pediatric or an adult health care professional, information regarding family stressors is an essential component of health care assessments.

Despite risks associated with growing up in a family with a depressed parent, some children are resilient, and their ability to adapt and function is not impaired. A protective factor for offspring involves early treatment of a parent's depression to decrease the severity of the depression and increase a parent's ability to function. Early treatment can buffer the effects of a depressed parent's social isolation through increasing community contacts, improving partner relations, and enhancing family relations. Harmful effects of a parent's depression can be diminished by having an unaffected parent, family member, or friend. Exposure to adults and siblings who provide diverse interactive experiences in caring, warm, and supportive ways can cushion the more negative influences of a depressed parent's low self-esteem, negative appraisals, and decreased socialization capabilities by promoting positive life experiences for children.

Depression in Children and Adolescents

The increased risk of depression in offspring of depressed parents and the increase in male and female adolescent suicide rates require that health care professionals recognize the symptoms of depression in children and adolescents.[56,57] In general, children and adolescents experiencing major depression display more than 1 of the following for 2 or more weeks: depressed mood with lack of reactivity, sadness and hopelessness, lack of interest and inability to experience pleasure or fun, decreased concentration, increased irritability and anger, fatigue, poor self-esteem, insomnia, withdrawal from friends and activities once enjoyed, missed school or a change in performance, psychomotor retardation, excessive guilt, anorexia, and suicidal ideations. Some further considerations when assessing for depression: young and prepubertal children also have somatic complaints, such as headaches or stomachaches; increased physical agitation; failure to thrive; separation anxiety; temper tantrums; fearfulness; sleep disturbances; injury proneness; and phobias and psychotic symptoms of delusions or hallucinations. Adolescents experience greater anhedonia, hopelessness, hypersomnia, weight changes (eating disorders need to be ruled out and can be comorbid disorders, as can substance-related disorders), use of alcohol and illicit drugs, and lethality of suicide attempts (gun shot, overdose). Drug and alcohol use is highly associated with adolescents' suicide attempts and completions and can frequently be associated with a conduct disorder, oppositional defiant disorder, and social and academic difficulties. To assess for depression in children and adolescents, it is necessary for health care professionals to inquire about the mental health histories of their patients' parents, and develop interviewing skills and questions that elicit information about children's and adolescents' family life, socialization patterns, and school performances.[58] Readers are referred to the *DSM-IV*[26] for a description and discussion of childhood and adolescent mental disorders.

Intervention Needs and Strategies

Depression tends to be a chronic disorder that continues to be unrecognized and untreated not only in adults but also in children and adolescents. Parents who do not recognize depression in themselves are apt not to identify depression in their child. In contrast, parents in whom depression has been diagnosed and treated understand the potentially debilitating condition that depression can be. The parent may be guilt ridden, fearful for their child, and reluctant to have a similar problem diagnosed and treated in their child.

Parents commonly are misinformed about treatment protocols for depression for themselves or a child, believing that pharmaceutical interventions are habit forming and hospitalizations are inevitable. Parents, in particular mothers, may be reluctant to discuss symptoms with a health care professional. Often, a parent does not characterize the child's symptoms as depression to a health care professional because of the stigma associated with a psychiatric disorder, fear that diagnosis may result in loss of employment, or embarrassment, resulting in a delayed diagnosis and treatment. A health care professional may underestimate a patient's depression, believing the "mood will lift" as a stressful situation remediates. Somatic symptoms associated with depression, such as fatigue, change in weight, headaches, gastrointestinal distress, or sleep disturbances, often become a health care professional's focus for treatment. The symptoms are treated while a depressive disorder is not diagnosed.[29] Regier et al[59] reported that 2 in 3 patients with depressive disorder did not identify themselves as depressed: 80% were seen for physical complaints, and of these individuals, a depressive disorder was correctly diagnosed by the primary health care professional in 1 in 8.

Hospitalization is required when there is a potential for suicidal behavior, regardless of age. It is essential for health care professionals to be knowledgeable about the inpatient psychiatric facilities in their community. There is variability between admission and payment criteria between agencies. Admissions are expedited during times of crisis if health care professionals remain up-to-date on treating facilities' health care policy changes that affect admission, treatment, and discharge protocols.

Hospitalization can be a concern for a mother whether she has a partner or not. In difficult domestic situations, women's hospitalizations are usually shortened, regardless of psychiatric and medical needs, because of their desire to care for offspring or to pacify an abusive partner.[60] Limited financial and health care resources can interfere with treatment plans and need to be addressed. Assisting with child care and financial issues can help alleviate the added stress of hospitalization and create a supportive environment that will allow parents to concentrate on their own treatment rather than be preoccupied with a home situation. If a woman has been involved in a self-help group, church, or community organization, support with child care and transportation is often available to her while in the hospital and after discharge. Unfortunately, depression and domestic violence generally isolate families, and a social network often has not been maintained.

Pharmacologic therapy is effective in the treatment of depression irrespective of etiology. Monoamine oxidase inhibitors, tricyclics, and selective serotonin reuptake inhibitors are antidepressants with different structural characteristics, pharmacologic effects, adverse effects, and therapeutic implications. It is beyond the scope of the present discussion to elaborate on age-related and gender-related pharmacokinetics, pharmacodynamics, and clinical management of depression with antidepressants. Readers are referred to the many available articles and books regarding psychotropic drugs for an extensive review.

A great challenge for health care professionals is the pharmacologic treatment of depression in women during pregnancy and the potentially adverse effects on the fetus. Although to date there is no definitive evidence that psychotropic medications cause birth defects, health care professionals must weigh the risks of psychopharmacologic use against the complications that the symptoms of depression may have on a fetus, such as poor nutrition related to changes in sleep and appetite, poor medical follow-up related to fatigue and hopelessness, and risk of suicide related to stress and hopelessness. Electroconvulsive therapy has been an alternative intervention to psychopharmacologic intervention when a mother is unable or unwilling to take medication.[29,30,61]

Women experience earlier onset, longer episodes, and increased recurrence of depression than do men, and there is growing evidence that differences in women's reproductive cycle and metabolic rates require variations in psychotropic medication management. Recent research investigations and health care professionals' accounts suggest that antidepressant use in women may work more slowly than in men, and women may experience more and different adverse effects.[29,30,61]

There is stronger research evidence for pharmaceutical treatment effectiveness with depressed adults than with children or adolescents, although this is rapidly changing.[57] Psychopharmacologic interventions are dependent on the severity of depression, the age of the child, what the health care professional assesses to be the cause, whether there are comorbid psychiatric and medical disorders, and whether a health care professional is sufficiently experienced in prescribing antidepressants to this population. There has been an increase in the use of antidepressants in the treatment of adolescent depression, and as more specific medications are approved for treatment by the Food and Drug Administration, it is expected that antidepressant use will increase. However, similar to adults, effectiveness is related to accurate dosing (many health care professionals undermedicate, and medications never reach clinical effectiveness) and adherence to administration schedules.[62]

The most successful intervention for depression, particularly in recurrent depression, involves a combined approach of antidepressant medications and psychotherapy. Psychotherapeutic approaches include family, group, and individual modalities. Health care professionals use these modalities in a variety of ways, across settings and with all age groups. Individual and group therapies that incorporate problem-solving approaches, such as cognitive-behavioral techniques that are more focused and structured, are particularly effective with women.[30,61,63] Cognitive-behavioral therapy and relaxation training are effective and implemented in group or individual therapeutic settings for children and adolescents. A cognitive, psychoeducational family-based approach has demonstrated sustained changes in parents by providing nondepressed family members greater understanding of a depressed member and increasing emotional closeness between partners and family members.[63] The content of sessions is modified to meet the needs of an individual, group, or family and includes subject matter that includes a definition and description of the nature of depression, the importance of following treatment plans, how to identify and develop resiliency-promoting characteristics in oneself and offspring, assertiveness training, how to talk to family members and friends about depression, how to develop constructive functioning skills, interpersonal relationships and coping skills, how to prioritize and balance the demands of daily living, accessing specific community resources for assistance in managing finances, meal planning, and where to find better housing, job training, and education.

Group settings provide members with mutual support while providing a forum to discuss differences and similarities. Diversity in perspectives broadens members' knowledge and understanding. Members offer support to each other to follow treatment protocols and explore new coping strategies and lifestyle changes. Opportunities in role modeling and sharing experiences and information decreases feelings of isolation and despair while increasing hopefulness, self-confidence, and self-respect.

Family therapy increases family members' understanding of each other's thoughts, feelings, and experiences. Family members are encouraged to discuss their concerns and fears in an attempt to increase family affiliations. Members learn how to support each other and at the same time are encouraged to develop independent strengths and relationships outside the home in the face of a family members' depression. Partner or couple's therapy is indicated when a parental relationship is problematic or strained and children are continually affected by parents' inability to support each other in parenting. Couple's therapy attempts to develop and maintain parental relationships, when possible, to decrease social isolation and enhance parenting skills by building parenting competencies, self-confidences, and self-worth.

Intervention research at the Touch Institute has found massage therapy for infants[53] and interaction coaching for depressed adolescent mothers[44] to be effective interventions. Infants of depressed mothers who received massage therapy had more organized sleep patterns, improved emotional responses, were more sociable, were more easily soothed, had greater weight gain, and had a greater decrease in stress hormones than did infants who were rocked over a 6-week period. When depressed mothers received interaction coaching to improve their interactional behaviors with their infants, mothers became more animated when instructed to get their infants' attention and became more sensitive to their infant's signals when they were instructed to imitate their infants, and infants in turn became more responsive to their mothers. Although these research studies had small sample sizes and there is a need for study replication, the results demonstrate that role modeling and educational instruction for mothers that modifies mothers' interactional style with her infant not only influences a mother's mood but also alters her infant's responses to her and enhances her infant's physical and mental well-being.

School systems have integrated classroom educational programs that teach students about the symptoms and interventions associated with depression as well as other psychiatric disorders. Programs include information about where students can go for help in their school systems and communities. Nonadherence to medication plans and treatment follow-up is a common difficulty among adolescents. School educational programs are a nonthreatening way to educate children about depression in themselves, friends, and families; allay negative perceptions of psychiatric problems; and support adherence to treatment regimens. Many school programs offer group therapy settings for students. Group settings in a school environment can be helpful when a home situation discourages outside assistance to build a professionally facilitated peer support system that can offer corrective and educational experiences and to create a sense of community within the school setting for youths. Frequently, school counselors and teachers act as confidants to students, providing a safe, private setting for students to discuss their problems. School personnel who are able to form trusting relationships with students are in excellent positions to refer students and their families for professional services.[64]

Health care professionals concerned with the increase in depression within their communities have contributed their expertise in psychiatric disorders by providing community-based educational programs. These programs are frequently free or offered for a modest fee to the public through church, hospital, and school programs. Professional facilitated support groups are also available through community agencies, private and professional group practices, and outpatient hospital clinics.

In summary, the high prevalence of depression, early onset of depression during childbearing and child-rearing years, comorbidity of depression with medical illnesses and other psychiatric disorders, and profound effectiveness of treatment in decreasing suffering and health care costs while increasing employment productivity and family functioning support initiatives aimed at early detection and treatment of depressive disorders. It is an urgent task for health care professionals in all specialities to explore the possibility of depression with their patients while dispelling negative attitudes and the stigma surrounding depression in the pursuit of timely comprehensive treatment for this disabling familial disorder.

CHILDREN WHOSE PARENTS ABUSE SUBSTANCES

The terms substance abuse, drug dependency, and drug addiction are discussed interchangeably and represent the class of substance-related disorders described in the *DSM-IV*.[26] Research, assessment, and intervention literature usually refers to adults abusing 1 substance, typically alcohol, an opioid, or cocaine and to a lesser degree nicotine, caffeine, cannabis, amphetamines, sedatives, hypnotics, or anxiolytics. However, individuals tend to abuse more than 1 substance, and comprehensive clinical assessments and treatment strategies directed at polysubstance abuse are needed for health care professionals when treating children or parents.

Substance abuse is a multidimensional, elusive problem. Information in the area of substance abuse and parenting is variable and often conflictual. *DSM-IV* criteria are often not well understood by health care professionals, resulting in misdiagnoses and underdiagnoses of parents with substance abuse problems. Furthermore, self-reports of substance-abusing behaviors and influence on parenting behaviors are of questionable reliability. Research design issues have rendered replication of many projects troublesome and conclusions not generalizable. The role of the mother in child development has received significantly greater attention than that of fathers; therefore, comparisons in this area are tenuous at best. The most conclusive information comes from longitudinal studies focusing on the effects of substances prenatally and beyond.[65]

Substance abuse stereotypically has been viewed as a problem in men of low socioeconomic status. Although substance abuse is found more often in men than in women, the misperception that substance abuse is predominately an affliction in men of low socioeconomic status not only has influenced research investigations, program funding, and treatment models but also can affect primary health care professionals' assessments. When a woman is a known substance abuser, she more often than not is perceived as an uncaring, negligent, or incompetent caregiver. These perspectives are more apparent with women of color. Women of color not only encounter language and cultural barriers that interfere with them receiving need-specific assistance, but they must also negotiate welfare systems that erroneously assume they are more drug dependent and less capable than are their white counterparts. Women of color are disproportionately tested for drug use with consequent increases in child protective service interventions. Substance abuse has been a principal factor in the increase in out-of-home placements.[66,67] Interactive patterns between parents and children and the effects that parenting functions have on children generally are not included in health care professionals' assessments, and appropriate referrals for treatment and to community service organizations, therefore, often are overlooked.[68]

It is difficult to isolate genetic, teratogenic, and environmental effects of specific substances because of the inclination toward polysubstance abuse by parents and the tendency of chronic substance-abusing mothers to have inadequate prenatal health care, poor nutrition, and overall compromised maternal health. However, there are 2 dominant areas of concern regarding children affected by drug abuse. One focus is the immediate and long-term effects of prenatal substance abuse on children. A second concentration has been on the developmental effects on children of living with 1 or 2 substance-abusing parents. Prevention and prenatal intervention programs are pivotal to the enhancement of family functioning and well-being and, appropriately, are priorities in public health policy. Nevertheless, most women who abuse substances do not receive comprehensive prenatal treatment and tend to use substances before they know they are pregnant.[69,70]

Teratogenic and Genetic Effects of Substance Abuse

Fetal alcohol syndrome is characterized by preterm deliveries, craniofacial malformations, stunted growth, delayed psychomotor maturation, impaired intellectual development, and hyperkinetic disorders with poor attention, distractibility, impulsivity, and hyperactivity. Fetal alcohol effects demonstrate less serious effects from in utero alcohol exposure and occur more frequently than fetal alcohol syndrome.

Children with fetal alcohol effects exhibit a less severe picture of the symptoms of fetal alcohol syndrome. Heavier alcohol consumption during pregnancy is associated with more severe physical and intellectual impairments. Although craniofacial malformations can appear less noticeable over time, more enduring effects include having physical difficulties with short stature, being underweight, and having delayed development, disturbed sleep patterns, hyperactivity, intellectual and cognitive deficits with slow language development, poor school performance, and emotional difficulties such as social withdrawal, delinquency, and conduct disorders.[68,70,71] Sustained physical, intellectual, and social impairments create the greatest challenges for parents, schools, and community resources.

Newborns whose mothers abuse alcohol and other substances demonstrate postnatal withdrawal symptoms days to weeks after delivery. In general, these infants are more easily aroused, highly irritable, and hypertonic; cry excessively; have tremors; experience sleep disturbances; and may have increased sensitivity to light, sounds, and touch, gastrointestinal difficulties, and respiratory distress. Prematurity, low birth weight, and microcephaly as well as an increased incidence of sudden infant death syndrome commonly result from prenatal opiate use. During the first year of life, poor motor coordination, poor attention, and hyperactivity have also been attributed to prenatal opioid exposure. Characteristic symptoms of increased arousal and irritability often diminish within the first year. More enduring characteristics include higher activity levels, impulsivity, decreased attention span, and an increased incidence of attention-deficit/hyperactivity disorder. Whether prenatal opiate exposure is responsible for longer-term outcomes of childhood and adolescent hyperactivity, conduct problems, oppositional behaviors, delinquency, criminal behavior, and increased suicide rates or whether these difficulties are more representative of family dysfunction and interpersonal discord remain unclear. When parents abstain from abusing substances and engage in treatment programs and fetal alcohol syndrome or fetal alcohol effects are not central to a diagnosis, children's school performances improve and behavioral problems lessen.[68,71-73]

More recently, human immunodeficiency virus transmission has brought new challenges to the substance-abusing population. Early diagnosis and treatment prolongs life. However, treatment of chronic medical problems associated with human immunodeficiency virus infection frequently requires hospitalizations and lifestyle modifications. In addition, the pervading threat to a child's family life through the loss of a parent or parents, family members, and friends is a stark reality.

In summary, substance abuse occurs as a family pattern across generations. Specific explanations for the transmission and genetic nature of substance abuse within families have not been identified. Regardless of which substance or substances a parent abuses, their children are at risk of repeating the substance use behavior and perpetuating the complications. The ubiquitous question of nature verses nurture continues.

Family Functioning, Impact on Children, and Assessment Requirements

In general, the highest incidence of substance abuse occurs during childbearing and child-rearing years. Children whose parents abuse substances are at high risk of physical, social, emotional, and educational challenges. Parent-child relationships are affected, and a child's relationships outside the home are influenced. The effects on children and family life are confounded when parents suffer from mental illnesses and abuse alcohol and illicit substances to self-medicate for symptom relief. Domestic violence, child abuse, child neglect, and subsequent out-of-home placements as well as homelessness are the more serious issues occurring among substance-abusing families.[68,73] Failure to thrive, anxiety, depression, somatic difficulties (headaches, sleeping problems, gastrointestinal complaints), truancy, aggressive behaviors, running away, and low self-esteem are common psychiatric and emotional problems for children. Evaluation of a child, therefore, needs to include inquiries about the child's developmental progress; sleep, eating, and physical activity patterns; school performance and activities; language development; family history of mental illness; family history of substance abuse; and family history of sexual, emotional, and physical abuse.

Misuse of substances impacts family structure and functional abilities. Denial, shame, and secrecy prevent accurate assessments and isolate family members in their attempts to hide the problem. Family disharmony, conflict, and unpredictable and inconsistent parental behaviors are characteristic. What was expected one day changes the next. Routines, promises, and plans are broken and changed. Parents are preoccupied with obtaining substances and are frequently physically ill. Family boundaries and roles are not clear, and some children are expected to assume adult responsibilities, while others become family scapegoats or get lost in the "shuffle." Parents frequently are autocratic, domineering, and overcontrolling with their children. There is a tendency to exclude outside assistance in parenting issues and family problems, thus restricting parents from corrective experiences and potential learning about age-appropriate developmental behaviors. Communication with children typically is verbally aggressive and demeaning through yelling, threatening, and disparaging remarks. When children try to communicate their needs, they are seen as demanding, poorly behaved, or ungrateful.[68,71,74-79] Health care professionals' evaluations of children should include parents' attitudes toward parenting and their children, family stressors, the way parents interact with their children, parents' own experiences with their parents and siblings, and family social networks and resources.

Women who abuse substances, particularly single mothers, experience economic hardships, social isolation, and high rates of depression, guilt, worry, and stress. Feelings of extreme guilt are common as a result of diverting family funds for substance procurement instead of better housing, clothing, and food and leaving children unattended or in less desirable situations. Drugs are used as a way to cope with demoralizing and difficult circumstances. Use of substances is also a way to socialize with peers and drug-abusing male partners.[80] Substance use is an attempt, although inevitably disabling, to decrease unwanted emotions associated with self-condemnation, loneliness, and isolation.

Contrary to popular belief, most parents who abuse substances value their parenting role. Children are viewed with deep pride and recognized as a stabilizing force. Only as a last resort will most mothers relinquish custody of their children to the care of a relative or foster care. Not wanting children to witness and repeat their behavior and ultimately to preserve their children's safety, mothers may decide to separate from their children. Substance-dependent mothers often enter treatment to function more effectively for the sake of their children's well-being and to keep their families intact.[65,81]

Despite compromised family environments, at-risk children have demonstrated an ability successfully to cope and adjust. Children whose temperament is more affectionate and "appealing," and who are socially active and engaging are more resilient and less vulnerable.[74] Family structures can also provide protective processes that promote successful life adjustment. For example, in family situations in which 1 parent is unaffected and a child maintains satisfying social support networks, the influence of a substance-abusing parent is cushioned.[82] Positive social networks, such as a nurturing grandmother, older sibling, teacher, or neighbor, can provide constructive self-esteem building attachments that balance the more negative consequences of family life. Further, many families struggle to preserve cohesive family and social relationships and strive to provide a sense of security and caring for children despite parents' substance abuse.[74]

Treatment and Prevention Issues

Substance abuse is a chronic and relapsing condition. Women with substance abuse problems, in particular, seek health care through emergency centers. Most men and women are referred to treatment facilities through primary health care professionals. Treatment is also sought after legal problems, pressure from spouses, or financial difficulties. This suggests that parental health and family circumstances may be seriously compromised before a parent seeks professional assistance. The stigma surrounding abuse of substances and fear of losing custody of children prevents parents, particularly single parents, from seeking treatment. Embarrassment, a desire for anonymity, fear of further humiliation, threats of financial loss from spouses or significant others, fear of prosecution, fear of unemployment, demands and needs of a family, and lack of accurate information are barriers to treatment.[83] Treatment facilities frequently do not accommodate women with their children and may not treat pregnant women. Families in which both parents abuse substances often necessitate mothers making living arrangements for children to participate in a treatment program.

Treatment facilities providing all-female treatment programs that address the distinctive needs of women and mothers and maintain accommodations for children have been the most successful. Such programs help interrupt detrimental parenting and interacting styles. Therapeutic communities and halfway houses that provide child care and have self-help groups, such as Alcoholics Anonymous and Narcotics Anonymous, help to build social support networks. Programs that create socialization with peers, a sense of hope, feelings of self-confidence, and a beginning for decreasing distress, guilt, and fear offer positive recovery opportunities that contrast with previous substance abuse experiences.[66,83]

Assistance for young children includes programs focusing on physiologic and psychosocial needs and family life. For example, preschool Head Start services for children have provided parent education, early childhood education and intervention, meals, and heath care monitoring. Head Start continues to work with community-based family support and education programs to provide comprehensive child development programs and comprehensive health screening and care.

Children of school age and beyond need education- and prevention-oriented programs. School-based education programs and youth services, through school counseling, can provide experiences for children that build confidence, self-esteem, and self-control. They also allow for early assessment of emotional and psychiatric problems. School programs, such as the Drug Abuse Resistance Education (DARE) program, are aimed at children who are at risk. They are designed to improve decision-making skills through education and positive peer support. High schools have developed programs focusing on adolescent substance abusers as well as peer support groups for adolescents who struggle with family situations that place them at risk of physical or emotional abuse by parents. Schools are attempting to work more closely with child welfare agencies that provide home visitation and more comprehensive case management programs. Many school systems work in coordination with self-help groups, such as Alateen for older children, and provide information regarding available self-help groups for all family members. Grandparents who are primary caregivers for children and adolescents in the absence of parents need emotional support and assistance with parenting skills and home instruction. School-based supportive services for children and families that are coordinated with community-based family treatment facilities are better able to provide comprehensive services. Collaboration between schools and treatment services decreases fragmentation, duplication of services, and role confusion among professionals.

Families need assistance in many areas of their lives. Parent education regarding typical child development and child-rearing practices introduces parents to new possibilities for interacting with their children and more effective parenting. Assertiveness training, development of new coping skills for frustration and anxiety, and interpersonal skills training to manage family stresses and conflicts are necessary to manage living without the use of substances. Public assistance is frequently necessary, as are vocational education and training. Comprehensive health screening for children, community based well-baby and well-child care programs, and prenatal and postpartum care as well as vocational education and training are frequently necessary for families. Often neglected is adequate transportation to services, which prevents children and parents from participating in available programs.

More often than not, families in which substances are abused are not known to child welfare services and legal agencies. Respect by health care professionals for family members' rights to privacy and confidentiality increases parents' trust and willingness to participate in treatment programs and community resources. It is important for families not to feel unprotected and intruded on by the same organizations and services that have the purpose of assisting during difficult times and circumstances.

To adequately meet the needs of families and children, health care professionals need greater knowledge and expertise in substance abuse and the treatment trajectory. Knowledge about the child welfare system and its services is also necessary, not only for reporting cases of suspected child abuse and neglect but also to provide more comprehensive health care and follow-up. When health care professionals are seen as compassionate, assistive, and knowledgeable, receiving health care for children and treatment for substance abuse is not as threatening for parents. Parents are more willing to discuss health and family problems when they know that a health care professional is sensitive to their needs and life circumstances.

Knowing that children from substance-abusing families are at risk for domestic violence, abuse, and neglect can engender negative responses in health care professionals. For example, as a result of prejudice on the part of health care professionals, African American women have been reported to legal authorities 10 times as much as white women have, despite similar rates of prenatal substance abuse. Awareness of biases and misconceptions helps to promote more equitable access to health care, health care resources, and treatment and helps to enhance communication between health care professionals and patients.[66,84]

In conclusion, family isolation and fear hinder collaboration between services and the development of comprehensive, family-oriented services. More consolidated efforts between community outreach programs, social service agencies, schools, primary health care professionals, and emergency treatment centers will help monitor family members' health care needs and provide more cost-effective comprehensive prevention and intervention programs.

CHILDREN OF ADOLESCENT PARENTS

Adolescent parenthood in the United States continues to be a challenge to the individuals and families directly involved in the phenomenon, to health care professionals, to educators, to communities, and to policy makers. Although adolescent pregnancy occurs across all demographic sectors of our society, adolescent parenthood continues to be a pattern that is more prevalent in lower socioeconomic groups.[85,86] Recent figures confirm that there are slightly fewer than 500 000 births to adolescents each year and that almost all the children, especially among families of ethnic minorities, are raised by the adolescents.[86-88] When an adolescent has a baby, the young parent needs to negotiate the transition to parenthood along with the developmental demands of adolescence.[19,89,90] Adolescent issues, such as identity formation, individuation, a changing body image and emerging sexuality, and especially cognitive immaturity (including egocentric and concrete operational thinking) often make it difficult for adolescent parents to assume the roles and responsibilities of parenthood.[89]

There are 3 critical issues that are central to the adjustment and outcomes of adolescent parents and their children.[91,92] These issues include whether the adolescent mother will be able to stay in school and go on to complete her educational and occupational training plans, how well the adolescent mother is able to assume the parenting role and develop a positive parent-child relationship, and the roles the family and community play in supporting the young mother and child during the transition to parenthood.

Protective Factors

There is much variability in the experience and outcomes of adolescent parents and their children, in part because there are many personal and environmental variables that mediate the process of adolescent parenthood. There are some consistent findings in the research literature concerning factors that buffer adverse outcomes and foster better outcomes for adolescent parents and their children.[91,93] These factors include social support (often provided by the maternal family, perhaps in combination with the baby's father), completion of an educational plan, limiting subsequent fertility, maternal self-esteem, infant intelligence, and an "easy" temperament in the infants of adolescent mothers.[94-96] Other researchers have consistently found that maternal depression has significant negative effects on the parenting process and the developmental and behavioral outcomes of children.[97-99]

The children of adolescents are at higher risk of problems if the mother lives alone and raises her child as a single parent.[100] Reviews of existing literature on outcomes studied in children of adolescent parents find increased rates of infant morbidity and mortality, less verbal interactions between mothers and children, few recognized developmental and behavioral problems until the children reach school age, and higher incidence of school and behavioral problems during adolescence.[86,91] It appears that emotional, behavioral, and cognitive problems in children of adolescent parents become more pronounced as the children develop beyond the preschool years.[97,101] There is evidence to support a link between child abuse and adolescent parents, and often these incidents of neglect or injury are related to insufficient supervision and anticipation of safety hazards. Despite methodologic problems with many of the earlier studies, there does seem to be a greater likelihood that children of adolescent parents will be abused or neglected, especially if the mother has more than 1 child during adolescence.[102] Steir et al[13] reported double the incidence of child maltreatment and a higher incidence of failure to thrive and change in primary caregiver by 5 years of age in children born to adolescent mothers, compared with children born to adult mothers. There is also more evidence in the clinical and research literature that documents that adolescent mothers themselves are more likely to have been physically or sexually abused in their recent or distant past.[86,103]

Family support is critical to successful outcomes for adolescent parents and their children. Often, grandmothers in families with adolescent mothers and infants have "first order" and "second order" effects on the infant's health and development, because they often provide daily direct care and provide the young mother with emotional and functional support in her new role.[104,105] There is some evidence that a shared or apprentice model is a family strategy that seems to benefit not only the new mother but also the child in the early periods of attachment.[97,104] There are some conflicting findings concerning the importance of mother-grandmother coresidence. Among many adolescent mothers, the age of the mother, the health status of the child, and the length of the period of mother-grandmother coresidence are all related to adolescent parenting competence.[106] The finding that young single parents with young infants and children who reside with extended family have better educational outcomes is consistent across several studies using differing methodologies. Although there may be adverse parent-child effects and mother-grandmother conflicts that occur as a result of this coresidence, these problems may be less important in the long term if the young mother is able to complete her education and then go on to obtain employment and establish her own household and family system.[96]

There is some evidence that a shared or apprentice model is a family strategy that seems to benefit not only the new mother but also the child in the early periods of attachment.

There appears to be a window of opportunity that exists during the first 2 years after the birth of the adolescent's child, when the benefits of mother-grandmother coresidence, including better parenting outcomes in adolescent mothers and better child developmental outcomes in infants and toddlers, are maximized.[96] Similar benefits are seen if the adolescent mother resides with the baby's father; however, coresidence with her partner is also related to higher rates of repeat pregnancy and childbearing and less educational attainment in the adolescent mother.[96,105,107,108]

Many of the partners of adolescent mothers are not adolescents themselves. Furstenberg et al[95] reported that for their sample of urban adolescent mothers, at least 50% of fathers were older than 20 years. Similar findings regarding paternal age are also reflected in national data.[109,110] Among fathers who are adolescents, constraints of poverty, incomplete education, unemployment, and involvement with crime, drugs, and incarceration limit the presence and support they can offer to their young child. Many fathers (young and old) who cannot afford to support their child may become discouraged and remove themselves from the child's life. Other fathers may be forced away by the maternal family, who may withhold visitation privileges in the absence of material contributions to the child's support.[22]

Despite the lower frequency of marriages and the more transient nature of the couple relationship among adolescent parents, Furstenberg et al[95] report that after 17 years of follow-up in a longitudinal research project of urban adolescent mothers and their offspring, one sixth of the children were living with their fathers and one sixth were seeing their fathers weekly. The remaining two thirds of the sample were living with a stepfather or someone like a stepfather. Toledo-Dreves and Zabin,[111] in a study of the duration of sexual relationships in 307 urban African American adolescent women, surveyed a subgroup of 80 young women who had given birth. At 2 years after the birth, two thirds of the women reported that they were still in a relationship with their baby's father, and 5% were married.

Parental Competence in Adolescent Parents

Because many adolescent parents are also single parents who commonly live in poverty, the studies that describe their poorer parenting practices and attitudes may actually be confounded by the effects of poverty rather than young age alone.[85,106] There are fewer studies that have followed their parenting styles and behaviors as their children reach preschool age and beyond. Chase-Lansdale et al[112] studied a sample of 99 African American adolescent parents and their 3-year-old children and found some patterns of harsh parent-child interactions across grandparent, parent, and child generations. Leadbeater et al[98] found that adolescent mothers, especially those who were depressed, manifested increased maternal-child conflict when observed with their preschool-aged children.

The mother's level of cognitive developmental maturity has great implications for her ability to understand the needs of her child and to interact with her caregiving helpers for negotiating necessary child care. Maternal role adjustment in adolescent mothers has been examined from various cognitive developmental perspectives.[113,114] Just as the cognitive developmental stage of concrete operational thinking limits decision making regarding sexuality (sexual activity patterns, compliance with contraception), it also influences the planning, anticipation, and decision making involved in daily parental roles and responsibilities. If the adolescent mother is thinking at a concrete operational level (focused in the present and reasoning more about objects and behaviors that can be directly observed), it may be difficult for her to consider future plans or implications of child-rearing techniques. It may also be difficult for her to anticipate the safety needs and hazards for a rapidly growing and changing child.

The mother's own egocentrism of adolescence may interfere with her ability to understand and appreciate the unique needs and perception of her child.[115] She may confuse her own needs, desires, and cognitive abilities with those of her child and, therefore, may hold inappropriately high expectations for her child's behavior and thought processes.[116] Her ability or inability to hypothetically see perspectives other than her own has implications for how she negotiates important relationships in her life, such as those with her child, partner, mother, or child care provider.

Areas of Assessment and Intervention

An assessment of the adolescent mothers' developmental and cognitive level is an important first step for meaningful assessments and educational and counseling strategies. Chronologic age may provide a starting point in the assessment, but there is much individual variation in maturity that may be assessed by spending time talking with the adolescent about her social and developmental history (family, school, peers, activities) as well as her impressions and thoughts about her child and behavioral issues to determine where she is on the spectrum of adolescent developmental issues (early, middle, or late adolescence).[117] Many adolescent parents who manifest a concrete operational orientation indicate that they would be less likely to think abstractly, plan for the future, or consider and anticipate future implications of their parenting styles or behaviors. Concrete thinking styles are also more likely to be accompanied by egocentrism in this group of young parents, making them less likely to view and understand the infant or young child as a separate and unique being with many nurturing needs rather than someone who can provide nurturing to the adolescent mother herself.

Supportive and educational programs for adolescent mothers need to be based on the understanding of the developmental and cognitive developmental vulnerabilities of these young women. Adolescent parents benefit from information that is focused on the day-to-day care and behaviors needed to safely manage the care of their babies without too much detail given to behaviors and issues coming up in the future. The information, whether presented in a group setting or in an individual clinical encounter, needs to incorporate concrete hands-on experiences to reinforce the behaviors or knowledge being taught. For example, describing a parenting skill like taking the baby's temperature is much less effective than is coaching the young mother as she performs the actual skill and providing her with praise as she masters the skill.

The issue of the young mother's egocentrism regarding her infant or young child also needs to be gently worked through. This can often be accomplished by demonstrations of various ways in which the infant is a separate individual with unique needs, capabilities, and thought processes different from the mother's. Demonstrating the infant's very short memory by hiding a rattle in sight of the infant (who then immediately forgets about it and does not look for it) is one way to make this abstract concept more concrete for young mothers. Trad[118] suggests strategies of previewing and rehearsing with young mothers what developmental stages their babies will be entering next as a way of helping concrete thinkers to begin to peer into the immediate future and plan for parenting behaviors that would match their baby's changing capabilities. This is especially important in the area of anticipating infant and toddler safety issues. Similarly, the strategy of role playing with adolescent mothers is useful for them to rehearse difficult or new kinds of negotiations in which they may need to engage with family members or child care providers.

The second critical area of assessment for adolescent parents is the nature and extent of their support network. This includes areas of family, partner and peers, and school. The adolescent's support network has direct implications for success with parenting, being able to provide for the essential daily living and safety needs of the child, the parent's emotional well-being, and meeting the developmental, academic, and occupational challenges necessary for the young parent to be able to grow into a self-sufficient adult. It is important to learn about the housing arrangements, the person the adolescent defines as her primary helper with her child and how she gets along with that person, and what her relationship is with her baby's father and her own mother or mother-figure. Peers, including new partners other than her child's father, may be a source of support, primarily emotional, for the young mother or a source of distraction from her parenting roles and responsibilities.

The ability of adolescent parents (mothers especially) to stay in school and complete their educational plans is linked with important long-term outcomes for themselves and their children.[95,97] Staying in school is linked to the ability to delay subsequent childbearing beyond adolescence and to the availability of child care. Not only is it important to assess that the adolescent mother is linked to teen-friendly health and reproductive health services, but it is important to keep checking periodically on the adolescent mother's consistent use of contraception (if she is sexually active) and whether she is able to keep appointments for her contraceptive follow-up visits.

It is very difficult for adolescent parents to attend school on a regular basis because of the competing demands on their time and attention placed by child care for their infants and toddlers.[101] Historically, daily child care arrangements commonly have been provided by family members during school hours, and often, these infant care providers were also working split shifts or had changing job shifts and other family responsibilities that interfered with their ability to provide consistent infant child care.[22,92] With the advent of changes in the welfare system, families are less available to provide that support, because more parents (mostly mothers) of adolescent parents are working at several jobs as single parents (often because of fewer publicly funded safety net programs) or because some families have become more disrupted by community influences of drugs, poverty, illness, alcohol, crime, and incarceration. Few of the infants or toddlers of adolescent parents are enrolled in child care centers. In addition to the chronic shortage of available child care centers serving infants and toddlers, it is often difficult for adolescent parents to negotiate the requirements for admission into these centers.[91,92]

Adolescent-Friendly Child Care

For adolescent parents who need daily child care for their infants and toddlers, high school-based child care centers offer a creative solution to this challenge. The school-based child care center is a dual-generational intervention model that provides social support, a source of accomplishment for parents (that may help buffer depression), safe child care, a learning environment for children, modeling of positive parenting skills, high school dropout prevention, and the structure to help young mothers stay organized about their own health care and needs as well as those of their child. The high school-based child care center is an important source of support for adolescent parents and their children and may also contribute to parental competence in young parents, more positive parent-child interactions, and better child developmental outcomes in these young families.

One such child care center located in New Haven, Connecticut is a high school-based infant and toddler center providing child care for student parents and their children during the school year. Parents take a daily parenting course and each week spend at least 1 hour in the center, where they care for and interact with their child with the guidance of the professional child care staff. This aspect of the program provides the young parents the chance to practice new skills and creates a valuable early childhood developmental and parent-child interaction laboratory setting within the child care center. A collaborative multidisciplinary team of high school teachers, child care providers, a pediatric nurse practitioner, an attorney, and a director of student services provide outreach services, including transportation, legal services, home visitation, and meetings with family members.

An evaluation of the first 3 years of the child care center determined that the 52 parents and children served by the center experienced a significant increase in grades, no repeat childbirths, and a 100% rate of high school graduation or continuation to the next grade level. Children's health records (immunization rates and percentages of pediatric health visits) demonstrated that they were being seen regularly for their pediatric primary care visits.[119]

This is an example of a 2-generational model. Current research indicates that longer-term effects of 2-generational child care interventions may be more significant than may short-term effects.[16,120]

Adolescent parents and their children constitute high risk and are vulnerable young families. However, there are several important support factors that seem to buffer many of the adverse outcomes for young parents and their children. Consistent family and social network support, continuing educational and occupational plans, delaying subsequent child births, and multiservice intergenerational programs for adolescent parents seem to provide some of these essential supports. School-based child care centers or other community child care centers that are staffed by individuals who understand some of the unique developmental and parenting needs of adolescent parents bring together the necessary components for the success of these young families during the transition to parenthood.

CHILDREN OF PARENTS WITH MENTAL RETARDATION

There is relatively little information in the clinical and research literature concerning families in which 1 or both parents are mentally retarded. Existing studies often have extremely small samples or report surveys of health care professionals caring for individuals with mental retardation.[121] There are very tentative estimates of the numbers of parents with mental retardation, largely because the condition is often masked or poorly diagnosed, and epidemiologic studies of prevalence are difficult and expensive to conduct.[122] The understanding and classification of mental retardation has changed from a system of categorizing individuals with mental retardation solely by their IQ to a system that includes IQ (approx 70 or lower) in combination with impairment in at least 2 domains of adaptive functioning.[123] The domains include communication, self-care, home living, social and interpersonal skills, use of community resources, self-direction, functional academic skills, work, leisure, health, and safety. The age of onset of mental retardation is defined as being younger than 18 years.[26,123,124]

Although health care professionals recognize that there are significant numbers of families with parents who are mentally retarded living in most communities, there are no reliable or current statistics estimating the national or regional prevalence.[125] In addition, there are no reliable estimates for the number of marriages or single-parent families or degree of cultural and economic diversity that characterize these families. In one study conducted in the St Louis area in the late 1980s, a sample of 402 parents with mental retardation were identified by community social and health agencies.[122] A subsample of 37 parents were studied in greater detail and were found to have an average age of 29 years, to be mostly female, to have an intellectual age of about 8 years, and to have between 2 and 3 children. Twenty-five percent of these families experienced a child being removed from the home by child protective agencies. Most parents relied on family members (their own mothers, fathers, and siblings) for emotional and functional support for living and raising their children. This study and others reported in the literature focused on the identified needs and problems experienced by parents with mental retardation. These problems included inadequate parenting skills, poverty, housing, daily living skills, child neglect, transportation, family conflict, lack of vocational skills, lack of adequate health care, lack of social and communication skills, and child abuse.[122]

The cause of the parents' mental retardation will determine whether their offspring are likely to have limited or normal intelligence. If the parent's mental retardation is caused by genetic factors, then there is a greater chance the child will also be affected, and if both parents have genetic retardation, then each child has a 42% chance of being affected.[126] Children of parents with mental retardation may have problems with speech and language and often do have school or learning problems that may be related more to their home environment and ability of their parents to provide them with appropriate stimulation rather than any inherent cognitive deficits.[122,127] Parents with mental retardation often have concurrent speech and language disorders, hearing loss, dental problems, and difficulty with organizing and sequencing tasks and schedules. They suffer from related problems of low self-esteem, homelessness, previous or current history of abuse, recurrent crises that wear down family support systems, and an inability to understand social and nonverbal cues.[128]

Problems with the parent-child interaction and, specifically, child abuse and neglect, have been reported in greater frequency in families in which there is a wider difference between parental and child IQ.[129] This trend is magnified when there are concurrent conditions of poverty, large family size, and absence of a family or other support network.

Areas of Assessment: Risks and Strengths

As with any parent, it is important to assess the individual characteristics of the parent with mental retardation, as well as the context within which they and their children live. The first area that requires thoughtful assessment includes the parent's own personal resources, including mental and adaptive functioning, comprehension, personal style, and problem-solving ability. Data from standardized testing provide some starting points, as do any educational assessments that may be available concerning the parents' experience with schooling, reading and comprehension level, and particularly their learning style. Special education teachers are particularly good resources for assistance with the planning of interventions (parenting support or classes) with parents who are mentally retarded. Individual characteristics of the parent will shape any interventions, such as whether they respond to tactile (pat on the shoulder or back) reinforcement in positive or negative ways, when they are more open to learning, when they are overloaded and need to be given some time and space without stimulation, and what their capacity is for using written cues or pictures to help with memory or multistep tasks they need to accomplish. It is important for health care professionals to assess how the parent is able to identify and solve problems related to the care and safety of their child. This can often be assessed through simple "what would you do if..." scenarios.

The level and supportiveness of family involvement also needs to be given careful consideration in terms of partner or spousal support as well as extended (most often maternal) family and community support. Families of parents with mental retardation may provide a supportive structure by providing positive modeling of parenting and help with daily living. However, they may also exploit the mentally retarded individuals for financial benefits or reject them and their children from the larger family.[128] In addition to identifying who the supportive individuals are, it is important to determine (from both parties, if possible), how they get along in general and, particularly, in response to collaboration with child care and supervision. If the mother with mental retardation is the child's primary caregiver, then it is important to identify who her support person is (mother, father, sister, grandmother, guardian, aunt, etc), how they share child-rearing roles and tasks, and how they negotiate decision making concerning areas that affect the child and the child's safety and well-being. If possible, it is useful to know what kind of teaching or coaching style the support person uses with the mother and the effectiveness of that style.

Whitman et al[128] have designed and implemented successful parent skills training programs for parents with mental retardation (IQ 40–50) who have infants and young children. The multimethod program included center-based classes, home visitation by parent aides, and much repetition, modeling, and reinforcement of skills taught. Classes were focused on issues of self-care for parents at the same time parenting skills were taught. A primary goal of the program was to repair and improve parental self-esteem. Parenting skills classes included child development, children's basic needs (safety, physical, and emotional), parent-child interactions, personal and child hygiene, daily routines for meeting the family's needs, time concepts, and health care.[128] Lessons from this model program were reinforced with picture books, group activities, much repetition, modeling of behaviors, use of songs and rhymes to help with remembering tasks, role play situations, and rehearsal of skills with props.

Although there are very few formal resources for parents with mental retardation, the national and local chapters of The Arc are useful for identification of existing programs for individuals with mental retardation. Parents with mental retardation often come in contact with many social services, but few communities have been able to integrate services into programs for these families.[130] Parent outreach programs and parent aid programs, often sponsored by child guidance agencies or child protective services, may be able to provide home visitation services and on-site help with family and home management issues while at the same time monitoring the family for child safety and parental competence.

Although few communities have specifically identified parenting programs for parents with mental retardation, it may be easier to find existing parent support programs that may be able to be modified for parents with mental retardation, and support groups or respite care programs for the extended family members, particularly grandparents, who are involved in care on a daily basis.

CONCLUSIONS/RECOMMENDATIONS

Health care professionals and child care providers who care for children living in families with special needs have the challenge of assessment of the child, the family system, and the context in which the family lives. Although each specific family condition described in this chapter includes specific risks and potential resiliencies, there are some general guidelines for the assessment and intervention concerning these families.

Recommendations for Health Care Providers

- Health assessment information should include a child's developmental progress; sleep, eating, and physical activity patterns; school performance and activities; language development; family history of mental illness; family history of substance abuse, duration of use, and specific substances used; family history of sexual, emotional, and physical abuse and incarceration; family social networks and resources; parents' knowledge level and attitudes toward parenting and children; family stressors; parental interaction patterns with children; and current use or involvement with supportive services (Special Supplemental Nutrition Program for Women, Infants, and Children [WIC], Temporary Assistance for Needy Families, Parent Aide Programs, visiting nurse services, etc).
- Networking needs to occur among primary health care professionals, school programs, treatment facilities, child welfare agencies, and legal agencies.
- Referrals should be made by health care professionals to appropriate community-based networks: churches, outreach programs, shelters, school programs, and vocational education and training programs.
- Referrals should be made to family-oriented treatment programs and specialized support programs that provide child care services throughout a treatment or intervention trajectory.
- Referrals should be made to issue-specific treatment programs (eg, smoking cessation, nutritional practices, 12-step programs, methadone maintenance programs, prenatal addiction programs, parenting classes, etc).
- Referrals should be made for psychiatric and family evaluations when substance abuse and psychiatric disorders are suspected or evident.

RESOURCE AND TREATMENT INFORMATION

Medical Home

National Center of Medical Home Initiatives for Children With Special Needs
American Academy of Pediatrics
141 Northwest Point Boulevard
Elk Grove Village, IL 60007
Phone: 800/433-9016
Web site: http://www.medicalhomeinfo.org

Depression and Substance Abuse

National Alliance for the Mentally Ill
Web site: http://www.nami.org

National Mental Health Services Knowledge Exchange Network (KEN)
Mental Health Information Phone: 800/789-2647
Web site: http://www.samhsa.gov/look3.htm
E-mail: Ken@mentalhealth.org

National Depression Screening Day's Primary Care Outreach Program
National Mental Illness Screening Project/NDSD
One Washington Street, Suite 304
Wellesley Hills, MA 02181-1706
Phone: 781/239-0071
Fax: 781/431-7447

The National Clearinghouse for Alcohol and Drug Information
Web site: http://www.health.org/

The Office of the Surgeon General
Web site: http://www.osophs.dhhs.gov

The Suicide Prevention Advocacy Network
Web site: http://www.spanusa.org

Treatment Organizations

The National Directory of Drug Abuse and Alcoholism Treatment and Prevention Programs
Developed by Substance Abuse and Mental Health Services Administration (SAMHSA)
Web site: http://www.health.org

National Council on Alcoholism and Drug Dependence Inc (NCADD)
Web site: http://www.ncadd.org

Treatment Referral Service
Phone: 800/662-HELP

Alcohol Treatment Referral Hotline
Phone: 800/ALCOHOL

Cocaine Hotline
Phone: 800/COCAINE

Alcoholics Anonymous World Services Inc
Phone: 212/870-3400

Families Anonymous
Phone: 800/736-9805

Al-Anon/Alateen Family Group Headquarters, Inc
Phone: 800/344-2666

Narcotics Anonymous
Phone: 818/773-9999

NAPARE Alcohol, Drug, and Pregnancy Hotline
Phone: 800/638-BABY

Nar-Anon Family Groups
Phone: 310/547-5800

Adolescent Parents

National Organization on Adolescent Pregnancy, Prevention, and Parenting
Web site: http://www.noappp.org
Phone: 202/783-5770

Office of Adolescent Pregnancy Programs
Web site: http://opa.osophs.dhhs.gov/titlexx/oapp.html

Morning Glory Press (books and videos on adolescent parenting)
Web site: http://www.morningglorypress.com

Children and Families Living in Poverty

Children's Defense Fund
Web site: http://www.childrensdefense.org

The David and Lucille Packard Foundation: The Center for the Future of Children
Web site: http://www.packfound.org

Single-Parent Families and Family Policy

National Council on Family Relations
Web site: http://www.ncfr.org

Parents With Mental Retardation

Smith R. *Children With Mental Retardation.* Bethesda, MD: Woodbine House; 1993

The ARC
Web site: http://www.thearc.org

Assessment Instruments

(These instruments are brief self-reports. Parents can fill them out in the waiting room before appointments or as part of a health care professional's interview. They can be used by health care professionals to screen parents for substance and alcohol problems for treatment referrals.)

Alcohol Use Disorders Identification Test[131]

CAGE[131]

Alcohol Dependence Scale (ADS)[131]

Michigan Alcohol Screening Test (MAST)[131]

Beck Depression Inventory (BDI)[132]

Beck Depression Inventory-11[132]

Zung Self Rating Depression Scale[132]

Center for Epidemiologic Studies-Depression Scale (CES-D)[132]

Edinburgh Postnatal Depression Scale[132]

REFERENCES

1. Bronfenbrenner U. Ecology of the family as a context for human development: research perspectives. *Dev Psychol.* 1986;22:723-742
2. Anderson SA, Sabatelli R. *Family Interaction.* Boston, MA: Allyn & Bacon; 1998
3. Luthar SS, Zigler E. Vulnerability and competence: a review of research on resilience in childhood. *Am J Orthopsychiatry.* 1991;61:6-18
4. McCubbin H, McCubbin M. Typologies of resilient families: emerging roles of social class and ethnicity. *Fam Relat.* 1988;37:247-254
5. Children's Defense Fund. *Number of Poor Children in America Rises Second Straight Year.* Washington, DC: Children's Defense Fund; 2003
6. Bronfenbrenner U, McClelland P, Wethington E, Moen P, Ceci S. *The State of Americans.* New York, NY: The Free Press; 1996
7. Federal Interagency Forum on Child and Family Statistics. *America's Children: Key National Indicators of Well-being.* Washington, DC: Federal Interagency Forum on Child and Family Statistics; 1999
8. Brooks-Gunn J, Duncan G. The effects of poverty on children. *Future Child.* 1998; 7:55-71
9. Berne AS, Dato C, Mason DJ, Rafferty M. A nursing model for addressing the health needs of homeless families. In: Wegner GD, Alexander RJ, eds. *Readings in Family Nursing.* Philadelphia, PA: Lippincott; 1993:109-121
10. Children's Defense Fund. *The State of America's Children: Yearbook 2000.* Washington, DC: Children's Defense Fund; 2000
11. Lewit E, Kerrebrock N. Childhood hunger. *Future Child.* 1997;7:128-137
12. Elder G, Eccles J, Ardelt M, Lord S. Inner city parents under economic pressure: perspectives on the strategies of parenting. *J Marriage Fam.* 1995;57:771-784
13. Steir D, Leventhal J, Berg A, Johnson L, Mezger J. Are children born to young mothers at increased risk of maltreatment? *Pediatrics.* 1993;91:642-648
14. Campbell DW. Family paradigm theory and family rituals: implications for child and family health. In: Wegner GD, Alexander RJ, eds. *Readings in Family Nursing.* Philadelphia, PA: Lippincott; 1993:122-130
15. Olds D, et al. Prenatal and infancy home visitation by nurses: recent findings. *Future Child.* 1999;9:44-65
16. St Pierre R, Layzer J, Barnes H. Two generation programs: design, cost and short term effectiveness. *Future Child.* 1995;5:76-93
17. Weinraub M, Gringlas MB. Single parenthood. In: Bornstein MH, ed. *Handbook of Parenting.* Vol 3. Mahwah, NJ: Lawrence Erlbaum Associates; 1995:65-87
18. Patterson CJ. Lesbian and gay parenthood. In: Bornstein MH, ed. *Handbook of Parenting.* Vol. 3. Mahwah, NJ: Lawrence Erlbaum Associates; 1995:255-274
19. Belsky J. The determinants of parenting: a process model. *Child Dev.* 1984;55:83-96
20. Hetherington E, Stanley-Hagan M, eds. *Parenting in Divorced and Remarried Families.* Mahwah, NJ: Lawrence Erlbaum Associates; 1995
21. Wallerstein J, Lewis J, Blakeslee S. *The Unexpected Legacy of Divorce.* New York, NY: Hyperion; 2000
22. Cherlin A, Chase-Lansdale P, McRae YC. Effects of parental divorce on mental health throughout the life course. *Am Sociol Rev.* 1998;63:239-249

23. Anderson CM. Single parent families: strengths, vulnerabilities and interventions. In: Carter B, McGoldrick M, eds. *The Expanded Family Life Cycle: Individual, Family, and Social Perspectives.* Boston, MA: Allyn & Bacon; 1999:399-416

24. Stack CB, Burton LM. Kinscripts: reflections on family, generation and culture. In: Glenn EN, Chang G, Forcey LR, eds. *Mothering: Ideology, Experience and Agency.* New York, NY: Routledge; 1994:33-44

25 Jackson J. Multiple caregiving among African Americans and infant attachment: the need for an emic approach. *Human Dev.* 1993;36:87-102

26. American Psychiatric Association. *Diagnostic and Statistical Manual of Mental Disorders, Fourth Edition (DSM-IV).* Washington, DC: American Psychiatric Association; 1994

27. American Academy of Pediatrics. *The Classification of Child and Adolescent Mental Diagnoses in Primary Care. Diagnostic and Statistical Manual of Mental Disorders for Primary Care (DSM-PC), Child and Adolescent Version.* Wolraich ML, Felice ME, Drotar D, eds. Elk Grove Village, IL: American Academy of Pediatrics; 1996

28. Downey G, Coyne J. Children of depressed parents: an integrative review. *Psychol Bull.* 1990;108:50-76

29. Weissman MM, Olfson M. Depression in women: implications for health care research. *Science.* 1995;269:799-801

30. Meagher D, Murray D. Depression. *Lancet.* 1997;349(Suppl 1):S117-S120

31. Areias MEG, Kumar R, Barros H, Figueiredo E. Correlates of postnatal depression in mothers and fathers. *Br J Psychiatry.* 1996;169:36-41

32. Beeber LS. Pattern integrations in young depressed women: part 1. *Arch Psychiatr Nurs.* 1996;3:151-156

33. Field T. Psychologically depressed parents. In: Bornstein MH, ed. *Handbook of Parenting. Vol 4. Applied and Practical Parenting.* Mahwah, NJ: Lawrence Erlbaum Associates; 1995:85-99

34. Inoff-Germain G, Nottelmann ED, Radke-Yarrow M. Relation of parental affective illness to family, dyadic, and individual functioning: an observational study of family interaction. *Am J Orthopsychiatry.* 1997;3:433-448

35. Kessler RC, Davis CG, Kendler KS. Childhood adversity and adult psychiatric disorder in the US National Comorbidity Survey. *Psychol Med.* 1997;27:1101-1119

36. Radke-Yarrow M, Klimes-Dougan B. Children of depressed mothers: a developmental and interactional perspective. In: Luthar SS, Burack JA, Cicchetti D, Weisz JR, eds. *Developmental Psychopathology: Perspectives on Adjustment, Risk, and Disorder.* New York, NY: Cambridge University Press; 1997:374-389

37. Lehman AF. Heterogeneity of person and place: assessing co-occurring addictive and mental disorders. *Am J Orthopsychiatry.* 1996;66:32-40

38. Kessler RC, Christopher BN, McGonagie KA, Edlund MJ, Frank RG, Leaf PJ. The epidemiology of co-occurring addictive and mental disorders: implication for prevention and service utilization. *Am J Orthopsychiatry.* 1996;66:17-29

39. Regier DA, Farmer ME, Rae DS, Locke BZ, Keith SJ, Goodwin FK. Comorbidity of mental disorders with alcohol and other drug abuse: results from the epidemiologic catchment area (ECA) study. *JAMA.* 1990;19:2511-2518

40. Ross HE, Glasner FB, Germanson T. The prevalence of psychiatric disorders in patients with alcohol and other drug problems. *Arch Gen Psychiatry.* 1988;45:1023-1031

41. Weissman MM, Myers JK, Harding PS. Prevalence and psychiatric heterogeneity of alcoholism in a United States urban community. *J Stud Alcohol.* 1980:672-681

42. Lamberg L. Treating depression in medical conditions may improve the quality of life. *JAMA.* 1996;276:857-858

43. Packard NJ, Haberman MR, Woods NF, Yates BC. Demands of illness among chronically ill women. *West J Nurs Res.* 1991;13:434-457

44. Malphurs JE, Field T, Lorraine C, et al. Altering withdrawn and intrusive interaction behaviors of depressed mothers. *Infant Ment Health J.* 1996;17:152-160

45. Field T. Maternal depression effects on infants and early interventions. *Prev Med.* 1998; 27:200-203

46. Laing C, Field T, Pickens, et al. Preschoolers of dysphoric mothers. *J Child Psychol Psychiatry.* 1996;37:221-224

47. Field T, Fox NA, Pickens J, Nawrocki T. Relative right frontal EEG activation in 3-6 month-old infants of depressed mothers. *Dev Psychol.* 1995;31:358-363

48. Billings AG, Moos RH. Children of parents with unipolar depression: a controlled 1-year follow-up. *J Abnorm Child Psychol.* 1985;14:149-166

49. Weissman MM, Gershon ES, Kidd KK, et al. Psychiatric disorders in the relatives of probands with affective disorders. *Arch Gen Psychiatry.* 1984;41:13-21

50. Weissman MM, Warner V, Wickramarqatne P, Moreau D, Olfson M. Offspring of depressed parents. *Arch Gen Psychiatry.* 1997;54:932-939

51. Weissman MM, Fendrich M, Warner V, Wickramaratne PA. Incidence of psychiatric disorder in offspring at high and low risk for depression. *J Am Acad Child Adolesc Psychiatry.* 1992;31:640-648

52. Boyle MH, Pickles AR. Influence of maternal depressive symptoms on ratings of childhood behavior. *J Abnorm Child Psychol.* 1997;25:399-412

53. Field T, Estroff DB, Yando R, del Valle C, Malphurs J, Hart S. Depressed mothers' perceptions of infant vulnerability are related to later development. *Clin Psychiatry Human Dev.* 1996;27:43-53

54. Fendrich M, Warner V, Weissman MM. Family risk factors, parental depression, and psychopathology in offspring. *Dev Psychol.* 1990;26:40-50

55. Nilzon KR, Palmerus K. The influence of familial factors on anxiety and depression in childhood and early adolescence. *Adolescence.* 1997;32:935-943

56. Block DS. Adolescent suicide as a public health threat. *J Child Adolesc Psychiatry Nurs.* 1999;12:26-38

57. Keller MB, Lavori PW, Beardslee WR, Wunder J, Ryan N. Depression in children and adolescents: new data on 'undertreatment' and a literature review on the efficacy of available treatments. *J Affect Disord.* 1991;21:163-171

58. Melnyk BM, Moldenbauer Z. Childhood depression. *Adv Nurs Pract.* 1999;97:4, 29, 97

59. Regier DA, Hirschfield RM, Goodwin FK, Burke JD, Lazar JB, Judd LL. The NIMH depression awareness, recognition, and treatment program: structure, aims, and scientific basis. *Am J Psychiatry.* 1988;145:1351-1357

60. Pound A. Parental affective disorder and childhood disturbance. In: Gopfert M, Webster J, Seeman MV, eds. *Parental Psychiatric Disorder: Distressed Parents and Their Families.* New York, NY: Cambridge University Press; 1996:201-218

61. Pajer K. New strategies in the treatment of depression in women. *J Clin Psychiatry.* 1995; 56(Suppl 2):30–37

62. Keltner NL, Folks. *Psychotropic Drugs.* 3rd ed. New York, NY: Mosby; 2001

63. Beardslee WR, Salt P, Versage EM, Gladstone TRG, Wright EJ, Rothberg PC. Sustained change in parents receiving preventive interventions for families with depression. *Am J Psychiatry.* 1997;154:510–514

64. Barnes GG. The mentally ill parent and the family system. In: Gopfert M, Webster J, Seeman MV, eds. *Parental Psychiatric Disorder: Distressed Parents and Their Families.* New York, NY: Cambridge University Press; 1996:42–59

65. Luthar SS, Cushing G, McMahon TJ. Interdisciplinary interface: developmental principles brought to substance abuse research. In: Luthar SS, Burack JA, Cicchetti D, Weisz JR, eds. *Developmental Psychopathology: Perspectives on Adjustment, Risk, and Disorder.* New York, NY: Cambridge University Press; 1997:437–456

66. Azzi-Lessing L, Olsen LJ. Substance abuse-affected families in the child welfare system: new challenges, new alliances. *Soc Work.* 1996;41:15–23

67. Goldberg ME. Substance-abusing women: false stereotypes and real needs. *Soc Work.* 1995;6:789–798

68. Mayes LC. Substance abuse and parenting. In: Bornstein MH, ed. *Handbook of Parenting. Vol 4: Applied and Practical Parenting.* Mahwah, NJ: Lawrence Erlbaum Associates; 1995:101–125

69. Mayes LC, Bornstein MH. The development of children exposed to cocaine. In Luthar SS, Burack JA, Cicchetti D, Weisz JR, eds. *Developmental Psychopathology: Perspectives on Adjustment, Risk, and Disorder.* New York, NY: Cambridge University Press; 1997:166–188

70. McMahon TJ, Luthar SS. Bridging the gap for children as their parents enter substance abuse treatment. In: Hampton RL, Senatore V, Gullotta TP, eds. *Substance Abuse, Family Violence, and Child Welfare. Bridging Perspectives: Issues in Children's and Families' Lives.* Vol 10. Thousand Oaks, CA: Sage Publications; 1998:143–187

71. Johnson JL. Forgotten no longer: an overview of research on children of chemically dependent parents. In: Rivinus TM, ed. *Children of Chemically Dependent Parents: Multiperspectives from the Cutting Edge.* New York, NY: Brunner/Mazel Publishers; 1991:29–54

72. Steinhausen H-C. Children of alcoholic parents: a review. *Eur Child Adolesc Psychiatry.* 1995;4:143–152

73. Nadel M, Straussner SLA. Children in substance-abusing families. In: Phillips NK, Straussner SLA, eds. *Children in the Urban Environment: Linking Social Policy and Clinical Practice.* Springfield, IL: Charles C. Thomas; 1997:154–174

74. Logue ME, Rivinus TM. Young children of substance-abusing parents: a developmental view of risk and resiliency. In: Rivinus TM, ed. *Children of Chemically Dependent Parents: Multiperspectives from the Cutting Edge.* New York, NY: Brunner/Mazel Publishers; 1991:55–73

75. Nield Anderson L. Family process alteration related to dysfunctional behavior. In: Dyer JG, Sparks SM, Taylor CM, eds. *Psychiatric Nursing Diagnoses: A Comprehensive Manual of Mental Health Care.* Springhouse, PA: Springhouse Corp; 1995:78–81

76. Velleman R, Orford J. The adult adjustment of offspring of parents with drinking problems. *Br J Psychiatry.* 1993;162:503–516

77. Velleman R. Alcohol and drug problems in parents: an overview of the impact on children and the implication for practice. In: Gopfert M, Webster J, Seeman MV, eds. *Parental Psychiatric Disorder: Distressed Parents and Their Families.* New York, NY: Cambridge University Press; 1996:233–243

78. Wegscheider S. *Another Chance: Hope and Health for the Alcoholic Family.* Palo Alto, CA: Science and Behavior Books Inc; 1981

79. Wellisch DK, Steinberg MR. Parenting attitudes of addict mothers. *Int J Addict.* 1980; 15:809–819

80. Nelson-Zlupko L, Kauffman E, Dore MM. Gender differences in drug addiction and treatment: implications for social work intervention with substance abusing women. *Soc Work.* 1995;40:45–54

81. Kearney MH, Murphy S, Rosenbaum M. Mothering on crack cocaine: a grounded theory analysis. *Soc Sci Med.* 1994;38:351–361

82. Williams OB, Corrigan PW. The differential effects of parental alcoholism and mental illness of their adult children. *J Clin Psychol.* 1992;3:406–414

83. Lex BW. Alcohol and other psychoactive substance dependence in women and men. In: Seeman MV, ed. *Gender and Psychopathology.* Washington, DC: American Psychiatric Press Inc; 1995:311–358

84. Chasnoff IJ, Landress HJ, Barrett ME. The prevalence of illicit drug or alcohol use during pregnancy and discrepancy in mandatory reporting. *N Engl J Med.* 1990;322: 1202–1206

85. Coley RL, Chase-Lansdale PL. Adolescent pregnancy and parenthood: recent evidence and future directions. *Am Psychol.* 1998;53:152–166

86. Alan Guttmacher Institute. *Sex and America's Teenagers.* New York, NY: The Alan Guttmacher Institute; 1994

87. Moore K, Papillo AR, Williams S, Jager J, Jones F. *Facts at a Glance.* Washington, DC: Child Trends Inc; 1999

88. Ventura S, Curtin S, Mathews T. *Teenage Births in the United States: National and State Trends, 1990–1996.* Hyattsville, MD: National Center for Health Statistics, National Vital Statistics System; 1998

89. Sadler LS. Adolescent parents. In: Corbett M, Meyer JH, eds. *The Adolescent and Pregnancy.* Boston, MA: Blackwell; 1987:231–248

90. Schellenbach C, Whitman T, Borkowski J. Toward an integrative model of adolescent parenting. *Human Dev.* 1992;35:81–99

91. Brooks-Gunn J, Chase-Lansdale PL. Adolescent parenthood. In: Bornstein MH, ed. *Handbook of Parenting.* Vol 3. Mahwah, NJ: Lawrence Erlbaum Associates; 1995: 113–149

92. Sadler LS. *The Process of Intergeneration Child Rearing Among Urban African American Adolescent Mothers and Grandmothers During the Transition to Parenthood* [dissertation]; University of Connecticut; 1997

93. Osofsky JD, Hann DM, Peebles C. Adolescent parenthood: risks and opportunities for mothers and infants. In: Zeanah C, ed. *Handbook of Infant Mental Health.* New York, NY: The Guilford Press; 1993:106–119

94. Chase-Lansdale P, Brooks-Gunn J, Paikoff R. Research and programs for adolescent mothers: missing links and future promises. *Fam Relat.* 1991;40:396-403

95. Furstenberg F, Brooks-Gunn J, Morgan S. *Adolescent Mothers in Later Life.* Cambridge, MA: Cambridge University Press; 1987

96. Roye C, Balk S. The relationship of partner support to outcomes for teenage mothers and their children: a review. *J Adolesc Health.* 1996;19:86-93

97. Horwitz S, Klerman L, Kuo H, Jekel J. Intergenerational transmission of school age parenthood. *Fam Plan Perspect.* 1991;23:168-172

98. Leadbeater B, Bishop S, Raver C. Quality of mother-toddler interactions, maternal depressive symptoms, and behavioral problems in preschoolers of adolescent mothers. *Dev Psychol.* 1996;32:280-288

99. Panzarine S, Slater E, Sharps P. Coping, social support and depressive symptoms in adolescent mothers. *J Adolesc Health.* 1995;17:113-119

100. Hubbs-Tait L, Osofsky J, Hann D, Culp A. Predicting behavior problems and social competence in children of adolescent mothers. *Fam Relat.* 1994;43:439-446

101. McAnarney E, Lawrence R. Day care and teenage mothers: nurturing the mother-child dyad. *Pediatrics.* 1993;91:202-205

102. Miller B, Moore K. Adolescent sexual behavior, pregnancy, and parenting: research through the 1980's. *J Marriage Fam.* 1990;52:1025-1044

103. Boyer D, Fine D. Sexual abuse as a factor in adolescent pregnancy and child maltreatment. *Fam Plan Perspect.* 1992;24:4-19

104. Apfel N, Seitz V. Four models of adolescent mother-grandmother relationships in black inner city families. *Fam Relat.* 1991;40:421-429

105. Spieker S, Bensley L. Roles of living arrangements and grandmother social support in adolescent mothering and infant attachment. *Dev Psychol.* 1994;30:102-111

106. East PL, Felice ME. *Adolescent Pregnancy and Parenting.* Mahwah, NJ: Lawrence Erlbaum Associates; 1996

107. Pope S, Whiteside L, Brooks-Gunn J, et al. Low birth weight infants born to adolescent mothers. *JAMA.* 1993;269:1396-1400

108. Unger K, Cooley M. Partner and grandmother contact in black and white teen parent families. *J Adolesc Health.* 1992;13:546-552

109. Landry D, Forrest JD. How old are US fathers? *Fam Plan Perspect.* 1995;27:159-165

110. Pirog-Good M. The family background and attitudes of teen fathers. *Youth Soc.* 1995;26:351-376

111. Toledo-Dreves V, Zabin L. Durations of adolescent sexual relationships before and after conception. *J Adolesc Health.* 1995;17:165-172

112. Chase-Lansdale P, Brooks-Gunn J, Zamsky E. Young African American multi-generational families in poverty: quality of mothering and grand-mothering. *Child Dev.* 1994;65:373-393

113. Gordon D. Formal operational thinking: role of cognitive-developmental processes in adolescent decision making about pregnancy and contraception. *Am J Orthopsychiatry.* 1990;60:346-356

114. Panzarine S. Interpersonal problem-solving and its relation to adolescent mothering behaviors. *J Adolesc Res.* 1989;4:63-74

115. Elkind D. Cognitive development and adolescent disabilities. *J Adolesc Health Care.* 1985;6:84–89

116. VanCleve S, Sadler L. Adolescent parents and toddlers: strategies for intervention. *Public Health Nurs.* 1990;7:22–27

117. Higginson J. Competitive parenting: the culture of teen mothers. *J Marriage Fam.* 1999;60:135–149

118. Trad P. Mental health of adolescent mothers. *J Am Acad Child Adolesc Psychiatry.* 1995; 34:130–142

119. Williams EG, Sadler LS. Effects of an urban high school-based child care center on adolescent parents and their children. *J Sch Health.* 2001;71:47–51

120. Peisner-Feinberg S, Clifford RM, Culkin ML, et al. *The Children of the Cost, Quality, and Outcomes Study Go to School.* 1999. Available at: http://www.fpg.unc.edu/~ncedl/PDFs/CQO-es.pdf. Accessed March 19, 2004

121. Bakken J, Miltenberger R, Schauss S. Teaching parents with mental retardation: knowledge vs skills. *Am J Ment Retard.* 1993;97:405–417

122. Whitman BY, Accardo PJ. Mentally retarded parents in the community. In: Whitman BY, Accardo PJ, eds. *When a Parent is Mentally Retarded.* Baltimore, MD: Paul H Brookes Publishing Co; 1990:3–10

123. Luckasson R, Coulter D, Polloway E, et al. *Mental Retardation: Definition, Classification and Systems of Supports.* Washington, DC: American Association on Mental Retardation; 1992

124. King BH, State M, Shah B, Davanzo P, Dykens E. Mental retardation: a review of the past 10 years, part I. *J Am Acad Child Adolesc Psychiatry.* 1997;36:1656–1663

125. Ingram D. Parents who have mental retardation. In: *Position Statements of The Arc.* Arlington, TX: The Arc; 1993:1–5

126. D'Souza N. Genetics and mental retardation. In: Whitman BY, Accardo PJ, eds. *When a Parent is Mentally Retarded.* Baltimore, MD: Paul H. Brookes Publishing Company; 1990:31–47

127. Denfield R. Outgrowing your parents at 8. *New York Times Magazine.* 1998;March 22: 32–35

128. Whitman B, Graves B, Haynes G. Parents learning together II: selected modules from the curriculum. In: Whitman B, Accardo P, eds. *When a Parent is Mentally Retarded.* Baltimore, MD: Paul H Brookes Publishing Co; 1990:67–110

129. Accardo PJ, Whitman BY. Children of parents with mental retardation: problems and diagnoses. In: Whitman BY, Accardo PJ, eds. *When a Parent is Mentally Retarded.* Baltimore, MD: Paul H Brookes Publishing Company; 1990:123–131

130. Tymchuk AJ. Moving towards integration of services for parents with intellectual disabilities. *J Intellect Dev Disabil.* 1999;24:59–74

131. Fleming MF. Strategies to increase alcohol screening in health care settings. *Alcohol Health and Research World.* 1997;21:340–347. Available at: http://www.niaaa.nih.gov/publications/arh21-4/340.pdf. Accessed March 19, 2004

132. Sharp LK, Lipsky MS. Screening for depression across the life span: a review of measures for use in primary care settings. *Am Fam Physician.* 2002;66:1001–1008. Available at: http://www.aafp.org/afp/20020915/1001.html/. Accessed March 19, 2004

ADDITIONAL RESOURCES

Ahn N. Teenage childbearing and high school completion: accounting for individual heterogeneity. *Fam Plan Perspect.* 1994;26:17-21

Brindis CD, Berkowitz GB, Clayson Z, Lamb B. California's approach to perinatal substance abuse: toward a model of comprehensive care. *J Psychoact Drugs.* 1997;29:113-122

Brown TG, Kokin M, Seraganian P, Shields N. The role of spouses of substance abusers in treatment: gender differences. *J Psychoact Drugs.* 1995;27:223-229

Brown VB, Ridgely MS, Pepper B, Levine IS, Ryglewicz H. The dual crisis: mental illness and substance abuse. *Am Psychol.* 1989;44:565-569

Cohn JF, Matia R, Tronick EZ, Connell D, Lyons-Ruth K. Face-to-face interactions of depressed mothers and their infants. In: Tronick EZ, Field T, eds. *Maternal Depression and Infant Disturbance.* San Francisco, CA: Jossey-Bass Inc; 1986:31-45

Depression in children: part 1. *The Harvard Mental Health Letter.* 2002;18:8

El-Mallakh P. Treatment models for clients with co-occurring addictive and mental disorders. *Arch Psychiatr Nurs.* 1998;11:71-80

Glidden LM, Floyd FJ. Disaggregating parental depression and family stress in assessing families of children with developmental disabilities: a multisample analysis. *Am J Ment Retard.* 1997;102:250-266

Hossain Z, Field T, Gonzalez J, Malphurs J, Del Valle C. Infants of depressed mothers interact better with their nondepressed fathers. *Infant Ment Health J.* 1994;15:348-357

Lesseig DZ. Primary care diagnosis and pharmacologic treatment of depression in adults. *Nurs Pract.* 1996;21:72-85

Lyons-Ruth K, Zoll D, Connell D, Grunebaum DC. The depressed mother and her one-year-old infant: environmental, interaction, attachment, and infant development. In: Tronick EZ, Field T, eds. *Maternal Depression and Infant Disturbance.* San Francisco, CA: Jossey-Bass Inc; 1986:61-82

Marcus AM, Tisne S. Perception of maternal behavior by elementary school children of alcoholic mothers. *Int J Addict.* 1987;22:543-555

Martinez A, Malphurs J, Field T. Depressed mothers' and their infants' interactions with nondepressed partners. *Infant Ment Health J.* 1996;17:74-80

Masten AS, Coatsworth JD. Competence, resilience, and psychopathology. In: Cicchetti D, Cohen DJ, eds. *Developmental Psychopathology: Risk, Disorder, and Adaptation.* Vol 2. New York, NY: Wiley & Sons; 1995:715-752

McFarlane WR, Link B, Dushay R, Marchal J, Crilly J. Psychoeducational multiple family groups: four-year relapse outcome in schizophrenia. *Fam Proc.* 1995;34:127-144

Seitz V. Adolescent pregnancy and parenting. In: Zigler EF, Kagan SL, Hall NW, eds. *Children, Families, and Government: Preparing for the Twenty-First Century.* Cambridge, MA: Cambridge University Press; 1996:268-287

Seitz V, Apfel N. Adolescent mothers and repeated childbearing: effects of a school based intervention program. *Am J Orthopsychiatry.* 1993;63:572-581

Seitz V, Apfel N. Effects of a school for pregnant students on the incidence of low-birthweight deliveries. *Child Dev.* 1994;65:666–676

Shea MT, Elkin I, Imber SD, et al. Course of depressive symptoms over follow-up: findings from the National Institute of Mental Health Treatment of Depression Collaborative Research Program. *Arch Gen Psychiatry.* 1992;49:782–787

Silverstone PH. Depression increases mortality and morbidity in acute life-threatening medical illness. *J Psychosom Res.* 1990;34:651–657

US Department of Health and Human Services. *Child Health USA '94.* Rockville, MD: US Department of Health and Human Services; 1995

Warner V, Weissman MM, Fendrich M, Wickramaratne P, Moreau D. The course of major depression in the offspring of depressed parents. *Arch Gen Psychiatry.* 1992;49:795–801

CHAPTER 21

Children With Special Health Care Needs

Carol Cohen Weitzman, MD

LEARNING OBJECTIVES

At the completion of this section, the reader will be familiar with:

- General principles in incorporating children with special health care needs into child care settings.

- An understanding of important information so that children with asthma, diabetes, cancer, and human immunodeficiency virus (HIV) infection can be successfully integrated into child care programs.

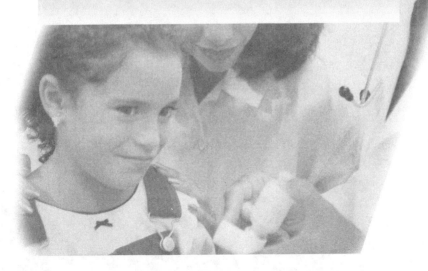

INTRODUCTION

A chronic health condition is defined as one that lasts or is expected to last for 3 months or longer and affects the child's usual age-appropriate activities or results in extensive hospitalization, home health services, or use of medical care in excess of that generally considered appropriate for a child of the same age. The category of chronic illness encompasses a wide range of diagnoses. Conservative estimates are that at least 10% to 15% of children have some chronic health condition, and some surveys report a prevalence of up to 30%. Approximately 10% of all children with chronic health problems or 1 million US children have physiologically severe conditions that impair functioning or require regular or daily intervention. Up to 18% of all children will have greater needs in school and in child care settings than will a typically developing child as a result of developmental, health, or behavioral reasons.

CHRONIC ILLNESS AND CHILD DEVELOPMENT

Regardless of whether they have a chronic illness, all young children need to develop positive self-identity, warm reciprocal relationships with other adults and children, and feelings of confidence, curiosity, and competence. When children with chronic illness enter child care settings, it is often difficult for child care providers to understand the disease and its management and the impact of caring for a child with illness in the center. It is equally difficult for parents to place their child in a child care setting, unsure of the medical risks and the emotional implications for their child in attending a group care program. Thus, there are many reasons why children with chronic illness may have difficulty accomplishing the developmental tasks of early childhood and developing a healthy sense of self and others. Depending on the severity of illness, children's lives may be characterized by multiple disruptions and hospitalizations. Early or prolonged separations from caregivers may threaten a young child's developing sense of security or interrupt formation of secure attachments. Some children will have experienced painful procedures, possibly on a daily basis, threatening their basic sense of trust. Physical or sensory disabilities may interfere with a young child's ability to fully explore his or her environment. Medications, dietary or activity restrictions, and parental grief and anxiety may restrict a child's abilities to interact successfully with others in the environment and to achieve increasing self-control, mastery, and autonomous functioning.

CHILDREN'S REACTIONS TO ILLNESS

Children's understanding of illness varies with age and cognitive development. Young children often associate causation of illness with misbehavior or not following rules, and therefore, having a chronic illness may be confusing and difficult for them to understand. During periods of sickness or stress, children may regress, and this may be characterized by loss of milestones, such as increased dependency on oral behaviors, wetting in a previously toilet-trained child, etc. Children may exhibit more difficulty with separation and express a greater need for an important adult nearby; less willingness to interact with peers; affective lability, including increased irritability; internalizing behaviors, such as depression, anxiety, or withdrawal; or externalizing behaviors, such as aggression, tantrums, and oppositionality.

Is It Worth It?

Taking the time and effort to successfully integrate children with special health care needs into child care settings is worthwhile for everyone. The child with a chronic illness is provided an opportunity to develop healthy peer relationships and gain exposure to a range of activities. Children without special needs learn about diversity and tolerance. Children will learn about the range of needs and capacities of others from an early age and in a loving, supportive manner. For child care providers, integrating children with diverse needs demonstrates that, often, only small modifications are required to meet a child's needs. More importantly, child care providers can appreciate the value and strengths of each and every child.

Key Components to Integrating Children With Chronic Illness Into Child Care Settings

Regardless of the particular chronic illness, certain fundamental principles in effective planning and communication exist that will facilitate a smooth transition to child care and a positive experience for the child with special health care needs.

Early communication

When a chronic illness is diagnosed in a child who is already in or planning to begin a child care program, a meeting should be initiated to exchange information and ideas. Optimally, the parents of the child, the child care staff, the child care director, the child's health care professional, and the health consultant to the center should be present. At this meeting, it is important to define the illness and answer the following types of questions:

- What is this disease and how is it being treated?
- Will treatment be required while the child is in the center, and what are potential adverse effects of medications and complications of the illness?
- Does this illness pose any risk to staff or other children, and do specific precautions need to be taken?
- Does this illness limit the child's activities?
- What has been explained to the child about his or her illness?
- What would the family like classmates and staff to know, and how would that best be accomplished?
- How much absence and disruption in the child's life is to be anticipated?
- Does the child require special equipment, or do the child care providers need special training?

The center can provide the following information:

- What is the center's experience in caring for a child with this chronic illness?
- Are staff trained in rescue breathing and first aid for choking or in administering medication?
- What restrictions exist in administering medications or performing blood tests (such as blood glucose tests)?

In addition to exchanging the above information, this is an important time for members of the team who will be participating in the care of the child to express their concerns and worries about caring for a child with chronic illness and to develop a support network. Because parents and staff may be experiencing grief, anger, and anxiety, it is important for frank and honest discussions to occur at the onset of care.

Emergency plans

From the outset, a specific written plan should be established to manage any emergencies that may occur while the child is in the center (see Appendix H). Any medications or treatments the child may require need to be available and accessible to child care providers. Providers must also be trained in the specifics of how to administer the medication or perform the needed treatment (suctioning, catheterization, glucagon administration, etc). Providers must also be trained to evaluate or judge whether a specific intervention is necessary. For example, the child with chronic asthma who has worsening symptoms may require a "rescue" medication. The provider would need to know the indications for use of an inhaled bronchodilator, such as increasing cough or wheeze, increased respiratory rate, presence of retractions, or other evidence of increased work of breathing. The child care provider would also need to be taught to enter a memo in the daily log regarding indication for intervention or treatment, what treatment was given, and what the result was. The health care professional can assist greatly by being available to the center for questions, support, and guidance and by giving clear guidelines for specific issues about which he or she needs or wishes to be notified.

Effective planning

Planning must be initiated to develop specific, thoughtful classroom strategies that will optimize and normalize the experience of the child with chronic illness and encourage healthy peer interactions. Therefore, it is important to:

- Incorporate an understanding of the child's illness into the entire class's experience in a clear and appropriate way for children of that age group and in a manner that respects the specific child's needs.
- Use strategies, such as advanced planning, to minimize situations in which the child may feel isolated or different.
- Promote opportunities for the child with chronic illness to develop autonomy and positive self-esteem, particularly surrounding the illness.

- Dispel myths about children with illness. Most children with chronic illness, when they are maintained on proper medications and treatments, can participate in a full range of activities.

Continued surveillance

Once the child has been successfully integrated into child care, it is important for the health care professional to maintain contact with the center. Periodic exchange of information will allow the health care professional to understand:

- How the child has adjusted
- How well the illness is being controlled
- What complications or questions have occurred
- Whether the staff needs additional training
- Whether the staff feels comfortable caring for this child
- How much absence there has been as a result of the illness and what strategies have been developed to help the child maintain a sense of continuity and trust with the caregivers

CHILDREN WITH CHRONIC ILLNESS

The next section of this chapter will highlight 4 distinct chronic illnesses that have been chosen to illustrate a spectrum of clinical issues. These include 2 chronic diseases with a range of daily care requirements (asthma and diabetes) and 2 life-threatening illnesses (malignancy and HIV infection).

Asthma

Definitions and Epidemiology

Asthma affects more than 1 in 20 American children (higher in certain subpopulations) and is the most common chronic illness of childhood. Asthma is defined as a reversible inflammatory airway disease triggered by a variety of immunologic and nonimmunologic factors. The onset of asthma typically occurs early in life, with approximately 75% of children developing the illness within the first 3 years of life.

History to Be Provided to Child Care Centers

There can be a wide range in the severity of asthma symptoms, varying from mild cough with frequent upper respiratory tract infections to chronic, continuous symptoms that can be severe or even life threatening. During the initial meeting with the child care center staff, the child's asthma needs to be clarified as to the degree (eg, mild to severe) and chronicity (eg, intermittent or chronic).

- What is the child's usual medication requirement?
- What known triggers exist for this child's asthma?
- When was the last asthma exacerbation? Was the child hospitalized at that time?
- How often does this child have asthma exacerbations?
- How often has this child had to miss school or activities because of illness?

● Depending on age and cooperation, what is the child's typical peak flow meter reading?

Challenges That May Occur in Child Care

The main problem that will affect a child with asthma in child care is an acute exacerbation of disease. Health care professionals need to educate child care staff to recognize when a child may have a worsening of symptoms. Young children, in particular, may not be able to articulate feelings of discomfort, and therefore, staff must rely on such signs as an increase in cough, presence of wheeze, increased respiratory rate or effort, chest retractions, and possibly, changes in peak flow meter readings. In addition, staff may note changes in a child's behavior, such as increasing agitation or, conversely, listlessness. If the child is older than 5 years, the health care professional should train the child and the child care providers in the use of a peak flow meter. This will provide important information about the child's clinical status, and management guidelines can be developed for specific peak flow rates.

It is important for health care professionals to help child care providers identify and prevent possible triggers for each child, such as:

● Allergens (eg, pets, dust, molds, and grass)
● Odors from paint, perfume, etc
● Smoke (eg, cigarette, fireplace)
● Strenuous exercise
● Cold outdoor temperatures
● Respiratory illness

It is important to emphasize to child care providers that, in general, exercise is important and should not be limited. If the child develops symptoms during exercise, the activity can be interrupted and medication can be administered. Some children may require medication before exercise.

Management Strategies

Because asthma exacerbations can be frightening for young children, child care providers should remain calm and sensitive during these episodes. The child should be brought to a quiet place, maintained in an upright position, and assessed for the severity of the exacerbation.

The child's health care professional can train child care providers to:

● Administer medication using appropriate device (eg, nebulizer or a metered-dose inhaler with a spacer device).
● Recognize the different categories of asthma medications, including preventive treatments and medications used to treat an acute event. The onset of action of various medications and possible adverse effects need to be explained.
● Support the child by helping to identify and articulate feelings, such as fear, that they may experience during an acute episode. When providers execute a predetermined plan in a calm manner, they communicate to the child their willingness and ability to help, which will diminish the child's anxiety.

- Enhance regular communication between health care professional, child care provider, and parent. One means of accomplishing this communication is by developing an asthma diary or log in which episodes and patterns of coughing or wheezing, management provided and outcome, and identified triggers are recorded. Additionally, when a child and family have a written plan outlining peak flow zones and listing all the medications and indications for taking each one, symptoms can be more effectively controlled on a day-to-day basis.

Diabetes

Definitions and Epidemiology
Type 1 diabetes mellitus (insulin-dependent diabetes mellitus) is one of the most common chronic diseases with onset in childhood; 1 in 400 to 600 children younger than 18 years in the United States are affected. Type 1 diabetes mellitus is a disease that destroys the islet cells of the pancreas and is characterized by a deficiency in insulin production. It is considered to be an autoimmune disease. By definition, type 1 diabetes mellitus requires the lifelong use of insulin injections to prevent ketoacidosis.

History to Be Provided to Child Care Provider
Diabetes is a chronic illness that requires daily planning and careful supervision. When these are in place, a child with diabetes can participate and enjoy a full range of activities. At the first meeting, child care providers need to learn the following information.
- How long has this child lived with diabetes?
- What is the typical range of blood sugars that the child has in a day and the goal set by the family and the child's health care professional?
- What strategies has the family developed to help the child cope with the disease?
- What is the daily insulin regimen for this child and the food and exercise routine?
- What is the frequency of blood sugar testing?

Challenges That May Occur in Child Care

Hypoglycemia
The most serious problem that may occur in a child with type 1 diabetes mellitus in a child care setting is hypoglycemia. This must be managed immediately. Young children will often not be able to articulate that they are experiencing hypoglycemia. Therefore, child care providers must become skilled at recognizing the following symptoms:
- Sweating
- Fatigue
- Poor coordination

- Irritability
- Confusion, disorientation
- Shakiness
- Pallor
- Unusual crying (especially in babies)

It is important to learn from parents about the child's most typical responses to low blood sugar.

Hypoglycemia is often attributable to failure to eat enough before exercise, a delayed or missed meal or snack, or too much insulin. Staff should remain calm and quickly help the child. A source of rapidly absorbed glucose should be supplied, such as juice, soda, or glucose tablets. When the child has improved, this needs to be followed by additional carbohydrate snacks, such as crackers and cheese, peanut butter on bread, etc. Before exercise or outdoor time, a backpack of snacks and rapidly absorbed sugar products should be assembled. During an episode of hypoglycemia, it is advisable to test the blood sugar; however, if this is not readily available or the child is rapidly decompensating, treatment should be instituted immediately. All hypoglycemic episodes should be recorded and reviewed with parents and health care professionals. If a child becomes unconscious, this is a medical emergency that requires a specific and efficient plan that staff and the director have reviewed in detail. Most centers cannot administer glucagon for severe hypoglycemia. Insta-Glucose (ICN Pharmaceuticals, Costa Mesa, CA) or Glutose (Paddock Laboratories Inc, Minneapolis, MN), which are glucose gels, can be squeezed inside the cheeks. This method is effective, and the child does not experience significant nausea. Child care staff must be instructed in the recognition of hypoglycemia and its treatment.

Hyperglycemia

High blood sugar poses less of a problem to child care providers, because difficulties with high blood sugar often develop over hours. The signs a child care provider may notice are:

- Increased thirst
- Increased urination
- Fruity odor to a child's breath
- Nausea and vomiting

Hyperglycemia can lead to ketoacidosis and significant morbidity or even mortality. In addition, the Diabetes Control and Complications Trial demonstrated a relationship between better control of blood sugar and fewer long-term complications. Child care providers should strive for "tight control" even in young children to prevent long-term complications but should also remain flexible to the limitations that may exist from being in a group care setting.

Management Strategies

Successful integration of a child with diabetes into a child care setting requires attention to 3 domains: insulin and testing of blood glucose, food, and exercise.

Insulin

Although most children in child care will not require insulin injections during their day at the center, it is important for child care providers to be aware of the daily regimen. Children should have their blood tested before lunch and when symptomatic. Regulations may vary from state to state, so health care professionals should be aware of the regulations in their state and local area. If prohibitions to testing exist, health care professionals should advocate for change to ensure that children with chronic illness may be provided appropriate testing (eg, blood glucose for children with diabetes) and treatments (eg, nebulizers for children with asthma). A designated place for blood testing within the child care center needs to be identified so the child's room in the center remains secure and nonthreatening. As soon as they are able, children should be encouraged to participate in their care by selecting the finger for testing or the strip from the vial. Children should never be tested when they are not prepared, because this will instill a sense of fear and anxiety within the child.

Food

Feeding young children in the early years can be challenging, and for the child with diabetes, it takes on special significance. Although children with diabetes need to have regular meals and snacks to avoid hypoglycemia, a flexible approach works best. Infants often have variable intake and may not be regular in their feeding habits, which can cause child care providers to feel anxious when caring for an infant with diabetes. Offering frequent small feedings will usually result in an adequate supply of carbohydrates and nutrition. Toddlers and preschoolers may refuse meals or become more selective in their choices of foods to exert their autonomy. Child care providers, to get these children to eat, may resort to cajoling, poor limit setting (such as not asking the child to maintain classroom table manners), scolding, threatening, etc. It is important that mealtime does not become a battleground at child care. Instead, simply offer the child a choice of foods and positively reinforce desired behaviors. For an older preschooler, reviewing his or her diabetes and meal plan may be helpful. Child care providers and parents must collaborate on how to manage the child's special dietary needs, including extra snacks and unexpected treats or special events in the classroom.

Exercise

Exercise is important for the emotional and physical health of children with diabetes. Without planning, however, hypoglycemia can result, which may discourage the child and the child care provider from further attempts. If strenuous exercise is anticipated, a snack should be eaten before activity. Careful supervision will help child care providers detect when the child becomes symptomatic from hypoglycemia during exercise, in which case a break may be needed. Snacks and a quick glucose source should always be readily available.

Malignancy and HIV

Definitions and Epidemiology

Of all pediatric malignancies, leukemia is the most common and is often diagnosed between 2 and 4 years of age. More than two thirds of children in whom leukemia is diagnosed will remain in remission at 5 years of age. In addition to the leukemias, a variety of other cancers present during childhood, including neuroblastoma, rhabdomyosarcoma, Wilms tumor, Hodgkin disease, brain tumors, Ewing sarcoma, and lymphoma. Each of these requires varied treatments and procedures, with differing prognoses.

It is estimated that 10 000 to 20 000 children in the United States have HIV infection. However, because of the recent decrease in transmission of the infection from mothers to their children attributable to the use of certain medications during pregnancy, there are now fewer children being born with the infection. As new medications and treatments become available to children and pregnant women, these figures will need to be revised. The rate of perinatal infection and progression to symptomatic disease may be altered by new recommendations about managing pregnancies in HIV-infected women and the use of new generations of antiretroviral drugs.

History to Be Provided to Child Care Centers

A child with a cancer will undergo a lengthy series of treatments. Parents and health care professionals can furnish important information for child care providers regarding current therapy and specific concerns, including the following:

- What type of cancer does the child have, and what is the prognosis?
- Where is the child in the course of treatment, and what is the total anticipated length of treatment?
- What are potential complications of the cancer and of the treatment?
- Does the child have any current limitations?
- Does the child have any indwelling catheters that require special attention?

Challenges That May Be Encountered in Child Care

Changes in the child

The child with cancer may have varying changes in physical appearance, stamina, and symptoms. These include:

- Fatigue
- Nausea and vomiting
- Weight loss or gain
- Hair loss

- Mood changes
- Surgical scars

Children may be worried about relapse or the discomfort of continued treatments. Therefore, for these children, the energy needed to master basic developmental skills may be channeled into surviving their disease and its treatment. It is important to help the child maintain self-esteem, present the illness to the class in a manner that is comfortable and acceptable to the child, and prevent the child from experiencing isolation or overprotection.

Infection

During periods of immunocompromise, children are highly vulnerable to life-threatening infection, and most will not attend child care. When a child is not immunosuppressed, he or she often can participate in a full range of activities. Three special precautions are required, however. These are exposure to varicella (chicken-pox) virus by an adult or child contact who has shingles (herpes zoster), chicken-pox, or measles. Actual or suspected exposure should be reported immediately to the parents because of the child's vulnerability to life-threatening illness and the need for rapid treatment. (These are the same precautions required for children who are infected with HIV.)

Medical crises

Although it is uncommon for young children to have medical crises in the classroom, symptoms should be reported to parents, and the center should be aware of whether the presence of fever requires special attention. Fever is particularly important if the child has an indwelling catheter for the administration of medication.

Frequent absences

The child with malignancy or HIV infection may have multiple absences because of hospitalizations for treatment or because of immunosuppression. It is important for the child to still feel a part of the class, and efforts should be directed toward helping other children in the class understand these absences. Classmates may send letters and pictures, and child care providers can telephone or make home or hospital visits.

Management Strategies

It is important for child care providers to have an opportunity to discuss caring for a child with a life-threatening disease. Although the child's prognosis may be excellent, it is unavoidable to consider that the child could die from the disease. This may create overwhelming, discouraging, or frightening feelings, which may lead to an overprotective, or conversely detached, relationship with the child. Providing a forum to discuss these feelings will ultimately benefit everyone.

It is important that child care providers make significant efforts to maintain open and direct communication and a supportive relationship with parents who are managing the stress and anxiety of caring for a child with cancer. Parents may at times appear to be angry, sad, or fearful, and it is important for providers to recognize that these emotions are being displaced onto the providers but are not truly caused by them.

Special Considerations for HIV-Infected Children
The reader is referred to Chapter 17, which includes a discussion of how staff can ensure protection from bloodborne diseases and institute standard (universal) precautions.

Confidentiality
Children with HIV infection have been discriminated against in school settings, despite the fact that transmission does not occur through casual contact and infection from child to child has never occurred in a child care or school setting. It is important for child care providers to know the confidentiality laws in their state. Most states do not require parents to reveal their child's HIV status. It is recommended that only a few child care staff members be aware of the HIV status of the child and that the child's HIV status not be included in the educational records unless the parents feel differently.

Neurologic disease
Before the recent advances in treatment, a large number of HIV-infected children showed evidence of central nervous system dysfunction and infection. This manifested itself as language difficulties, attention problems, and learning difficulties. However, with current treatments, such problems are likely to be less prevalent.

Family stress
Because most children become infected through vertical transmission, their mothers are usually infected, as other family members may be. Therefore, these children may experience profound loss, early separation, and significant illness within their families. Sensitive caregiving is especially necessary to provide stability for these children and to help them with their grief.

Pervasive Developmental Disorders

Definitions and Epidemiology
Pervasive developmental disorder–not otherwise specified (PDD-NOS) is the diagnostic category used when the criteria for autism are not fully met, but the child possesses many similar features and has impaired functioning. It is characterized by significant deficits in reciprocal social interaction and communication skills and stereotypical behaviors and interests. Most of these children have various underlying problems in sensory processing and in the organization of their response. Although the prevalence of autism is now thought to be 1 to 2 per 1000 (4.5 per 10 000),

the prevalence of PDD-NOS may be higher. Many of these children, especially those with mild to moderate impairment, good cognitive functioning, and language skills, will be enrolled in age-typical child care programs.

History to Be Provided to Child Care Centers

Because the spectrum of presentation and disability is so variable, specific information for each child needs to be obtained, including the following:

- Is the child receiving special services (eg, occupational and speech and language therapy, etc)?
- Will these services be received at the center?
- What is most helpful in engaging the child?
- Does the child have unusual anxieties or sensitivities?
- Does the child have behaviors or behavioral patterns stereotypical or characteristic of PDD-NOS?
- What helps when the child is having difficulty relating to others or managing situations?

Management Strategies

Working with a child with PDD-NOS often requires significant classroom planning and provider training. Child care providers are strongly encouraged to work with other professionals caring for the child to develop an individualized plan. Provided are a few basic strategies to help integrate a child with PDD-NOS successfully. It is often beneficial when service providers, such as speech or occupational therapists, provide treatment in the center. They can often provide training and guidance to child care providers.

Caregivers' responses

Children with difficulties in their capacity to relate are in especially great need of warm and consistent relationships in the context of predictable and often highly structured environments. Child care providers often have difficulty developing and sustaining these relationships because of misperceptions about the child's behaviors and intentions. Children may avert their gaze or have difficulty communicating their needs and reading social cues. This may be interpreted as an aloof, unfriendly, or unmanageable child. In addition, a child may have sensitivities, such as touch or sound, and may become anxious, avoidant, withdrawn, or aggressive when overwhelmed by these sensations. Caregivers must understand that these behaviors are attempts to manage overwhelming feelings experienced by the child. This understanding will foster more empathic ways to work with and engage the child.

Listen to the child

The goal of working with children with PDD-NOS is to help them to develop purposeful and intentional interactions. Over time, this will lead to the development of higher functions and greater adaptive behaviors. It is important for child care providers to follow the lead of the child and use natural opportunities to continually elicit adaptive and communicative responses. If a child is repetitively lining up cars, a provider can slowly join this activity by following the child's cues and begin to expand the child's repertoire. It is important for child care providers to treat the child's responses and behaviors as if they are intentional and then work to stretch the child's capabilities and interest, enjoyment, and joint attention in mutually pleasurable social interactions.

CONCLUSIONS AND RECOMMENDATIONS

Health care professionals are in an important position to provide valuable information and guidance to child care providers and parents about chronic disease so that they can optimize the child's experience and diminish anxiety about incorporating these children into a child care setting. Effective planning, communication, and sharing of knowledge about specific chronic diseases between health care professionals and child care providers will enhance the ability of a child with a chronic illness to enjoy normative experiences. This will help children derive gains from enrolling in quality child care so they may flourish and develop to reach their greatest capacities.

Confidentiality must always be considered when individual health information is shared. The Health Insurance Portability and Accountability Act of 1996 (HIPAA) includes a privacy rule, which took effect April 14, 2003. Health care professionals must be particularly diligent in preserving confidentiality with respect to any individually identifiable health information, whether oral or recorded in any form or medium. Disclosure of personal health information requires authorization by the individual, parent, or guardian except in special instances, such as suspected abuse or neglect or certain issues relating to public health.

RESOURCES

American Cancer Society. *Back to School: A Handbook for Teachers of Children with Cancer*. Atlanta, GA: American Cancer Society; 1988. Publication No. 88-20M No. 2640-LE

American Diabetes Association. *A Word to Teachers and Child-Care Providers*. Alexandria, VA: American Diabetes Association; 1990

Brackenridge BP, Rubin RR. *Sweet Kids: How to Balance Diabetes Control and Good Nutrition with Family Peace*. Alexandria, VA: American Diabetes Association; 1996

Centers for Disease Control and Prevention. HIPAA privacy rule and public health. *MMWR Early Release*. 2003;52:1-12

Cohen HJ, Papola P, Alvarez M. Neurodevelopmental abnormalities in school-age children with HIV infection. *J Sch Health*. 1994;64:11-13

Crocker AC, Lavin AT, Palfrey JS. Supports for children with HIV infection in school: best practices guidelines. *J Sch Health*. 1994;64:32-34

Dominguez KL. Management of HIV-infected children in the home and institutional settings. Care of children and infections control in schools, day care, hospital settings, home, foster care, and adoption. *Pediatr Clin North Am*. 2000;47:203-239

Greenspan SI, Kalmanson B, Shahmoon-Shanok R. Assessing and treating infants and young children with severe difficulties in relating and communicating. *Zero to Three.* 1997;17(5)

Jenkins M. Human immunodeficiency virus type 1 infection in infants and children. In: Rudolph AM, Hoffman JE, Rudolph CD, eds. *Rudolph's Pediatrics.* 20th ed. Stamford, CT: Appleton & Lange; 1996;655-660

Larsson EV, Luce SC, Anderson SR, Christian WP. Childhood autism. In: Levine MD, Carey WB, Crocker AC, eds. *Developmental-Behavioral Pediatrics.* 2nd ed. Philadelphia, PA: Saunders; 1992;533-542

National Cancer Institute. *Students with Cancer: A Resource for the Educator.* Bethesda, MD: National Cancer Institute; 1990. NIH Publication No. 91-2086

Perrin JM. Chronic illness. In: Levine MD, Carey WB, Crocker AC, eds. *Developmental-Behavioral Pediatrics.* 2nd ed. Philadelphia, PA: Saunders; 1992:335-345

Plaut TF. *One Minute Asthma—What You Need to Know.* Amherst, Pedipress Inc; 1995

Schonfeld DJ. The child's cognitive understanding of illness. In: Lewis M, ed. *Child and Adolescent Psychiatry.* 2nd ed. Baltimore, MD: Williams & Wilkins; 1996

Schulz CM. *Why Charlie Brown, Why? A Story About What Happens When a Friend is Very Ill.* New York, NY: Topper Books; 1990

CHAPTER 22

Children With Developmental Disabilities

Carol Cohen Weitzman, MD, and Desmond P. Kelly, MD

LEARNING OBJECTIVES

From this section, the reader will gain:

- Improved understanding of the spectrum of disorders and the related special needs of children with developmental disabilities.

- Appreciation of the challenge of incorporating children with disabilities into child care centers.

- Knowledge of special services that can benefit children with disabilities.

- Understanding of professional roles in the provision of appropriate, accessible, and safe child care for children with disabilities.

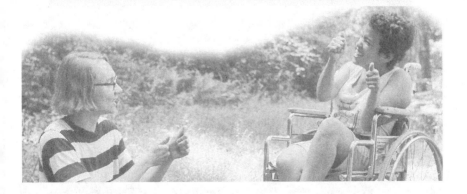

INTRODUCTION

Developmental disability is defined as a chronic condition attributable to mental or physical impairment that manifests in childhood, is likely to continue indefinitely, and results in substantial functional limitation in major life activities, such as self-care, language, social skills (eg, autism), learning, or mobility. In addition to the predicted incidence of children with disabilities related to syndromes and natal and perinatal insults, there are an increasing number of children who have survived extreme prematurity or critical illnesses and who are faced with complex medical needs and developmental challenges. Many of these children have benefited from early developmental interventions and are succeeding in mainstream settings at school. There are often delays in identification and diagnosis of developmental disorders, and problems are frequently encountered in securing child care services for children with disabilities. Children with disabilities should have access to child care services that meet their special needs, offering them the opportunity for inter-action with their peers without disabilities and exposure to activities that promote their physical, intellectual, and social development. It is incumbent on primary care physicians and other health care professionals to be familiar with the special medical and developmental needs of their patients and to advocate for the provision of appropriate child care services.

The impact of disabling conditions has been eloquently described.[1] The "differentness" that is created has an impact on performance, services required, ability to participate in activities, and engagement or connectedness (interrelationships and interactions with other persons). Some families are assuming a more primary role as advocates and team members in meeting the medical and educational needs of children with disabilities, and in turn, they need increased levels of support. Many of these families bear heavier financial, physical, and emotional burdens. Child care services have added benefits for these families not only by allowing parents to pursue employment but also by providing support, referral to other resources, and respite from the stress of caring for a child with special needs.

THE SPECTRUM AND IMPACT OF DEVELOPMENTAL DISABILITY

Developmental disability can vary in presentation from a readily recognizable condition with clear-cut impairment of function to subtle disorders with which the impairment is not apparent and may initially be overlooked. All health care and education professionals working with young children need to be alert to any signs suggesting delayed or atypical development.

Developmental disorders that might be encountered in child care settings can be categorized by the developmental domain of primary disability.

Neuromotor Disorders

Motor disabilities range from poor coordination or dyspraxia (difficulties with planning motor movements) to severe dysfunction of neuromotor systems. Some motor disabilities result from specific defects in development of neural structures, such as myelomeningocele, and others might be related primarily to muscular problems, such as muscular dystrophy. The term cerebral palsy denotes a group of conditions in which damage to the central nervous system during the early developmental period (prenatal, perinatal, or infancy) results in neuromotor impairment. The insult to the central nervous system is static (not progressive), although the effect on function can vary with increasing physical size and more complex demands. Terms used to classify cerebral palsy reflect the pattern of impairment: spastic (with increased muscle tone); dyskinetic or athetoid (involving the basal ganglial or thalamic regions of the brain, resulting in involuntary movements); or ataxic and tremor (with primarily cerebellar dysfunction affecting balance and coordination). Other terms relate to the pattern of dysfunction by region: quadriplegic (all 4 extremities and oral-motor skills involved); diplegic (all 4 extremities but lower extremities more involved); or hemiplegic (extremities on 1 side). Children with neuromotor problems are prone to associated health problems, including feeding difficulties; seizures; orthopedic problems, including joint contractures or hip dislocation; vision and hearing problems; constipation; and pressure sores. It is important to note that although children with cerebral palsy frequently have cognitive or learning difficulties, these are not directly proportional to their neuromotor dysfunction.

Language Disorders

Developmental language delays or disorders can predominantly involve receptive skills (language processing and comprehension), expressive abilities (translating ideas into spoken words), or speech articulation and fluency and intelligibility. Communication problems are frequently associated with behavioral challenges because of frustration with not being able to understand language or to express one's needs, thoughts, and feelings.

Pervasive Developmental Disorder

Children with autistic disorder and Asperger syndrome manifest atypical patterns of function in the 3 key areas of language and communication, social relatedness, and repetitive or stereotypical behaviors and interests. These children have a particular dependence on routine and predictability in their daily experiences and frequently have difficulty adjusting to transitions. Their physical appearance is usually normal, and their unusual behavioral patterns can be perplexing to parents and health care professionals, with resultant delays in diagnosis (see Chapter 21).

Attention Disorders

Much has been written about attention-deficit/hyperactivity disorder (see Chapter 8), the most common neurobehavioral disorder of childhood, which affects 3% to 5% of children in the United States. Although the functional impairment related to attention problems is seen most acutely at school age, many of the behavioral challenges will manifest earlier. There is a risk of premature or inaccurate diagnostic labeling in this disorder, because the cardinal manifestations of inattention, distractibility, impulsivity, and hyperactivity can also be symptoms of other underlying medical disorders, learning difficulties, mental illness, and social dysfunction.

Cognitive Impairment

Children with cognitive impairment or mental retardation manifest delays in all developmental domains. Those with specific genetic syndromes or disorders, such as Down syndrome or fragile X syndrome, might have a family history of developmental disorders or show unusual physical features. These children quite often have distinct behavioral styles that are characteristic of the condition.

Sensory Impairment

Sensory impairments can have a profound influence on development. Visual impairment is more readily apparent and can affect motor skills and mobility as well as social interaction. Hearing loss can be subtle and might only be detected when a child is delayed in acquiring language skills. The move toward universal screening of newborns for hearing loss will decrease the age of diagnosis of hearing loss from the previously unacceptable average of 2.5 years. A significantly better outcome has been demonstrated in children who are diagnosed and receive intervention before 6 months of age.

Although detailed discussion of developmental disabilities is beyond the scope of this chapter, it is important that the child care provider be well informed regarding the specific risks for medical problems or the expected behavioral difficulties of children with disabilities who might be enrolled in their programs. In turn, there should be a clear plan for monitoring and intervening if new medical problems emerge (see Appendix H). Prerequisites of such a plan should include communication with the child's health care professional and planning of activities to maintain health and promote physical and psychologic development.

GOALS AND BARRIERS

Legislation, such as the Individuals With Disabilities Education Act (Pub L No. 101-476), underscores the significant national commitment to the concept that early services are critical if children with disabilities are to reach their full potential.[2] Such services should focus on promoting the child's acceptance into the family, stabilizing health problems, building interpersonal skills, and maximizing abilities that may heighten the potential for independence and productivity in each phase of development. There must be efforts to integrate the child into appropriate community supports and services used by all children and their families. Availability of appropriate child care services is a key component of such integration. There has been a long standing goal of enrolling 85% of all preschool-aged children with disabilities into regular child care programs with trained staff and an appropriately designed curriculum. This goal remains largely unattained.[3]

There are many challenges inherent to the incorporation of children with disabilities into child care settings. In a recent survey, more than half of a sample of mothers of children with disabilities reported that finding child care was difficult. Cost and quality of the programs were common barriers. Other predictors of difficulties were children with lower cognitive and adaptive abilities and those with more externalizing behaviors.[4] Another study cited primary barriers as lack of availability of resources and staffing, including health care professionals.[5] In that survey, 65% of the centers that responded indicated that they accepted children who were chronically ill or disabled, but the actual number of children with disabilities who were enrolled was low. There appeared to be a level of misunderstanding among directors of programs as to the nature and impact of various disabling conditions. Child care for children who are assisted by technology is rarely available outside the family.[5]

Efforts to increase the enrollment of children with disabilities in child care programs should focus on training, staff-child ratios, continuous availability of health consultants, and staff support. A key to success of such an objective is staff availability and competitive salaries.

THE ROLE OF THE CHILD CARE CENTER

Specific elements must be addressed by child care centers providing services for children with disabilities. These include the physical environment, daily programming to meet the developmental and emotional needs of the child, staff knowledge and skills to accommodate medical needs of the child, and access to special services that the child might require. Any entity providing care for infants, toddlers, or preschool or school-aged children on a regular basis must incorporate activities to promote their education and development.

Accessibility and safety are vital components. Rooms should be free of barriers (physical and sensory) and should be as clean and uncluttered as possible. There should be adequate room for children using adaptive equipment or those with limited mobility to move safely between activities. Developmentally appropriate materials should be available, including art equipment, play equipment, books, and tapes. Specific adaptations may need to be made on the basis of the needs of the child. For example, such materials might need to be brighter or amplified for children with sensory impairments. In contrast, children who have problems with integration of sensory input might benefit from accessibility to quieter areas in which there is less stimulation. Some children need special assistance with feeding and nutrition, necessitating access to support staff with knowledge and training regarding special feeding problems. The family and its needs should be addressed as the service plan is developed before, or early into, the child's registration, and they should continue to be included as ongoing programming evolves.

Programming is very important. Many young children with disabilities will experience difficulties transitioning from 1 activity to another. A predictable and consistent daily routine, reinforced by visual reminders and similar cues, will help in such transitions. Activities should be directed to the development of fine motor, gross motor, language, self-care, and social skills on the basis of updated comprehensive assessments incorporating results of medical and developmental examinations and assessments of cognitive and overall functioning. Written reports from involved specialists are strongly recommended. A wide variety of systems of communication should be considered to ensure that children understand the routine and expectations.

Many young children with disabilities will experience difficulties transitioning from 1 activity to another.

The availability of special services will depend on the location and setting of the child care facility. Programs have been developed in a number of states in which child care centers are located adjacent to large medical centers or have the services of medical specialists available to them. In such programs, children who are medically fragile or dependent on technology are cared for by staff including nurses and child life specialists. Speech and language, occupational, and physical therapists from hospital programs can provide individual therapy in the center and instruct staff regarding developmentally appropriate activities for the children. Similar services might be provided by home health care or area education agencies or other agencies from which children could receive their therapies at the child care center as well as in the home setting. In all situations, child care programs should strive to establish linkages with the agencies and other professionals in their community who provide services for children with disabilities. These organizations are potentially valuable resources with regard to staff and parent training as well as developmental screening and treatment. Health care professionals should be collaborators in the planning of child care services and the integration of specific therapies for on-site treatment of disabilities.

THE ROLE OF THE HEALTH CARE PROFESSIONAL

The health care professional has a large role to play in the health and development of children with disabilities. The American Academy of Pediatrics has stressed the importance of a "medical home" for all children with developmental disorders. The primary health care professional who has ongoing contact with the child and family bears an important responsibility with regard to early detection of developmental delays and coordination of interventions to treat problems that have been identified.

Depending on the degree of disability and availability of services, the physician can assist parents in selecting appropriate child care services. The primary health care professional should advise parents regarding staff-child interactions, staff-child ratio, group size, and an administrative structure that ensures the implementation of a physically, socially, and developmentally appropriate program. Caregivers in small facilities may require training regarding disabilities and how they affect the child's overall development.[6] The primary health care professional should review and monitor the child care services to ensure that they are appropriate and meet the medical and developmental needs of the child. For the more compromised child, the capacity of the program to initiate emergency services is critical.

Children with disabilities are prone to acute illnesses, and the primary health care professional should ensure that families and child care programs know how to judge when a child's illness requires medical evaluation or exclusion from the program. A brief medical summary clarifying the special needs of the child, treatments or interventions required within the child care program, and a specific emergency plan will be of great help to child care staff. The primary health care professional or an identified knowledgeable staff member should be available to answer questions relative to acute medical problems as they occur. Direct communication between the health care professional and the child care provider, with previous approval by parents can be very effective. The Health Insurance Portability and Accountability Act of 1996 (HIPAA) includes a privacy rule, which took effect April 14, 2003. Health care professionals must be particularly diligent in preserving confidentiality with respect to any individually identifiable health information, whether oral or recorded in any form or medium. Disclosure of personal health information requires authorization by the individual, parent, or guardian except in special instances, such as suspected abuse of neglect or certain issues relating to public health.[7] The health care professional should review the health policies on management of illness being used by the program.

The health care professional can also consult with programs by advising about the management of children with special needs, providing educational materials, training staff members, and linking the child care administration with other agencies and programs providing services for children with disabilities.

Advocacy efforts with licensing agencies and legislative bodies are vital for the implementation of a standard of care for child care facilities serving the child with disabilities. Allocation of funding and subsidies to cover the increased cost of care for children with disabilities should also be promoted.

CONCLUSIONS AND RECOMMENDATIONS

Children with disabilities should have access to child care services that meet their special needs, offering them the opportunity for interaction with their peers who do not have disabilities and exposure to activities that promote their physical, intellectual, and social development. It is incumbent on primary care physicians and other health care professionals to be familiar with the special medical and developmental needs of their patients and to advocate for the provision of appropriate child care services.

REFERENCES

1. Crocker AC. The impact of disabling conditions. In: *Mosby's Resource Guide to Children with Disabilities and Chronic Illness.* Wallace HM, Biehl RF, McQueen JC, Blackman JA, eds. St Louis, MO: Mosby Year-book Inc; 1997:22-29
2. American Academy of Pediatrics, Committee on Children With Disabilities. Pediatric services for infants and children with special health care needs. *Pediatrics.* 1993;92:163-165
3. Crowley AA. Integrating handicapped and chronically ill children into day care centers. *Pediatr Nurs.* 1990;16:39-44
4. Warfield ME, Hauser-Cram P. Child care needs, arrangements, and satisfaction of mothers with children with developmental disabilities. *Ment Retard.* 1996;34:294-302
5. Thyen U, Kuhlthau K, Perrin JM. Employment, child care, and mental health of mothers caring for children assisted by technology. *Pediatrics.* 1999;103:1235-1242
6. American Academy of Pediatrics, American Public Health Association, and Maternal and Child Health Bureau. *Caring for Our Children. National Health and Safety Performance Standards: Guidelines for Out-of-Home Child Care Programs.* 2nd ed. Elk Grove Village, IL: American Academy of Pediatrics; 2002
7. Centers for Disease Control and Prevention. HIPAA privacy rule and public health. *MMWR Early Release.* 2003;52:1-12

ADDITIONAL RESOURCES

Accardo PJ, Whitman BY. *Dictionary of Developmental Disabilities Terminology.* Baltimore, MD: Paul H. Brookes; 1996

American Academy of Pediatrics, American Public Health Association, and Maternal and Child Health Bureau. *Caring for Our Children. National Health and Safety Performance Standards: Guidelines for Out-of-Home Child Care Programs.* 2nd ed. Elk Grove Village, IL: American Academy of Pediatrics; 2002

American Academy of Pediatrics, Committee on Early Childhood, Adoption, and Dependent Care. The pediatrician's role in promoting the health of patients in early childhood education and/or child care programs. *Pediatrics.* 1993;92:489-492

Blackman JA. *Medical Aspects of Developmental Disabilities in Children Birth to Three.* Rockville, MD: Aspen Publishers; 1990

Kaiser B, Sklar-Rasminsky J. *HIV/AIDS and Child Care: Fact Book and Facilitators Guide.* Ottawa, Ontario: Canadian Child Care Federation/Health Canada; 1995

Rubin IL, Crocker AC. *Developmental Disabilities: Delivery of Medical Care for Children and Adults.* Philadelphia, PA: Lea & Febiger; 1989

Wallace HM, Biehl RF, McQueen JC, Blackman JA, eds. *Mosby's Resource Guide to Children with Disabilities and Chronic Illness.* St Louis, MO: Mosby Year-Book Inc; 1997

ORGANIZATIONS

National Association for the Education of Young Children
1509 16th Street NW
Washington, DC 20036-1426
Phone: 202/232-8777
Toll-free: 800/424-2460
Web site: http://www.naeyc.org

Zero to Three National Training Institute
2000 M Street NW, Suite 200
Washington, DC 20036
Phone: 202/638-1144
Web site: http://www.zerotothree.org

CHAPTER 23

School-Aged Child Care

Howard L. Taras, MD

LEARNING OBJECTIVES

This chapter will help the reader understand:

- The proportion of elementary school-aged children in self-care and the community resources available for the care of these children.
- The potential problems of self-care for children of different ages.

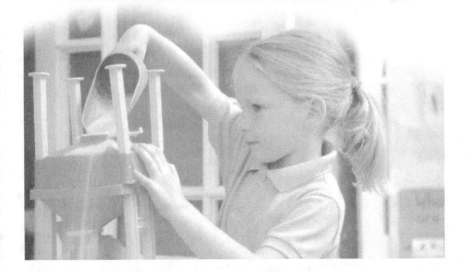

INTRODUCTION

Nearly 75% of children 5 to 13 years of age do not have an adult family member available to supervise them when school is not in session. This factor introduces 2 sets of important questions. First, where do these children go, who is supervising them, and what are they doing? Second, is the nature of children's after-school activities having an effect on their development, and what effect do after-school activities have?

These questions are difficult to answer, and data on these issues are not easy to interpret. The type of child care chosen for school-aged children varies with specific ages of children. These factors also vary with families' socioeconomic and socio-demographic characteristics. Although optimal solutions for school-aged child care are still not defined, there are some interesting trends emerging regarding child care for school-aged children. Pediatricians, along with other health care professionals, have a role in understanding these trends and in helping families find the solutions to best meet their child care needs.

WHERE CHILDREN GO AFTER SCHOOL

Nearly two thirds of school-aged children have 2 employed parents or a single employed parent. The most commonly reported arrangement is care by relatives, accounting for 25% of children. Child care centers and family child care homes served 14% and 7% of school-aged children, respectively. Three percent hired a child care provider to come to the home, and 7% used various other arrangements.[1] No arrangements were provided for 44% of the children in this population. This latter group is termed "children in self-care" or "latch-key children." Multiple child care arrangements are the norm, with 76% of children experiencing at least 2 different arrangements in a typical week.

Children in Self-Care

Self-care is the most common after-school option for children once they reach 11 years of age. It is very common for children as young as 7 or 8 years of age. By 10 years of age, as many as 60% of children are home alone for at least some portion of their after-school hours. About one third of all latch-key children are "supervised" by an older sibling. Most commonly, the sibling is only a couple of years older. Parents are not usually satisfied with self-care arrangements but have limited flexibility in meeting their children's needs in other ways. Other arrangements may not be easily accessible or age-appropriate. Transportation to off-site after-school programs is a major inhibiting factor to use of these programs. Paradoxically, self-care is most common among the highest socioeconomic quartile and least common among the lowest socioeconomic quartile.

Centers

Before- and after-school programs now receive most of the attention as a feasible alternative to less desirable arrangements for school-aged children. Currently, an estimated 50 000 programs providing care before and after school exist to serve 1.7 million children (5–13 years of age). More than one third of these programs are located in child care centers. Public schools with extended school-day programs house 28%, and 14% are in religious institutions. Before- and after-school programs are underused nationally. Average enrollment is estimated to be at 59% of capacity, and only one third of programs operate at 75% or more of their licensed capacity,[2] although some regions report long waiting lists for limited slots in after-school programs. Because after-school programs are typically subsidized by parent fees, they are often least available where they are most needed—low-income, high-crime neighborhoods.

Other Arrangements

Many children are enrolled in various types of after-school programs that are neither center- nor school-based. Some parks and recreation departments offer drop-in supervision. Similar arrangements have been organized by arts centers, cultural centers, ethnic minority centers, Boys and Girls Clubs, and YMCAs/YWCAs. Many children are enrolled in after-school athletic classes or teams. In some communities, public libraries are willing to provide a safe environment for children.

THE EFFECTS OF SUPERVISED CARE AND SELF-CARE

There are no conclusive data on the effects of self-care among school-aged children, and there have been no definitive research studies on the effects of various forms of supervised care. A review of the literature shows decidedly mixed reports.

On the positive side, some studies have shown that in the best of circumstances, children in self-care develop a strong sense of self-esteem and mature early.[3] Self-care was shown for 1 cohort of students to have no measurable negative implications for peer relationships, emotional well-being, report card grades, or standardized scores. Within a suburban middle-class sample, latch-key children functioned better than those in after-school programs for many of these characteristics.[4] Not surprisingly, latch-key children are better informed about handling emergencies than are supervised children.

Many negative effects of self-care also have been reported. Poor self-esteem, fewer opportunities for social development, and feelings of social isolation have been found when compared with children in supervised care.[5] Children in self-care are reported to be more headstrong and hyperactive.[4] Recurring nightmares and increased fear of noises, darkness, and intruders have been found among latch-key children. Some close themselves off in 1 room or will not answer the telephone as a method of coping.

Some of the biggest concerns for self-care are for adolescents and preadolescents. Children have more opportunity to experiment with deviant behaviors when left at home alone. Some studies show that many make use of these opportunities. Smoking, substance abuse, and earlier sexual experiences are more likely to occur in the absence of adult supervision. Delinquent behavior, gang activity, and other activities that make these adolescents feel that they "belong" are thought to be exacerbated by lack of any adult supervision at home or elsewhere when adolescents are not in school. There is greatest cause for concern for children who are younger, those left alone often and for long periods of time, and those living in unsafe neighborhoods. The highest risk time for youth to be perpetrators of violent juvenile crime or to be victims of violent crime is between 3 pm and 6 pm.[6-10] This is also the time when 16- and 17-year-olds are most likely to be involved in a car crash or be killed by a nonmotorized vehicle accident. Supervised care during this high-risk time can help protect these children from physical and emotional harm.

CHARACTERISTICS OF QUALITY IN SCHOOL-AGED CHILD CARE PROGRAMS

It has been shown that parents often enroll their children in the first program they investigate for their school-aged child. Health care professionals need to understand the characteristics of various programs so that they can knowledgeably discuss the options with parents.[11-13] Parents tend to purchase higher- and lower-quality care at similar costs, and convenience often supersedes quality in parent selection of school-aged child care. Barriers to use of after-school care include lack of availability, transportation, hours of operation, and inability to pay fees charged by programs.

Goals of before- and after-school programs vary. The main purpose of most is to provide adult supervision and a safe environment for children. Providing recreational activities and culturally enriching opportunities are common secondary goals. Prevention of risk-taking behaviors (drug or alcohol abuse, smoking, etc) and the provision of remedial help to children having difficulty in school are goals of certain programs.

Activities

Activities vary widely among programs. Socializing and free time are the most common activities provided in all programs. Many sites are equipped with board and card games, puzzles, building blocks, and Legos. Opportunities to read independently in a quiet environment or to do homework are provided in some but not all centers. Child care programs can have a positive impact on academic growth. This may occur because child care settings are less threatening than school for some children or there may be a lower child-adult ratio, making adults more accessible. Parents without good spoken or written English skills have difficulty helping their children with homework and may seek arrangements in which homework can be supervised by an adult who can better answer their child's questions. Videos, television viewing, and computer games are not uncommon. Children in some programs are encouraged to participate in unstructured physically active play, such as running.

Parents should explore the range of activities provided to children in different programs. Arts and crafts, dress-up play, music-making and appreciation, storytelling, field trips, science activities, computer stations, and even tutoring or psychologic guidance are provided in some programs. These activities and services can serve to make the hours in child care very productive. A high degree of structure is excellent for children who become problematic with free play or who simply watch hours of television when there is no direct supervision. Other children need a break from their structured school programs and seem happier directing themselves to various activities. Parents should look for balance in the age-appropriate activities that best suit their child's needs.

Parent involvement and interaction are key elements to a successful program. Some programs have insisted that parents have some presence either in the centers themselves as their children transition from and to parental care or on curriculum and policy advisory boards for the centers or programs.

Parent involvement and interaction are key elements to a successful program.

The location of a child care facility influences the opportunities available for various activities. Proximity and access to a playground, a cafeteria, or a gym offers more opportunity than do programs restricted to a classroom. Use of many community resources, consistent expectations of children, allowance for some spontaneity, and capitalizing on the special talents of staff, parents, and even children themselves are elements that optimize a program.

A Safe Environment

Staffing should be sufficient to properly supervise children. That includes always knowing the whereabouts of each child and how each is spending his or her time. Group sizes are optimal when small enough to allow each child to develop a relationship with a staff person. This is a primary index of quality that parents need to observe. The recommended average child-staff ratio is 8:1 for 5-year-olds and 10:1 to 14:1 for children 6 to 14 years of age.

Restricted indoor space is a common problem. Children need quiet places for naps, resting, and doing homework. Quiet spaces need to be separate from space where activities like dancing, cooperative art projects, drama, dressing up, and building block activity can take place. Because classrooms are commonly used, there are certain restrictions on rearranging space for optimal use. These problems can be alleviated to some extent when comfortable, ambient temperatures and adequate outdoor space are readily available.

Other safety factors are similar to those pertaining to child care for younger children. Playground equipment needs to be sound, free from hazards, and on safe surfaces. Snacks and meals need to be nutritious. Children with special needs (chronic and acute) require written routine and emergency plans that are authorized by their parents and doctors, and the center must have the resources to carry out those plans. Security must be maintained by documents that specify who is allowed to pick up each child and by strict child sign-in and sign-out procedures.

ASSESSING QUALITY

Before beginning work, child care staff require specific training and orientation including youth development, program policies, job responsibilities, behavior management, family interaction, curriculum planning, and first aid/cardiopulmonary resuscitation or First Response training. Background checks should be performed for all staff and volunteers. Involvement of families increases the quality of the program, and several options should be available (eg, family advisory board, volunteering on field trips, publishing newsletters). Positive, respectful relationships should be developed among staff and children. Youth should be able to choose among various quiet and physically active experiences, should be given opportunities for leadership, should help determine the rules that children will abide by at the program, and should develop positive character traits and competencies. Behavior should be guided through the use of positive techniques. Bullying should specifically not be allowed. Adult staff members need to spend their time working with groups or individual children rather than congregating in adult/staff groups.

The program director must provide strong leadership, supporting staff, giving feedback, holding regular meetings to plan activities, and assessing the effectiveness of the programs in meeting the needs of all children being served. In-service training should occur regularly.

The facility should have adequate storage space and adequate, safe indoor and outdoor space and equipment; should be well lit and in good repair; and should maintain a comfortable temperature. Written policies regarding child or staff illness, emergencies, disasters, staff responsibilities, etc should be available.[14]

HEALTH CARE PROFESSIONAL'S ROLE IN SCHOOL-AGED CHILD CARE

Remembering to ask about child care arrangements for the school-aged child is the first and most difficult hurdle for most health care professionals to overcome. Parents are likely to be more thoughtful of the ramifications of their arrangements if they know their health care professional is interested enough to ask about it.

For children in self-care, health care professionals may want to ask some of the questions in Table 23.1. Telephone hot lines or reassurance lines for children are increasingly common ways for children to feel connected with an adult even

TABLE 23.1. Questions to Ask Parents of Children in Self-Care[15]
1. What is the number of hours that the child spends at home alone per day (or per week)?
2. What in-home rules are used when the child is at home alone?
3. Is there an older sibling in the home of the person who cares for the child? What is the older sibling's age? What is the older sibling's sex?
4. How does the parent check on the child's safety when the child is at home alone?
5. What types of special entertainment devices (eg, television, video cassette recorder/player, video games, personal computer) have been purchased to keep the child entertained while at home alone?
6. What types of safety (eg, burglar alarm, cell phone) devices are in place to protect the child while at home alone?
7. What schedule does the child follow when at home alone?
8. What activities is the child allowed to take part in when at home alone?

when they are home alone. Some communities continue to sustain "block parent" programs, in which designated parents plan to be home and available during certain hours of the day so neighborhood children in self-care can reach them in emergencies. It is important to help make parents aware of these programs and ideas and to help prepare children for self-care (Table 23.2).

Children can be interviewed separately about their comfort with staying home alone. There are books, films, and brochures available in libraries that serve to educate children and parents on the latch-key or self-care experience. Children who are developmentally mature enough to follow nonurgent instructions may not be able to do so when there is an emergency. There are times when a child's chronologic age, developmental stage, personality traits, or medical conditions will be cause for a health care professional to advocate against self-care for children. For instance, the impulsive child with attention-deficit/hyperactivity disorder may not be ready for self-care at an age when many other children could successfully negotiate this arrangement. At these times, some of the other options mentioned in this chapter should be recommended as safer alternatives.

Child health care professionals may also assume an advocacy role for school-aged child care. The needs of all income groups need to be considered, as do the needs of a wide range of school-aged populations. Community and state policies that address child care issues for the school-aged child can be influenced by parents and health care professionals.

TABLE 23.2. How to Prepare Children for Self-Care

1. Be sure the individual child is mature enough to be left in self-care for an hour or 2 or for whatever length of time is necessary.

2. Ask about the child's wishes. If the child does not feel ready or is fearful, seek other arrangements.

3. Things to leave by the phone:
   A. Emergency phone numbers:
      1. Parents' work
      2. Neighbor who stays at home
      3. Extended family members or family friends who agree to assist
      4. 911 with a summary of when to call
      5. Hot line for homework
      6. Hot line for support if a child feels lonely or needs someone to talk with
   B. House rules: (expectations about)
      1. No friends over when parents absent
      2. Homework
      3. Chores
      4. Television/video games/computer time
      5. Instructions about whether child may leave the house, with whom, and to where
      6. Cooking
   C. Suggested and allowed activities
   D. Snacks and suggestions for snacks

4. Role play possible scenarios:
   A. How to handle phone calls. What should the child say when he or she answers the phone?
   B. What if someone comes to the door?
   C. What about strange noises or smells?
   D. What to do if the child is lonely, frightened, stuck on a homework problem, feels ill, etc?

5. Which children should not be in self-care?
   A. Those whose parents work late, resulting in the child spending many hours alone each day
   B. Those who live in unsafe neighborhoods
   C. Those who have medical, psychologic, or behavioral conditions that put them at increased risk of an adverse consequence
   D. Those who are not developmentally ready, usually younger than 11 years or younger than 14 or 15 years with a younger sibling. Remember, even though a 12- to 13-year-old may successfully baby-sit for a neighbor's child, sibling care presents different, more complex, and often more emotionally charged situations.

6. Arrange a specific time for "check-in calls," that is, the child calls the parent as soon as he or she gets home after school, or the parent calls home at a predesignated time. These calls serve as reassurance to the child and parent that all is well. Use this time to inquire about the child's day and planned activities, assigned homework, and review of house rules and to serve as a "verbal hug."

CONCLUSIONS AND RECOMMENDATIONS

Pediatricians and other health care professionals have a role in understanding trends in after-school child care and in helping families find the solutions to best meet their child care needs. Parents should be encouraged to choose care arrangements that include a safe environment and age-appropriate activities. If self-care is being considered for the school-aged child, the health care professional can help parents determine whether the child is ready to stay home alone and can help parents prepare for such an arrangement.

REFERENCES

1. Out-of-school time. *Child Care Bulletin*. 1997;17 [serial online]. Available at: http://www.nccic.org/ccb/ccb-so97/outtime.html. Accessed March 19, 2004

2. US Department of Education, Office of Policy and Planning. *National Study of Before and After School Programs, Final Report*. Portsmouth, NH: RMC Research Corporation; 1993

3. Rodman H, Pratto DJ, Nelson RS. Child care arrangements and children's functioning: a comparison of self-care and adult-care children. *Dev Psychol*. 1985;21:413–418

4. Vandell DL, Ramanan J. Children of the National Longitudinal Survey of Youth: choices in after-school care and child development. *Dev Psychol*. 1991;27:637–643

5. Berman BD, Winkleby M, Chesterman E, Boyce TW. After-school child care and self-esteem in school-age children. *Pediatrics*. 1992;89:654–659

6. Fight Crime: Invest in Kids. *America's After-School Choice: The Prime Time for Juvenile Crime, or Youth Enrichment and Achievement*. Washington, DC: Fight Crime: Invest in Kids; 2000

7. Kerrebrock N, Lewit EM. Children in self-care. *Future Child*. 1999;9:151–160

8. Peterson L. Latchkey children's preparation for self-care: overestimated, underrehearsed, and unsafe. *J Clin Child Psychol*. 1989;18:36–43

9. Richardson J, Dwyer K, McGuigan K, et al. Substance use among eighth-grade students who take care of themselves after school. *Pediatrics*. 1989;84:556–566

10. Snyder HN, Sickmund M, Bilchik S. *Juvenile Offenders and Victims. 1999 National Report*. Washington, DC: US Department of Justice and Delinquency Prevention; 1999

11. Ghazvini A, Mullis RL. Center-based care for young children: examining predictors of quality. *J Genet Psychol*. 2002;163:112–125

12. To T, Cadarette SM, Liu Y. Child care arrangement and preschool development. *Can J Public Health*. 2000;91:418–422

13. Phillips D, Adams G. Child care and our youngest children. *Future Child*. 2001;11:34–51

14. National Institute on Out-of-School Time for the Corporation for National Service. *Making an Impact on Out-of-School Time: A Guide for Corporation for National Service Programs Engaged in After School, Summer, and Weekend Activities for Young People*. Washington, DC: Corporation for National Service; 2000

15. Coleman M, Rowland B, Robinson B. Latchkey children and school-age child care: a review of programming needs. *Child Youth Care Q*. 1989;18:39–48

ADDITIONAL RESOURCES

American Academy of Pediatrics, American Public Health Association, and Maternal and Child Health Bureau. *Caring for Our Children. National Health and Safety Performance Standards: Guidelines for Out-of-Home Child Care Programs.* 2nd ed. Elk Grove Village, IL: American Academy of Pediatrics; 2002

Fink DB. *Latchkey Children and School-age Child Care: A Background Briefing. Policy Issues.* Washington, DC: Office of Educational Research and Improvement; 1986

The Urban Institute. *Child Care Patterns of School-Age Children With Employed Mothers.* Washington, DC: The Urban Institute; 2000

The Urban Institute. *What Happens When the School Year Is Over? The Use and Costs of Child Care for School-Age Children During the Summer Months.* Washington, DC: The Urban Institute; 2002

US Census Bureau. *Census Bureau Says 7 Million Grade-School Children Home Alone.* Washington, DC: US Census Bureau; 2001

US Census Bureau. *Who's Minding the Kids? Child Care Arrangements.* Washington, DC: US Census Bureau; 1995

Legal Issues: Serving Children With Disabilities in Child Care and Liability for the Child Care Health Consultant

Alice Bussiere, JD

LEARNING OBJECTIVES

By the end of this chapter, readers should be able to:

- Determine whether a child has a disability as defined by the Americans With Disabilities Act.

- List at least 4 actions that violate a child's rights under this law.

- Identify the factors that determine what accommodations are reasonable.

- Appreciate the importance of understanding liability issues in planning and conducting their work as child care health consultants.

- Understand the importance of adequate insurance coverage.

- Know what questions to ask their attorney and insurance carrier.

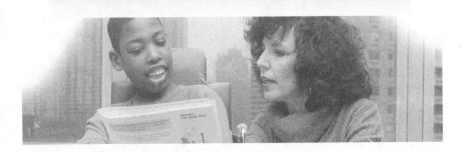

INTRODUCTION

Legal issues associated with child care most commonly involve concerns related to serving children with disabilities or those specific to the child care health consultant. This chapter will cover some of the basic questions relevant to these topics. However, for more detail or for current answers for specific questions, the reader is advised to consult a legal advisor.

Researchers estimate conservatively that 10% of the population of the United States has some form of disability.[1] With advances in medical technologies and changes in the business of medicine, children with disabilities increasingly are cared for not in hospitals or institutions, but rather in the same community environments in which so-called "typically developing" children are raised.

This fact, combined with the implementation of welfare-to-work programs and an economic environment that assumes most families will conform to a working-parent model means that parents of children with disabilities or special health care needs are seeking community-based care with increasing frequency. With 65% of women with children younger than 6 years and 78% of women with children between 6 and 17 years of age in the workforce, all families are struggling to find safe and affordable care for their children. In fact, approximately 13 million preschoolers are enrolled in child care, representing 3 in 5 children.[2] Parents of school-aged children often rely on laws, such as the Individuals With Disabilities Education Act (IDEA)[3]—which gives every child with a disability the right to a free and appropriate public education—to help them provide appropriate care during work hours. Although IDEA does apply to children younger than public school age, few parents are able to take advantage of this entitlement for their younger children. Even those who can do not necessarily obtain the full-day services that all kids—disabled or not—receive at school. However, parents of younger children with disabilities have more difficulty securing services to help them rear, and provide financially for, their family. As a result, these families are turning to child care programs to help fill the gap.

Although some providers are concerned about their ability to care for children with special needs, the Americans With Disabilities Act has encouraged many child care providers to break through their concerns to serve these children. Health care professionals who treat children with disabilities or work with child development programs can ensure that inclusion of these children occurs in a safe environment with well-informed providers and parents.

Malpractice liability is a significant issue for health care professionals, even in the role of child care health consultant. Health care professionals who serve as child care health consultants should be aware of their responsibilities in their role as health consultants and ensure that they have adequate insurance coverage, whether or not they charge for their services. Liability issues vary depending on the professional training and credentials of the health care professional, the type of work the health consultant performs, the relationship between the consultant and the child care provider, and the law in the state in which services are provided. However, there are basic issues relevant to all child care health consultants that should be considered before agreeing to provide services.

SERVING CHILDREN WITH DISABILITIES IN CHILD CARE

An Overview of the Americans With Disabilities Act

The Americans With Disabilities Act (ADA)[4] is a relatively new civil rights law. Passed by Congress and signed by President Bush in 1990, the ADA prohibits discrimination against persons with disabilities in a wide variety of public arenas. The ADA does not give special government benefits or subsidies to persons with disabilities. Rather, like other civil rights laws, the ADA simply requires that employers, local governments, and private businesses treat persons with disabilities in a nondiscriminatory manner. Specifically, the ADA requires that community members evaluate what reasonably can be done to meet the needs of a person with a disability to include that individual in community life.

Whom Does the ADA Protect?

The ADA protects any person who has "a physical or mental impairment that substantially limits one or more major life activities."[4] Major life activities include caring for oneself, performing manual tasks, walking, seeing, hearing, speaking, breathing, and learning. The ADA does not protect individuals with minor limitations in one of these areas; rather, the law covers persons with substantial limitations, such as individuals with long-term, chronic, or severe impairments.

Although it is not possible to list all the specific conditions the ADA covers, some of these impairments include visual, speech, and hearing impairments; cerebral palsy; epilepsy; muscular dystrophy; multiple sclerosis; mental retardation; emotional illness; specific learning disabilities; and human immunodeficiency virus infection (HIV). As mentioned above, the ADA does not protect children with temporary and minor conditions like chickenpox, mild allergies, or a broken finger.

Historically, persons with physical or mental impairments that substantially limit major life activities were not the only victims of societal fear of illness and disabilities. Thus, the ADA also protects individuals who:

- Have a history of this type of impairment (such as a child with cancer now in remission)
- Are "regarded" as having an impairment (such as a child with facial scarring, even though the child actually does not have any limitations in major life activities)
- Are "associated with" any of the persons described above (eg, children seeking admission to a child care program cannot be denied simply because a sibling has tested positive for HIV or because a parent uses a wheelchair); associated persons do not have to be relatives

Who Must Comply With the ADA?

As mentioned above, the ADA prohibits discrimination in many different areas of community life. Most relevant to families of children with disabilities, however, are the ADA provisions applying to public accommodations (called Title III) and to state and local government services (called Title II). Child care programs also must comply with the employment antidiscrimination provisions of the ADA (Title I) in regard to the hiring and treatment of employees, including teachers, assistants, and other staff. This chapter does not, however, deal with the unique requirements of those provisions.

Child care providers

Public accommodations are private businesses or establishments—both for-profit and nonprofit—that serve the community at large. They include privately operated programs, such as family child care homes, child care centers, nursery schools, preschools, or Head Start programs run by nongovernmental agencies. Hence, most child care programs—family child care homes and child care centers, regardless of size—may not discriminate on the basis of disability. As the ADA applies to private businesses, even child care programs that receive no government subsidies or funds must comply with the ADA.

Child care programs operated by religious entities are exempt from the public accommodations provisions of the ADA, which is a federal law. However, state and local antidiscrimination laws may cover these groups; hence, religious organizations that run child care programs should check local laws before refusing to serve a child with a disability.

State and local governments

Child care programs operated by state and local government agencies (school districts, park and recreation departments, etc) also must comply with the ADA. Additionally, if a private child care program rents space from a governmental entity, such as a school district, the private program must comply with the public accommodation provisions of Title III, and the school district will have coexisting obligations under the state and local government provisions of Title II.

A governmental entity also may run afoul of the ADA in the child care context by passing laws or regulations that have the effect of excluding children with special needs from child care. For example, if the state agency in charge of licensing child care providers enforced a rule that licensed child care providers may not serve children with HIV infection, the governmental entity would violate the ADA. Similarly, state agencies may not enact a blanket prohibition against licensed child care providing incidental health services—such as blood glucose monitoring tests or gastric tube feeding—in child care, as the effect of such a rule would be to deny a child with a disability services that are otherwise available to typically developing children.

What Acts Does the ADA Prohibit?

Like other civil rights laws, the ADA generally prohibits discrimination against an individual simply because that person has a disability. Discrimination can occur in a variety of ways, so specific violations of the ADA in the child care context may take the following forms.

Denial of participation

A child care program may not refuse to enroll a child in the program simply because that child has a disability. The only exception to the rule against banning children with disabilities from child care is if a child poses a "direct threat" to other children or staff when participating in child care. The "direct threat" exception is very narrow; only children posing a significant risk to others may be excluded, and that risk assessment must be based on objective medical opinion or other evidence. When evaluating whether a child poses a direct threat, consider the nature of the condition that poses the risk, the probable duration of that condition, the severity of risk, and the probability of actual harm. Furthermore, if the risk can be eliminated or mitigated by modifying policies, practices, or procedures, then the child should be permitted to enroll. Thus, an HIV-infected child will not pose a direct threat in the typical child care setting, because standard precautions make the risk of contracting HIV infection through casual contact negligible.

Limits on participation

Similarly, child care providers may not limit a child's participation in the program simply because of disability. Thus, children with disabilities should not be excluded from field trips, outdoor activities, or other program activities unless they pose a "direct threat," as discussed above, and that threat cannot be eliminated by reasonably modifying the program.

Segregation

Civil rights laws have long rejected the idea that segregated facilities can give people similar opportunities. Because "separate but equal" is illegal, segregating children with disabilities against the wishes of the child or their parents violates the ADA. Integrated services must be offered, although providers can create separate programs that are specifically designed to meet the needs of an individual with a disability, as long as the family can choose to participate in the integrated program instead of the segregated one.

The prohibition on segregation is particularly important to keep in mind when serving children with HIV infection or acquired immunodeficiency syndrome (AIDS). The rights of a child with HIV infection or AIDS to participate fully, equally, and not separately from the other children are very clear under the ADA. As mentioned above, a child's involvement can be limited only if the disability poses a "direct threat" to staff or other children. A child's HIV status alone will not pose such a risk to others through touching and normal play, although a child with AIDS who also has secondary infections could, in certain circumstances, pose a significant risk to others. Consequently, the law requires that a child with HIV infection be allowed to engage in normal activities with other children in the most integrated setting appropriate to the needs of the child.

Discouragement

Sometimes, discrimination takes less obvious forms, such as in the case of discouragement. Discouragement generally does not involve an outright refusal to serve, but rather consists of erecting barriers to service that nondisabled program participants do not face. Examples of discouragement include repeatedly suggesting that a child with a disability use another program or facility, requiring that the family of a child with a disability fill out excessive amounts of paperwork to enroll, or delaying a final decision on enrollment in an effort to get the family to give up efforts to obtain services. The ADA prohibits such discouragement to families of children with disabilities.

Higher charges

Child care providers generally cannot charge the family of a child with a disability more than they charge other families in the program. There are several important qualifiers to this general rule. First, if the child's care is subsidized by the government, the government can subsidize children with disabilities at a higher rate than other children. Furthermore, if the child receives a professional service that is billed separately (such as a physical therapist that comes to the child care facility to conduct physical therapy), the child care program can pass on the bill to the parents. Finally, if a child requires services that would not be reasonable for the program to absorb (see the discussion of "Reasonable Accommodations"), the parent can choose to pay for that extraordinary accommodation.

Unnecessary inquiries about a disability

Child care providers ask all families a variety of questions when enrolling children into the program. For example, state licensing laws sometimes require that providers obtain basic health information on each child in their program (eg, see California Department of Social Services, Community Care Licensing Division, *Evaluator Manual: Children's Day Care* Vol. I, §101220). Requesting such information is permitted under the ADA, but child care providers should not use this information as a device to screen for children with special needs. Moreover, child care providers should not require families of children with disabilities to give more information than is necessary to comply with licensing requirements or to ensure the child's safe participation in the program. If a family identifies the child as having a disability, the only additional information a child care provider should need concerns the special accommodations the child would require. Child care providers generally do not need the particular diagnosis a child has received to provide safe care if they have a list of necessary accommodations.

Often, parents will want to give the child care provider more information than is necessary to ensure safe participation in the program. If the parent is willing to provide this information voluntarily, the child care provider may put the information in the child's file. However, providers should be careful to protect the child's privacy. Children and their parents have privacy rights in their medical and educational records, and in some states child care licensing requirements specifically require that child care providers keep confidential all records concerning children in their care (eg, see California Code Regulations Title 22, §101221 (stating that "all information and records obtained from or regarding children [in child care centers] shall be confidential"). Thus, child care providers should not release any information about a child, including to health care professionals, unless the child's parent has given permission to do so.

Failure to reasonably accommodate

A unique provision of the ADA is the statute's requirement that private businesses (including child care providers) reasonably accommodate a person with a disability to avoid a discrimination claim. In other words, a child care program may have to modify its services to ensure that they are accessible to children with disabilities. As each program has different resources available to it, and as each child with a disability will require different types and intensities of accommodations, evaluating whether or not a particular accommodation for a specific child is reasonable is a highly individualized process and requires creative thinking. Good communication between the parents, treating health care professionals, and the child care program also is important when developing a plan for reasonable accommodations. This new way of thinking is explained below in greater detail.

What Are Reasonable Accommodations?

There are 3 types of accommodations that child care programs may have to make: 1) changes to policies, practices, or procedures; 2) providing special equipment or services to ensure effective communication; and 3) architectural modifications (see 28 CFR §§36.302 [modifications in policies, practices, or procedures], 36.303(c) [auxiliary aids and services to ensure effective communication], and 36.304 [removal of architectural barriers]). Whether or not accommodations are reasonable and, thus, are required under the ADA must be evaluated on a case-by-case basis.

First, programs may need to change their policies, practices, and procedures to accommodate an individual with a disability. Examples of this type of change might include:

- Providing alternative foods at lunch and snack time for children with severe food allergies
- Changing the program schedule for a child who takes medication and must sleep in the morning

- Waiving an immunization policy for a child who has HIV infection or AIDS and who cannot receive standard immunizations given to most children

A particular policy change is not reasonable if it fundamentally alters the nature of the program, as in the case of a child who is so medically fragile that her participation in a preschool program would be limited to watching other children work from a reclined position.

A child care program also may need to provide auxiliary aids and services to help with communication for persons with disabilities affecting hearing, vision, or speech. Examples of auxiliary aids and services include:

- Large-print books
- Sign language interpreting
- TTY phone capacity for communicating with parents who are deaf
- Braille labels on classroom objects for children who are blind

A program is not required to buy auxiliary aids if doing so either would impose an undue financial burden on the program or would fundamentally alter the nature of the program. An undue burden means a significant difficulty or expense. Factors to consider in determining whether a cost poses an undue burden include the cost of the auxiliary aid or service, the financial resources of the program, the number of employees needed, and whether other lower-cost alternatives exist. A child care program also is not required to provide an auxiliary aid for communications if it would fundamentally alter the nature of the program. For example, a program need not supply a sign language interpreter for a child with a hearing impairment during a parent-teacher conference if the program typically does not permit children to participate in these conferences.

Finally, programs must remove architectural barriers that prevent access to services. This type of accommodation might include rearranging furniture, installing ramps, or widening doorways. The ADA requires private child care providers to remove barriers only if removal is readily achievable, which means that it can be done without much difficulty or expense. Child care programs run by state or local governments must comply with the more stringent standard for architectural modifications established by Title II of the ADA. If one type of barrier removal is too difficult or costly, programs must explore other ways of making the services available. For example, if modifying the front door of a family child care home would be too costly but changing a side door would be inexpensive, the provider should make the side door accessible.

Liability for the Child Care Health Consultant

Actions a child care health consultant can take include:

- Educating child care providers about common childhood disabilities and diseases, such as describing the condition, explaining the care involved and complications that might arise, and answering questions

- Ensuring that policies developed by any medical associations or community groups with which he or she is affiliated protect the rights of persons with disabilities to participate in community life

Unfortunately, outlining the liability of a child care health consultant clearly and succinctly is difficult because a variety of factors must be taken into consideration to determine liability in any specific situation.

Professional Training and Credentials

The liability of the health care professional depends in part on professional training and credentials. For example, the law recognizes different duties of care for a medical doctor, a nurse practitioner, and a home health aide. Health care professionals should be aware of the duty of care they are expected to meet in their state and should not provide services outside their professional capacity.

Scope of Practice

State laws set out the appropriate scope of practice for certain professionals in statutes, such as a medical practice act or nurse practice act. Many of these laws also recognize that a health care professional may delegate certain duties to other individuals, such as child care providers. Health care professionals should be familiar with the permissible scope of their responsibilities under state law as well as the circumstances under which they may delegate those responsibilities to others. In general, the health care professional retains responsibility for oversight of these delegated duties or procedures.

Role of the Child Care Health Consultant

Child care health consultants may serve in a variety of roles. For example, the consultant may:

- Inform child care staff about general health care issues, such as infectious diseases common in child care
- Review and comment on child care policies, such as procedures for dealing with emergencies or infectious disease control
- Train child care staff to carry out specific procedures, such as emergency first aid, or to use specific equipment, such as nebulizers
- Analyze illness and injury logs to identify patterns and to recommend improvements in preventing and managing illness and injury
- Advise the child care staff about how to respond to a specific situation concerning a specific child, such as providing on-call advice when a child has a seizure
- Review staff safety issues with the child care program administrator, such as how to respond when a staff member comes into contact with blood
- Provide health care services to children in care, such as health screening exams
- Provide information and referrals, such as how to obtain Medicaid coverage, or how to find a health care specialist

Each of these roles has different implications. Liability of the health consultant will depend on what legal duty he or she has under the circumstances and to whom the duty is owed. Consent and confidentiality requirements also will vary.

It is important for the child care health consultant to clarify the scope of responsibility he or she is undertaking, preferably in a written agreement with the child care provider and any other involved parties. Child care health consultants also should clarify whether they are providing services to the child care provider, the family, or someone else. When the consultant is providing direct services to a child or advice on a particular child's situation, it is essential to obtain appropriate consent as well as to coordinate with the child's treating health care professional and clarify responsibilities with that professional.

Relationship Between the Child Care Health Consultant and Child Care Provider
Child care health consultants may be paid or volunteer. They may be private contractors, employees of the child care provider, or employees of someone else. Each of these arrangements may bring different implications to questions of liability for the health care professional or other parties. The relationship also will have implications for insurance coverage. The malpractice policy of the health care professional may not cover volunteer or consulting work done at another site, and the child care provider may not have coverage for medical malpractice.

The child care health consultant should ensure that there is agreement about what the relationship is, understand the implications of that arrangement under applicable state law, and determine whether insurance coverage will be effective in these circumstances.

Avoiding Liability Problems
Although liability issues vary, a child care health consultant can undertake a few common sense precautions to avoid problems.

Clarify Responsibilities
Come to an agreement about what services you will provide and to whom you will provide each type of service. Put the agreement in writing, and follow the agreement. You may be tempted to go beyond the scope of your agreement when your services are needed, but you should do so very cautiously and only with a complete understanding of the liability implications. For example, if you have agreed to provide general training to child care staff, you should be clear about whether you will accept follow-up calls seeking advice on how to deal with a particular situation or a specific child. If you agree to provide follow-up consultation, you should be sure to obtain appropriate consent and observe confidentiality requirements. You also should be aware that different liability issues arise when you give advice about a specific child.

Communicate Clearly

Be sure that child care providers, parents, and others know your role and any limits on the services you provide. When training or giving advice to child care staff, be sure that staff members understand what you are saying and what limitations exist on the advice you render. Clearly outline what the training qualifies the trainee to do. If your training provides continuing education certificates or other written evidence of completion, be careful about how you characterize the training results. For example, you may want to limit language on a continuing education certificate to a statement that the person completed training or demonstrated competence as of a specific date. More general language might be construed as certifying ongoing competency, thus expanding the potential liability of a trainer.

Provide High-Quality Service

Set a high standard and meet it consistently. Use the most current recommendations from national authorities, such as the American Academy of Pediatrics, the American Public Health Association, and the Centers for Disease Control as well as *Caring for Our Children: National Health and Safety Standards: Guidelines for Out-Of-Home Child Care Programs*. Stay abreast of developments by taking continuing medical education courses and reading relevant child care health and safety publications.

Be sure your working arrangements permit you to do your work in a professional manner. For example, be clear about whether and when you will be on call, and carefully evaluate whether you can respond to emergencies. Do not assume that the usual standard of care is inapplicable because you are volunteering your services. Do not take on more work than you can do adequately, regardless of the need for your help. Only render advice within your area of professional expertise.

Keep Good Records

Keep appropriate records. Keep a written description of all services you provide, including the date, the service provided, and the individual served. When providing direct services to a child or consultation concerning a specific child, keep a health record including the date of the service or consultation, the name of the child, the reason for the consultation, any advice you gave or action you took, and copies of signed consent and waiver of confidentiality forms.

Be Familiar With the Laws That Apply to Child Care

Child care providers must comply with laws that are specific to the industry, such as licensing requirements and staff training requirements, and general laws, such as child abuse reporting statutes, Occupational Safety and Health Administration (OSHA) standards, and the Americans With Disabilities Act (ADA). Some programs may have special requirements. For example, Head Start programs must meet Head Start Program Performance Standards. Some states have laws specific to health consultation, such as those that require regular visits to infant centers by a health care professional. To provide effective services, you need to be aware of these legal requirements and make sure that your advice is consistent with them. You must also be familiar with your own responsibilities under child abuse reporting laws and state requirements for reporting communicable diseases.

Know and Comply With Consent and Confidentiality Requirements

Obtain appropriate consent before providing any direct services to children. For example, in most circumstances you must obtain the parent's consent before providing treatment to a child or giving advice to child care staff concerning a specific child's medical condition. However, parental consent is not required to provide general training to staff or to consult with child care staff on general issues not related to a particular child.

The Health Insurance Portability and Accountability Act of 1996 (HIPAA) includes a privacy rule, which took effect April 14, 2003. Health care professionals must be particularly diligent in preserving confidentiality with respect to any individually identifiable health information, whether oral or recorded in any form or medium. Disclosure of personal health information requires authorization by the individual, parent, or guardian except in special instances, such as suspected abuse or neglect or certain issues relating to public health.[5] As a health consultant in child care, you may be required to follow the confidentiality requirements imposed on the child care provider as well as those imposed on you as a health care professional. Be sure that you understand which requirements apply and that you obtain appropriate releases before sharing information with any other party. For example, you should not discuss a child's situation with child care staff without obtaining permission from the child's parent.

These requirements also may affect the information that a child care provider can share with you. For example, confidentiality considerations require that the child care staff obtain permission from a parent before discussing a child's medical condition or behavioral problems with you.

Make Sure Your Insurance Coverage is Adequate

Determine whether your work as a health consultant is covered by your regular malpractice policy or by the insurance policy of the child care provider or agency with which you are working. Make sure that the policy covers all the work you will be doing at the location you will be providing services. Provide a written description of your responsibilities to your insurance carrier and ask for written confirmation that you will be covered, an explanation of any restrictions, and a description of any additional coverage that is necessary. If someone else maintains the coverage, make sure that continued coverage is part of your written agreement with that party. Ensure that the policy covers legal defense as well as paid claims. Even if you are not found liable, you may need to defend yourself in a lawsuit.

Consult an Attorney and Your Insurance Carrier

If you have an attorney, consult with him or her about the law in your state and how it applies to your situation. If you do not have a regular attorney, you can obtain a referral from your local bar association. Some communities have pro bono projects that provide free legal services to nonprofit organizations and individuals who cannot afford legal services. Check to see whether your services come within their priorities, especially if you are volunteering your services.

Your insurance agent or carrier also may be able to provide you with advice on how to avoid liability problems. Some carriers make free legal advice available to assist their clients in avoiding unnecessary claims.

CONCLUSIONS AND RECOMMENDATIONS

Given that health care professionals play such an important role in the health and welfare of children with disabilities, it should come as no surprise that the involvement of pediatricians is crucial to the successful inclusion of these children in child care programs. Actions a treating health care professional can take to ensure full inclusion include:

- Developing written protocols about how to perform incidental health care procedures, such as gastric tube feedings or nebulizer treatments for children with asthma, for parents and other caregivers of patients
- Training parents and child care providers about how to attend to the special health needs of a patient with a disability
- Being available to answer questions from child care providers about patients if the parents have consented to this exchange of information

Child care health consultants can improve the quality of child care services and impart significant benefits to children, their families, and their child care providers. Consultation also can be a rewarding experience for the health care professional. To minimize the risk of liability problems, the child care health consultant should think through potential liability issues before beginning to provide assistance and take some common sense steps to avoid potential problems.

REFERENCES

1. Gold B. Who will care for our children? A historical perspective of services for young children with disabilities. In: *Project Exceptional: A Guide for Training and Recruiting Child Care Providers to Serve Young Children with Disabilities.* Vols 1, 7, 10. Sacramento, CA: California Department of Education, Child Development Division; 1996
2. Children's Defense Fund. *Child Care Basics.* Available at: http://www.childrensdefense.org/childcare/childcare/basics.asp. Accessed March 19, 2004
3. Individuals With Disabilities Education Act. 20 USC §1400 (1999)
4. Americans With Disabilities Act. Pub L No. 101-336 (1990)
5. Centers for Disease Control and Prevention. HIPAA privacy rule and public health. *MMWR Early Release.* 2003;52:1-12

SUGGESTED READINGS

American Academy of Pediatrics, American Public Health Association, and Maternal and Child Health Bureau. *Caring for Our Children. National Health and Safety Performance Standards: Guidelines for Out-of-Home Child Care Programs.* 2nd ed. Elk Grove Village, IL: American Academy of Pediatrics; 2002

Child Care Law Center. *Caring for Children with Special Needs: The Americans with Disabilities Act and Child Care.* San Francisco, CA: Child Care Law Center; 1995

Project Head Start. *Mainstreaming Preschoolers Series.* Washington, DC: US Government Printing Office. DHHS Publication No. OHDS 783115 (emotional disturbance); OHDS 783114 (orthopedic handicaps); OHDS 7831111 (mental retardation); OHDS 7831111 (health impairments)

California Department of Education. *Project Exceptional: A Guide for Training and Recruiting Child Care Providers to Serve Young Children with Disabilities, Volume 1.* Sacramento, CA: California Department of Education, Child Development Division; 1996

OTHER RESOURCES

Child Care Law Center
973 Market Street, Suite 550
San Francisco, CA 94103
Phone: 415/495-5498
Web site: http://www.childcarelaw.org

Disability Rights Education and Defense Fund Inc (DREDF)
2212 Sixth Street
Berkeley, CA 94710
Phone: 510/644-2555
TTY: 510/644-2626
Web site: http://www.dredf.org

Bazelon Center for Mental Health Law
1101 15th Street NW, Suite 1212
Washington, DC 20005
Phone: 202/467-5730
Web site: http://www.bazelon.org

Pediatricians and Public Health Collaborating to Support the Health and Safety of Children in Child Care

Peter Michael Miller, MD, MPH, and Phyllis Stubbs-Wynn, MD, MPH

LEARNING OBJECTIVES

The learning objectives for this chapter are:

- To define the public health mission and describe the 3 core functions of public health agencies at federal, state, and local levels.
- To identify the 10 essential public health services.
- To identify successful child care health and safety collaborations between the American Academy of Pediatrics (AAP) and the Maternal and Child Health Bureau (MCHB) addressing core functions and essential public health services at the federal level.
- To identify successful AAP-MCHB child care health and safety collaborations between pediatricians and public health at the state level.
- To help pediatricians perform day-to-day activities to improve child care services to their patients and to the community at the local level.

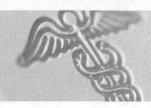

The clinical practice of pediatrics and the national, state, and local public health systems must work cooperatively to achieve maximum benefits for children in both in-home and out-of-home child care settings. Both pediatricians and public health professionals should be familiar with each other's activities and mutual interests and responsibilities.

Information is provided about MCHB activities regarding child care, interaction between the MCHB and the AAP, and ongoing efforts to improve services to pediatricians and child care providers to promote quality care to children and families.

THE PUBLIC HEALTH MISSION AND CORE FUNCTIONS

The public health mission has been defined as fulfilling society's interest in ensuring conditions in which people can be healthy.[1] As such, public health systems focus on the health of populations as opposed to the personal health care system, which focuses on the health of individuals. Although the public health system generally operates on 3 governmental levels (federal, state, and local public health agencies), all levels have assessment, policy development, and assurance as their core functions.

- Assessment involves the collection and analysis of data on the health status of the nation, state, or local community and the dissemination of that information.
- Policy development requires the active involvement of public health agencies in providing leadership to the development of public health policies based on the use of scientific, evidence-based knowledge.
- Assurance involves actions public health agencies take to provide the services necessary to achieve agreed upon goals. Assurance is accomplished by encouraging action by other entities (private or public sector), requiring such action through regulation, or providing services directly.[1]

In an effort to operationalize the core public health functions, the following 10 essential public health services were identified by the Essential Public Health Services Work Group[2]:

1. Monitor health status to identify community health problems.
2. Diagnose and investigate health problems and health hazards in the community.
3. Inform, educate, and empower people about health issues.
4. Mobilize community partnerships to identify and solve health problems.
5. Develop policies and plans that support individual and community health efforts.
6. Enforce laws and regulations that protect health and ensure safety.
7. Link people to needed personal health services and ensure the provision of health care when otherwise unavailable.
8. Ensure a competent public health and personal health care workforce.
9. Evaluate effectiveness, accessibility, and quality of personal and population-based health services.
10. Research for new insights and innovative solutions to health problems.

AAP AND MCHB COLLABORATIONS AT THE FEDERAL LEVEL FOR CHILD CARE HEALTH AND SAFETY

Achieving optimal health for children in child care settings requires a working partnership among child care providers, public health professionals, and pediatricians and other primary care clinicians serving children. The active involvement of the AAP with public health agencies such as the MCHB (part of the Health Resources and Services Administration) has paved the way for pediatricians to make much needed and valuable contributions to public-private partnerships promoting the health and safety of children in child care settings. The MCHB has a long-standing history of working with the AAP to support the health and safety of infants and young children in child care settings. This ongoing collaboration has supported MCHB child care health and safety core public health functions in the areas of public policy and assurance and supported the ability of the MCHB to deliver essential public health services.

Ensuring Quality in Child Care Settings

The work of the MCHB in the area of ensuring quality in child care settings was based on appreciation of the bureau's role as a federal agency to encourage the development of new knowledge. The MCHB, while recognizing the fact that standard setting was the role of state governments, was also aware through its state Title V needs assessment process and other indicators that an unmet need in many states was the development of the knowledge base from which health and safety standards could be developed for child care settings. In a 1990 report, the National Research Council called for "uniform national child care standards based on current knowledge from child development research and best practice from the fields of public health, child care, and early childhood education—as a necessary...condition for achieving quality in out-of-home child care. Such standards should be established as a guide to be adopted by all states as a basis for improving the regulation and licensing of child care and preschool education programs."[3]

The AAP has played a strong leadership role in working to develop guidelines for national child care health and safety standards. In 1987 and again in 2002, the AAP partnered with the American Public Health Association (APHA) and the MCHB in the development of guidelines for out-of-home child care programs titled *Caring for Our Children: National Health and Safety Performance Standards: Guidelines for Out-of-Home Child Care Programs.*[4] This publication made available new knowledge that states could use as guidance in their development of state standards and licensing regulations they determined to be most needed to promote and protect the health and safety of infants and young children in child care settings. The publication *Stepping Stones to Using Caring for Our Children: National Health and Safety Performance Standards: Guidelines for Out of Home Child Care Programs—Protecting Children from Harm*[5] was developed by a public-private partnership between the MCHB, AAP, APHA, and National Resource Center for Health and

Safety in Child Care Settings. The book was derived from the 981 standards contained in the first edition of *Caring for Our Children*. The focus of *Stepping Stones* is to identify those standards most needed for the prevention of injury, morbidity, and mortality in child care settings. *Stepping Stones* contains 180 standards and can be used by state licensing and regulatory agencies as well as child care, health resource and referral agencies, and a variety of other public and private organizations and parent and advocacy groups to promote and protect the health of young children in child care programs. AAP members played a leadership role in the development of both publications by serving as cochairpersons on the steering committees and providing invaluable review and feedback on early childhood. *Caring for Our Children* is today recognized as the leading authoritative tool for health and safety guidelines for child care and serves as the guidelines for child care providers, parents of children in child care, health professionals serving child care, and state officials responsible for monitoring health and safety in child care.[4]

Policy Development

Healthy Child Care America Campaign

In May 1995, secretary of the US Department of Health and Human Services, Donna Shalala, launched the Healthy Child Care America (HCCA) Campaign at the National Child Care Health Forum in Washington, DC. The HCCA Campaign is a federal program integration initiative to foster collaboration between health and child care systems. The campaign is the result of a partnership between 2 agencies of the US Department of Health and Human Services—the MCHB and the Child Care Bureau (CCB), which work to create and maximize linkages between health care professionals and the child care community.

The HCCA Campaign is based on the principle that families, child care providers, and health care professionals in partnership can promote the healthy development of young children in child care and increase access to preventive health services and safe physical environments for children. The MCHB and CCB believe that linking health care professionals, child care providers, and families maximizes resources for developing comprehensive and coordinated services and improves the quality of child care programs. The federal partnership between the MCHB and CCB was expanded to include more than 180 health and child care agencies, organizations, advocates, and parents at the National Child Care Health Forum, at which participants were asked to assist the Department of Health and Human Services in developing the HCCA Campaign's Blueprint for Action. The Blueprint for Action provides communities with steps they can take to expand existing public and private services and resources or to create new services and resources that link families, health care professionals, and child care providers. The HCCA Blueprint for Action can be found on the AAP Healthy Child Care America Web site (http://www.healthychildcare.org).

The AAP, with grant support from the CCB and MCHB, became the HCCA Campaign coordinator in October 1996. A valuable tool developed by the AAP early in the HCCA Campaign was a series of newsletters developed to help caregivers and health professionals share resources and strategies on ways to implement the concepts identified in the Blueprint for Action. There are 12 newsletters with articles about the physician's role in child care, nurses as health consultants, early brain development, medication administration, language development, infectious diseases, and other topics relevant to child development, health, and safety in child care. The newsletters may be accessed online (http://www.healthychildcare.org). Additional activities coordinated by the AAP include the development of national tribal child care health and safety standards, a national child passenger safety training program for child care providers (supported by the National Highway Traffic Safety Administration), funding to implement 30 regional child care initiatives, a national network of health and safety experts, and a comprehensive Web site that includes a state-by-state map of HCCA Campaign contacts, versions of the Healthy Child Care America newsletters available for downloading, and PowerPoint presentations. The AAP has established an important education group to encourage and support greater pediatrician involvement in child care issues, the Special Interest Group in Early Education and Child Care (SIGEECC). Pediatricians may join this group through membership in the AAP Section on Community Pediatrics and have access to information and resources to help their patients in early education and child care settings. The SIGEECC also provides tools to increase access to quality care in communities and states and across the nation. Future SIGEECC activities will include the HCCA Campaign speakers' bureau, a mentorship program that supports partnerships with pediatricians, and training meetings for pediatricians to become more involved in issues related to child care.

The HCCA Back to Sleep Campaign

The HCCA Back to Sleep Campaign is designed to build on the success of the HCCA Campaign and Back to Sleep campaigns by uniting child care, health, and sudden infant death syndrome (SIDS) prevention partners across the country to reduce the number of SIDS-related deaths in child care settings. Through this campaign, a variety of coalition partners offer technical assistance and resources to promote the Back to Sleep message in child care programs, raise awareness, and change practices in child care programs. The campaign also seeks to support inclusion of safe sleep practices within state child care regulations. The HCCA Back to Sleep Campaign was developed in 2002 by the MCHB and 13 partners from the public and private sectors. The campaign was officially launched in January 2003 at a congressional briefing sponsored by First Candle, the CJ Foundation, and the AAP. Before the 1992 recommendation by the AAP to place infants on their backs to sleep to reduce the risk of SIDS, more than 5000 babies in the United States died from SIDS every year. Since the introduction of the Back to Sleep Campaign, the rate of stomach sleeping has declined and the number of deaths of babies in the United States from SIDS has been reduced to fewer than 3000 each year.[6]

There have been reductions in the incidence of SIDS in all sectors of the population with notable exceptions for black and American Indian/Alaska Native populations and infants in child care settings. In the year 2000, it was reported that approximately 20% of SIDS cases occurred in child care settings.[7] The goal of the HCCA Back to Sleep Campaign is to reduce the risk of SIDS in child care settings. Campaign objectives are to educate child care providers, parents, and policy makers about practices to reduce the risk of SIDS and increase the number of states that include back-to-sleep positions in their child care licensing regulations.

With support from the CCB and MCHB, the AAP has taken the lead in the development and implementation of a training and technical assistance program to educate child care providers on Back to Sleep and other SIDS risk reduction practices for child care settings. The AAP has developed a speaker's kit on SIDS for pediatricians to use with parents in their child care consultation and has developed and disseminated the publication "Reducing the Risk of SIDS in Child Care: Caring for Our Children Supplement." Other AAP activities in support of this campaign have included participating in national conference calls focusing on "train the trainer" efforts to prevent SIDS in child care, educating policy makers on safe sleep practices, and including SIDS practice implementation in child care program evaluations.

AAP AND MCHB COLLABORATIONS AT THE STATE LEVEL FOR CHILD CARE HEALTH AND SAFETY

The HCCA Campaign proved to be a successful initiative in reaching communities with its message and supporting their efforts with resources from the Campaign's Blueprint for Action. Encouraged by this development, the MCHB launched the Health Systems Development in Child Care and the Healthy Child Care America 2000 programs. Both programs were grants to state MCHB and CCB agencies supporting their efforts to use the child care environment as a focal point for state planning around integration of health and child care service systems. The HCCA program has 3 objectives:

1. To strengthen the quality of child care through the dissemination, adoption, and use of *Caring for Our Children* standards and *Stepping Stones.*
2. To strengthen the child care health consultant infrastructure through the identification, training, and deployment of health and child care professionals as health consultants to child care programs.
3. To strengthen linkages between health care professionals and child care providers and the use of child care settings as access points to health insurance and medical homes.

The National Resource Center for Health and Safety in Child Care Settings (http://nrc.uchsc.edu/), based at the University of Colorado Health Sciences Center, serves as the national resource supporting the first objective. The National

Training Institute for Child Care Health Consultants (http://www.sph.unc.edu/ courses/childcare/) at the University of North Carolina School of Public Health serves as the resource for the second objective, and the AAP supports the third objective. The Committee on Early Childhood, Adoption, and Dependent Care of the AAP has produced a manual titled *The Pediatrician's Role in Promoting Health and Safety in Child Care*[8] to assist pediatricians to be better direct advisors to parents, to connect more effectively with child care programs, and to advocate to improve child care services in their states and local communities.

AAP chapters played a leadership role in Pennsylvania, New Jersey, and Arizona by becoming the State Healthy Child Care America grantee or by working in collaboration with the state grantee for HCCA 2000.

The Pennsylvania Chapter of the AAP expanded the focus of their ECELS program to create the ECELS-Healthy Child Care Pennsylvania program.[9] The goal of Healthy Child Care Pennsylvania is to implement the HCCA Blueprint for Action in Pennsylvania. The specific objectives carried out by the Pennsylvania Chapter of the AAP for HCCA include training and linking health consultants with child care programs; ensuring that children have up-to-date preventive health services; and improving support for care of children with special health care needs. The Pennsylvania Chapter of the AAP is also working to support the state's quality improvement initiatives by infusing the content of *Caring for Our Children* into the state's quality improvement activities.

The primary goal of the New Jersey HCCA project is to expand the development and implementation of a coordinated, collaborative, community-based, statewide system of child care health consultation to enhance the quality, accessibility, and availability of healthy, safe, developmentally appropriate, culturally sensitive child care services for all New Jersey children in various child care settings. The New Jersey Chapter of the AAP has worked to recruit and train child care health consultants to work in collaboration with the county child care health consultants and to develop a quality improvement program to evaluate their effectiveness. They have also completed an enhanced needs assessment of the child care community, including child care providers, children/families, and consultants, and assessed the pediatric primary care provider's involvement in child care consultation and their interest in increasing that involvement. They have worked to educate pediatricians and increase their awareness of child care issues as well as increase the number of child care providers that voluntarily request child care health consultation services.[10]

The Arizona Chapter of the AAP was asked to lead Arizona in the planning and implementation of the state's HCCA program. The goals of the Arizona HCCA program are to ensure the safety of children in child care; create infrastructure that provides consultation, coordination, and education for providers; and engage in outreach activities for insurance coverage and medical services.[11]

State Early Childhood Comprehensive Systems Initiative

In 2003, the MCHB launched the State Maternal and Child Health Early Childhood Comprehensive Systems (SECCS) grants to support states in planning, developing, and ultimately implementing collaborations and partnerships to support families and communities in their development of children who are healthy and ready to learn at school entry. State plans anticipate the implementation of systems that would include but not be limited to access to medical homes, mental health and social-emotional development, early care and education/child care, parent education, and family support. The MCHB is currently supporting 51 states/territories in their development of SECCS. AAP-supported pediatrician participation in HCCA and the National Center of Medical Home Initiatives for Children with Special Needs (http://www.medicalhomeinfo.org/) are 2 examples of how pediatricians are already working on early childhood initiatives that share the same goals as the SECCS initiative. Continued partnerships between pediatricians and their state MCHB programs can significantly advance the work of early childhood comprehensive systems building.

WHAT THIS MEANS FOR PRACTICING PEDIATRICIANS

Child Care Health and Safety Collaborations Between Pediatricians and Public Health at the Local Level

1. Care for your patient, but also think about group implications. A child may have an infection, but if he or she attends any type of child care, there can be risk of spread to other children, or the child's illness may be indicative of infection in other children in the child care program. A child in care may be well, but if a parent is ill with hepatitis, it may be indicative of subclinical infection within the program. A pediatrician can make a big difference in the containment of contagious diseases within the child care setting.
   - With parental consent, make contact as appropriate with child care providers when treating a child with an infectious disease.
   - Know how to contact public health nurses and child care health consultants to assist in managing infections in child care settings.
2. Utilize national, state, and county child care health and safety policies to improve infectious disease, playground safety, food management, etc.
   - Know the key county child health (eg, MCHB director) person(s) in the community to discuss public health implications for child care infections.
   - Be familiar with state and local groups setting infectious disease policies; participate in development of local policies. Many counties have developed infectious disease management manuals and protocols for infectious diseases. Nationwide guidelines will soon be published by the AAP and Centers for Disease Control and Prevention. The AAP has a manual, *Managing Infectious*

Diseases in Child Care and Schools: A Quick Reference Guide,[12] that is especially helpful.

- Be familiar with *Caring for Our Children, Stepping Stones,* Head Start, and national Tribal standards to ensure your patients are in safe and healthy child care settings. The Head Start performance standards can be found online (http://www.acf.dhhs.gov/programs/hsb/performance). The CCB Minimum Tribal Child Care Standards also can be found online (http://www.nccic.org/tribal/min-std.html).
- Be aware of local requirements for child abuse reporting and know local law enforcement and social services contacts.
- Be familiar with and apply AAP recommendations for specific issues, such as Back to Sleep policies in child care, safe transportation requirements, services for children with special needs, etc. Most of these are available online (http://www.healthychildcare.org).
- Consider sending an office health person to the National Training Institute for Child Care Health Consultants in North Carolina.
- Be aware of your state HCCA program and contacts to assist in local and statewide child care policy improvements. For example, states have been able to change laws to facilitate the delivery of medications to children in child care (eg, children with asthma, diabetes, allergies, etc). HCCA program grantees and AAP chapter child care contacts are listed online (www.healthychildcare.org).

3. Think about child development issues for children in child care as well as health and safety concerns.
   - Be familiar with literature regarding the importance of early social and emotional developmental support for young children (eg, *From Neurons to Neighborhoods: The Science of Early Childhood Development*[13]). Appropriate child care program staffing, training, and program activities are crucial in helping children prepare for interaction with their peers and with adults, adapt to their environments, and be ready for school.
   - Be familiar with national guidelines for early childhood developmental education, such as those from Head Start, the National Association for the Education of Young Children (NAEYC), the Child Welfare League of America, and Zero to Three, and in *Caring for Our Children.*
   - Consult with child care providers regarding behavioral issues that may affect patients and other children in the program (toileting, biting, temper tantrums, etc).
   - Be willing to work with the local MCHB director and other pediatricians to create uniform management policies for children within a child care program and across programs to facilitate consistency of management. Nearly every AAP chapter has a child care contact, and the list is available online (www.healthychildcare.org).

4. Advocate.

- Support local child care programs in your area. Work with local resource and referral agencies to improve guidelines and monitoring of child care programs.
- Support county programs, including interactions with county boards of supervisors, to increase and direct federal, state, and county funding to child care services.
- Join the AAP SIGEECC to receive guidance and assistance as you work within your state and also to offer advice and support for local and national child care activities. To join the SIGEECC, contact the AAP about becoming a member of the Section on Community Pediatrics.

REFERENCES

1. Institute of Medicine, Committee for the Study of the Future of Public Health. *The Future of Public Health.* Washington, DC: National Academy Press; 1988

2. Essential Public Health Services Work Group of the Core Public Health Functions Steering Committee. Essential public health services. Washington, DC: Public Health Foundation; 1994. Available at: http://www.phf.org/essential.htm. Accessed June 2, 2004

3. Hayes CD, Palmer JL, Zaslow MJ, eds. *Who Cares for America's Children? Child Care Policy for the 1990s.* Washington, DC: National Academy Press; 1990

4. American Academy of Pediatrics, American Public Health Association, and Maternal and Child Health Bureau. *Caring for Our Children. National Health and Safety Performance Standards: Guidelines for Out-of-Home Child Care Programs.* 2nd ed. Elk Grove Village, IL: American Academy of Pediatrics; 2002

5. American Academy of Pediatrics, American Public Health Association, and Maternal and Child Health Bureau. *Stepping Stones to Using Caring for Our Children.* Elk Grove Village, IL: American Academy of Pediatrics; 2004

6. Moon RY, Patel KM, Shaefer SJ Sudden infant death syndrome in child care settings. *Pediatrics.* 2000;106:295–300

7. Moon RY, Biliter WM. Infant sleep position policies in licensing child care centers after Back to Sleep Campaign. *Pediatrics.* 2000;106:576–580

8. American Academy of Pediatrics, Committee on Early Childhood, Adoption, and Dependent Care. *The Pediatrician's Role in Promoting Health and Safety in Child Care.* Elk Grove Village, IL: American Academy of Pediatrics; 2001

9. Pennsylvania Chapter of the American Academy of Pediatrics. Healthy Child Care America/ECELS Project Report. Rosemont, PA: Pennsylvania Chapter of the American Academy of Pediatrics; 2001

10. New Jersey Chapter of the American Academy of Pediatrics. Healthy Child Care America Project Report. Trenton, NJ: New Jersey Chapter of the American Academy of Pediatrics; 2001

11. Arizona Chapter of the American Academy of Pediatrics. Healthy Child Care America Project Report. Phoenix, AZ: Arizona Chapter of the American Academy of Pediatrics; 2001

12. Cotler J, ed. *Managing Infectious Diseases in Child Care and Schools: A Quick Reference Guide.* Elk Grove Village, IL: American Academy of Pediatrics; 2004

13. Shonkoff JP, Phillips DA, eds. *From Neurons to Neighborhoods: The Science of Early Childhood Development.* Washington, DC: National Academy Press; 2000

ADDITIONAL RESOURCES

Child Welfare League of America
440 First Street NW, Third Floor
Washington, DC 20001-2085
Phone: 202/638-2952
Fax: 202/638-4004
Web site: http://www.cwla.org

Head Start Bureau
Web site: http://www2.acf.dhhs.gov/programs/hsb/
National Association for the Education of Young Children (NAEYC)
1509 16th Street NW
Washington, DC 20036
Phone: 800/424-2460
Web site: http://www.naeyc.org

Zero to Three
National Center for Infants, Toddlers, and Families
2000 M Street NW, Suite 200
Washington, DC 20036
Phone: 202/638-1144
Web site: http://www.zerotothree.org

CHAPTER 26

Adoption and Foster Care

Mark D. Simms, MD, MPH, and Jerri Ann Jenista, MD

LEARNING OBJECTIVES

The goal of this chapter is to help the reader to:

- Understand that adopted children or children in foster care may present special, unique, and sometimes challenging issues for the child care provider. Although some of these issues are unique to the adopted or foster child, most are common to both groups of children. In fact, some children in foster care will already be in the process of adoption.

- Recognize that the child care setting can provide a source of social support for the adoptive or foster family and assist with parenting skills, particularly around issues of behavior, development, and socialization. It can also provide a safe, nonthreatening location for supervised visits by the birth parents.

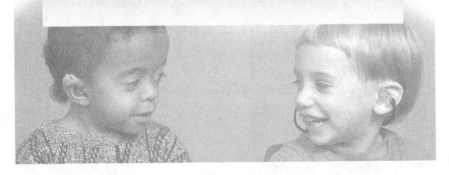

FOSTER CARE

In most respects, foster care is a form of child care, although children in foster care often have very special needs. The number of children in the foster care system in the United States is increasing, particularly the proportion of preschool-aged children. In September 2001, the last year for which accurate statistics are available, approximately 542 000 children lived in licensed foster homes. As a result of the difficult circumstances that led to their placement, most children entering the foster care system have chronic and complex physical, developmental, and emotional problems. Regrettably, the degree of preparation and training of foster parents to care for children with these types of problems has not kept pace. As a result, foster parents and social workers have a great need for assistance in understanding and managing these children. In addition, since the 1980s, the number of foster mothers who are employed full- or part-time outside the home has increased to nearly two-thirds, making the availability of high-quality child care an important component of foster care. Fortunately, many children in foster care attend organized child care, early intervention, or early childhood education programs, and many more might benefit from these experiences.

This chapter presents a brief description of the foster care system, describes the common health and mental health problems of these children, and discusses ways in which health care professionals and child care providers can assist social workers, foster parents, and birth parents to care for these special children.

THE FOSTER CARE SYSTEM

Preservation and support of families has been the cornerstone of child welfare policy in the United States throughout the 20th century. The Promoting Safe and Stable Families Amendments of 2001 (Pub L No. 107-133) was the last major federal legislation to guide current practices. This bill was initiated because of the continued need to protect children and strengthen families. The goal is to encourage and enable states to develop or expand programs of family preservation services, community-based family support services, adoption promotion and support services, and time-limited family reunification services. In recent years, as part of an effort to keep children within their family, ethnic, and cultural surroundings and in response to the decreasing availability of other foster homes, social service agencies have made a strong effort to recruit extended family members to provide "kinship" foster care. Once a child has been placed in foster care, the social worker's energy should be directed toward returning the child to his or her family's care as soon as possible. It is only after these efforts have failed that the parents' legal rights are terminated and the child may become eligible for adoption.

Although they are dedicated to ensuring the safety and well-being of vulnerable children, public child welfare systems are often poorly structured to carry out these goals. Once children have been removed from their parents' care through a court order, it is often unclear who has the legal authority to provide specific aspects of the children's care. Social workers change frequently, sometimes as a planned part of the system. For example, a child may enter foster care through the efforts of a protective services worker who may then transfer the case to an "intake" worker. The child may next be assigned to a caseworker, followed by a permanency planning worker, and finally to an adoption worker. The child may also live in multiple settings. For example, the first placement may be in an emergency shelter setting, followed by a "receiving home," and then a foster home. Approximately 25% of children live in 3 or more foster homes during their tenure in out-of-home placement, because foster parents cannot manage the child's problems or needs or because they become ill, move, or otherwise close their home to the agency. Clearly, this can be a very disruptive and confusing experience for young children who may have great difficulty adapting and coping with changes.

FOSTER PARENTS

Foster parents are licensed by a private or public social service agency, receive monthly stipends to cover the basic costs of raising the children in their care, and have responsibility for day-to-day care of the children in their home. They do not have legal custody, and they do not have legal standing in making decisions about the child's placement or treatment. There are 2 broad categories of foster parents: nonrelative ("traditional") and relative ("kinship"). Nonrelative foster parents often become involved in fostering because of an interest in helping needy children, a personal or family experience with foster care (eg, a relative or friend is or was a foster parent or the individual may have been in foster care during childhood), or because of a desire to adopt—so-called "fost-adopt" or "high-risk" or "legal-risk" adoption placements. On the other hand, relative foster parents step forward to care for their extended family member's children or are recruited by social workers. They, too, are supervised by agency social workers and receive a stipend to care for the children in their care.

HEALTH PROBLEMS

Children entering foster care placements have many of the same types of health problems as do other children from similar socioeconomic backgrounds; however, the number and severity of illnesses is greater. Health problems that often require immediate attention at the time of initial placement in foster care include acute infections (eg, otitis, respiratory infections, or on rare occasions, sexually transmitted diseases) and communicable diseases (eg, scabies or head lice, tinea, impetigo), skin lesions related to trauma or abuse (eg, burns, cuts, scars) or poor hygiene, anemia, lead poisoning, poor nutrition, dental problems, and inadequate immunizations. As many as one third of children in foster care continue to have chronic physical and developmental disorders and require care from medical specialists or rehabilitation therapists (see Table 26.1).

> ### TABLE 26.1. Common Health Problems of Children in Foster Care
>
> - Asthma and chronic respiratory diseases
> - Dermatologic diseases
> - Musculoskeletal problems
> - Dental diseases
> - Neurologic disorders: cerebral palsy, post-traumatic brain injury, and epilepsy
> - Genitourinary: enuresis
> - Gastrointestinal: encopresis
> - Birth anomalies and birth defect syndromes
> - Human immunodeficiency virus infection
> - Technology dependence
> - Poor physical growth: height and weight
> - Developmental delays

Although the American Academy of Pediatrics and the Child Welfare League of America have developed specific guidelines for the health care of children in foster care, health, dental, and mental health services for this population of children vary widely among states. A recent report from the US General Accounting Office revealed that many children in foster care do not receive even basic health services while in placement. In many parts of the country, pediatricians may have to take the initiative to develop and coordinate health and educational services for this population by working directly with public and private social service agencies.

COMMON BEHAVIORAL PROBLEMS

Placement in foster care offers children a new supportive family setting and the opportunity to receive nurturing and love, to develop positive relationships with caring adults, and to be exposed to the world in a developmentally appropriate fashion. In most instances, these goals are accomplished and the children show dramatic improvement in their overall well-being. Unfortunately, some children who experienced abuse or neglect before placement develop maladaptive behaviors and coping strategies that can be very challenging and difficult for their foster parents to manage. The health care professional may be able to assist the foster parents, social workers, and child care providers to help these children by interpreting their behaviors and offering suggestions for appropriate management. Table 26.2 lists some of the common behavioral problems observed in this population and relates them to particular aspects of the child's experiences in foster care.

TABLE 26.2. Common Behavioral Problems of Children in Foster Care

Problems Originating Before Placement

- Aggressive or hyperactive behavior
- Excessive fear, withdrawal, or passivity
- Extreme negativity or self-abusive behavior
- Polyphagia (excessive eating) or polydipsia (excessive drinking)
- Hiding or hoarding food
- Sleep disturbances (chronic night waking or wandering)
- Attachment disorders
- Sexualized behaviors (precocious or solicitous)
- Poor peer interactions or play behaviors
- Aggressive behaviors/foul language
- Fire setting
- Poor hygiene

Stress of Separation From Birth Parents and Adjustment to the Foster Home

- Excessive crying
- Inconsolability (rejection of foster parents' or social worker's efforts to comfort)
- Feelings of loneliness, abandonment, guilt, or longing for parents, siblings, or other family members
- Regression in development (bedwetting or soiling)
- Anorexia (refusal to eat)
- Denial of concerns (overly friendly, nonchalant behavior)

Ongoing Stresses of Foster Care Placement

- Behavior problems that are related to visits with:
  ~ The birth parent(s)
  ~ Siblings living in different foster homes or with the birth parent(s)
  ~ Child's social worker
- Behavior problems related to other foster children entering or leaving the foster home
- Inability of the child to "settle in" to the foster home (accept "rules" or "authority" of the foster parents)
- Lack of improvement in maladaptive behavior

Nearly all children experience behavioral and adjustment problems during foster care. To a large extent, a child's initial reaction to placement will be affected by the circumstances under which he or she was removed from the previous home. For example, a "planned" move to a foster home after a trial of family preservation services may be perceived by the child as less disruptive and traumatic than placement resulting from a middle-of-the-night drug raid. The child's reaction will also depend on his or her previous relationships with adults (eg, the mother or other primary caregivers), experiences of being left in the care of others (eg, friends of the family or relatives), age, overall level of development, and whether he or she is placed together with siblings. Shortly after placement in their new home, many children feel a mixture of fear, loneliness, guilt, abandonment, and anger. They may cry for their parents and reject the advances of social workers or foster parents to comfort them. Such initial adjustment reactions often subside by the second or third month. Alternatively, some children may be overwhelmed or in a state of emotional "shock" and denial, acting as if nothing unusual has happened to them. They may be friendly, outgoing, and agreeable to their new caregivers. After a period of several days or weeks of placement, an initially placid or cooperative child may pass through this "honeymoon" phase and begin to show some signs of behavioral difficulty.

Children who are placed in foster care may not have had many of the "normal" experiences of other children their age. Thus, they may not be familiar with popular television characters, nursery rhymes, or games, such as playing "house" or "store." They may be very passive and may not know how to make choices about food or activities or even how to make their immediate needs known, such as hunger or toileting. Conversely, some children are very aggressive about "getting their share," because this may have been a useful survival strategy in the past. Foster parents should be counseled that these behaviors, although clearly distressing, disruptive, and different, are more likely attributable to the child's past stresses than to problems within the current placement. It is important to keep in mind that most young children have a very limited understanding of their circumstances. These children usually perceive the separation from their parents or former caregivers as a punishment for being bad and blame themselves for their predicament. When disciplined, these children may feel that they are being scolded because of their foster status. In most cases, children respond well to a consistent, nurturing, positive approach to discipline that teaches new sets of expectations and more appropriate social behavior.

Foster parents may benefit from knowing that the child's adjustment problems are common and that these behaviors serve a useful purpose by calling attention to the child who is feeling distressed and insecure. However, if the behavior problems do not seem to resolve in 2 or 3 months with reassurance and common behavioral management approaches or if the problems appear to become worse over the first few months, the foster parents may need more specific assistance and the child should be referred to a child psychologist, psychiatrist, or developmental/behavioral pediatrician for further evaluation and treatment.

THE ROLE OF CHILD CARE PROGRAMS FOR CHILDREN IN FOSTER CARE

High-quality child care programs can be very helpful to children entering foster home settings and their foster parents. The goal of these programs should always be to complement the efforts of the new caregivers and to support the children's positive adjustment to their new home.

Child care programs can provide a structured schedule and predictable environment for children. The staff can observe and evaluate the child's overall development, social interactions, and emotional reactions and work with foster parents to develop strategies that promote the child's healthy development and adjustment.

Frequently, foster parents have to cope with many conflicting demands, without adequate or appropriate support or resources from the child welfare agency or community. More often than not, they are given little information about the child and are expected to provide for his or her special needs. It is important for child care providers to assess the foster parents' need for assistance in caring for children in their home. These needs may become apparent once the child enters a child care program. For example, if child's attendance is poor or irregular, the staff should determine whether the foster parents need assistance with transportation or if there are other children in the home with extraordinary needs. Alternatively, the child may be ill frequently or may have multiple chronic medical and behavioral problems, and the foster parents may need help gaining access to appropriate health care services or referrals for rehabilitation or mental health treatment.

PARENTAL VISITS

Although active involvement of birth parents with their children during placement, through visits or phone calls, is an excellent predictor of the child's eventual return home, these visits are frequently associated with behavior problems and other signs of emotional distress. Some children are simply afraid of seeing parents who may have abused or neglected them, and others may be angry with a parent who they feel abandoned them. Many children feel a conflict of loyalty between their birth mother and their foster mother, both of whom they love and depend on. This sense of conflict and the resulting behavior problems are often exacerbated when there are disagreements between the birth mother and foster mother. More often than not, parental visits take place in settings that are not conducive to supporting or improving the parent-child relationship and may inadvertently contribute to the stress of the foster care experience.

A child care setting can be an ideal place to conduct parent and child visits while the child is in foster care placement. Child care programs offer many potential advantages over the common visiting alternatives, such as rooms at the social service agency, the foster home, or unstructured sites at restaurants or parks. These programs are child centered, with appropriate activities and equipment for the child; the professional staff can model appropriate parenting and behavior management skills; and parents have the opportunity to observe other children in addition to their own. During these visits, the center staff can provide parents with instruction on many aspects of basic child care and normal child development. Even if the birth parent is unable to attend a particular visit, the child can participate in the regular schedule of activities and programs. Finally, if the child is returned home to live with his or her birth parents, the child care program can continue to be a valuable resource to the family, offering stability, predictability, ongoing support, and guidance.

If visits occur at a different site and the child leaves from or returns to the child care center, the child care staff can help to prepare the child for visits or help the child adjust after visits. Some children have difficulty before the visits because they may be afraid, excited, or anxious. Others may have difficulty after the visits because they are sad or angry or miss their birth parents. If visits are very unstructured for the child or the birth parent is encouraging defiant behavior, the child may engage in more deviant behaviors on return to the child care center.

ADOPTION

Although most children in foster care will eventually return to their families of origin, approximately 16% of them eventually will be adopted. Approximately two thirds will be adopted by the foster parents with whom they have been living, 15% to 20% will be placed with an extended family member, and the rest will be placed with new families. In addition, a growing number of children from countries around the world are being adopted by US citizens, with an estimated 20 099 children adopted internationally in 2002. Because there is no central collection of adoption statistics, there are an unknown number of private agency and independent adoptions each year; it is estimated that there are approximately 120 000 total adoptions annually in the United States. It is estimated that approximately 1 million children live with adoptive parents, representing 2% to 4% of all families.

Although adoption provides the stability of a loving, permanent family for children, it can also create unique issues for children in child care settings. Children who have recently joined their new families may not have developed secure attachments to their new parent(s) and may have more separation anxiety than other children their age. These children will need extra comforting at transition times and may benefit from extra reminders (eg, photographs or audiotapes) of their new parents' continued presence. Those who have previously lived in institutional settings may be very comfortable in the routine of a child care center, even as their new parents report significant difficulties at home. Children who have had multiple changes in caregivers or who have never developed an attachment to a special caregiver may show indiscriminate friendliness toward all adults, eagerly seeking warmth and attention whenever they can find it. Child care providers should be aware of these needs and work with the child's new family to promote a sense of security for the child and strong attachments to the new parents.

Newly adopted children may bring with them special health needs as well. In addition to the health issues already described for children in foster care, children who have been adopted internationally are known to be at high risk of a variety of infectious diseases, including tuberculosis, intestinal parasites, and hepatitis B. All internationally adopted children should be screened according to the guidelines listed in Table 26.3. In addition, newly adopted children may not have started or completed immunizations and many need to be caught up according to established guidelines (see Fig 17.1).

TABLE 26.3. Screening Tests for Infectious Diseases in International Adoptees

- Hepatitis B virus serologic testing: hepatitis B surface antigen, hepatitis B surface antibody, and hepatitis B core antibody
- Hepatitis C virus serologic testing
- Syphilis serologic testing (nontreponemal and treponemal tests)
- Human immunodeficiency virus 1 serologic testing
- Complete blood cell count with red blood cell indices
- Stool examination for ova and parasites (3 specimens)
- Stool examination for *Giardia lamblia* and *Cryptosporidia* antigen (1 specimen)
- Tuberculin skin testing

Reprinted from American Academy of Pediatrics. *Red Book: 2003 Report of the Committee on Infectious Diseases.* Pickering LK, ed. 26th ed. Elk Grove Village, IL: American Academy of Pediatrics; 2003:175

OTHER SPECIFIC ISSUES FOR THE CHILD CARE PROVIDER

Administrative Issues

1. Guardianship may be a question for some children, especially before an adoption is finalized. Permission for field trips, authorization for medical care, etc may be required from a social service agency, the court, or another court-appointed person who may hold legal guardianship. Specific details and updates about who is allowed to grant what sort of permission should be included in the child's file at the center. Communication between child care center and foster care agency staff is the best way to resolve issues of permission and consent. This may become a delicate issue in some foster care situations in which the foster care agency may be holding guardianship and, yet, the family from which the child was removed may still have contact with the child and may come to the child care center. Once an adoption is finalized, the adoptive parents have the same legal rights and authority as any other parents.

2. Payment for child care services may be different for the child in an adoptive or foster care situation. For children with special needs who hold an adoption subsidy or who are receiving some other state or federal support, the source of payment may be some other agent than the adoptive or foster parent. Care should be taken not to allow any positive or negative comment or judgment on the basis of where the child's support originates. Similarly, different children within the same foster or adoptive family may have different funds supporting them and, thus, differing payment plans.

3. Occasionally, an adopted child is not a US citizen. Questions may be raised as to whether the child is eligible to participate in federally or state-funded activities, such as Head Start or food supplementation programs. Funding sources, programs, and qualifications for participation vary from state to state. Although

some states restrict access for illegal immigrants to certain programs, alternative funding may be available. Social services should be able to assist families to obtain needed services.

Curriculum

1. Care should be taken to ensure that adopted or foster children do not feel excluded from specific activities. For example, when making Mother's Day cards, an adopted child in an open adoption relationship should not be discouraged or prevented from making 2 cards—one for the adoptive mother and one for the birth mother. Similarly, a foster child may desire to make a card for foster and birth mothers. For Grandparent's Day or Father's Day, a foster or adoptive child may have no relatives fitting those traditional categories. The child should be encouraged to make the card for or invite the guest who fills that role in his life, even if it is a nonrelative.

2. Activities focused on families or relatives should always allow for nontraditional family settings and composition. There should be an acknowledgement and acceptance of the fact that there are different kinds of families, all valid.

3. Adopted or foster children may have come from different cultural, social, or ethnic backgrounds. As with family composition, differences in experience, religion, and culture should be acknowledged and accepted.

Behavioral and Developmental

1. Children placed in foster or adoptive situations past infancy may have had very deprived or abusive past experiences. They may not have had exposure to "typical" childhood experiences. It is important to include adoptive or foster parents' strategies for discipline and behavior modification to ensure consistency at home and in child care.

2. Distressing, disruptive, or different behaviors are more likely to be attributable to past experiences and stresses than to the current adoptive or foster care placement. However, emotionally or behaviorally impaired children in adoptive or foster care may be at higher risk of abuse because of the emotions their behavior evokes in the adoptive or foster family (parents and siblings). Thus, worrisome behavior should not automatically be dismissed as a sequela of the child's past or automatically attributed to the current placement. If the child or family is in counseling or other therapy, it may be helpful to have the child care staff involved in some way. Communication with the foster care agency caseworker, when concerns arise regarding the child's behavior, is advisable.

3. Newly adopted children may still be very insecure in their attachment to their new parent(s) and may need extra reassurance after their departure that they will indeed return. Children often function at a significantly lower level emotionally than their age or other capabilities would suggest, and it can be helpful

for caregivers to think of them and respond to their needs as they would for a much younger child. Every effort should be made to have a consistent caregiver help the child through transitions, and caregivers should work closely with parents to promote strong attachments to parents along with a healthy adjustment to child care.

Personal

1. Adopted or foster children frequently come from different ethnic and cultural backgrounds and do not look like their adoptive families. This may create problems when comments are made to the child directly by other children, staff, or parents or when the child inadvertently overhears a conversation or comment made about this difference. Child care staff must be sensitive to these issues, educate all of the children about cultural and familial differences, and not engage in or condone remarks that may hurt or embarrass a child. When these incidents do occur, it is important to validate the child's feelings about being labeled as different. This may also create an embarrassing situation if a new or temporary provider is not aware of the status of the child when an adult who does not resemble the child arrives to pick the child up.

2. Children may have very negative or disturbing histories. They may tell some of these events or experiences to other children or to staff, sometimes without distinguishing past from current events. Child care staff should have some knowledge of the child's background and may need special counseling or instruction to be able to respond to distressing or violent accounts that may be disturbing to the child or other children in the classroom. Providers need to be comfortable dealing constructively with feelings of grief, loss, fear, or anger. Resources in the community can be identified, and a plan of response can be put into place before the child's admission if a special needs care plan has been developed for the child.

3. Foster or adopted children may not have baby pictures or other mementos of their early childhood and may be upset when asked to bring these to the child care center for a special project.

4. Some foster or adopted children will be in placement because of a disabling condition. Not only do these children have the issues of dealing with the condition itself, but the child also may have to deal with the confusion about whether the disability is related to the foster or adoptive placement.

CONCLUSIONS AND RECOMMENDATIONS

Child care providers and health care professionals need to understand that adopted children or children in foster care may present special, unique, and sometimes challenging issues for caregivers. Although some of these issues are unique to the adopted or foster child, most are common to both groups of children. The child care setting can provide a source of social support for the adoptive or foster family and assist with parenting skills, particularly around issues of behavior, development, and socialization. It can also provide a safe, nonthreatening location for supervised visits by birth parents.

RESOURCES

Adoption and Foster Care Analysis and Reporting System. Data submitted for the FY 2001, 10/1/00 through 9/30/01. Washington, DC: Administration for Children and Families, US Department of Health and Human Services; 2003

American Academy of Pediatrics, Committee on Early Childhood, Adoption, and Dependent Care. Developmental issues for young children in foster care. *Pediatrics*. 2001;106:1145-1150

American Academy of Pediatrics, Committee on Early Childhood, Adoption, and Dependent Care. Health care of young children in foster care. *Pediatrics*. 2002;109:536-541

Flango V, Flango C. *The Flow of Adoption Information From the States*. Williamsburg, VA: National Center for State Courts; 1994

Saiman L, Aronson J, Zhou J. Prevalence of infectious diseases among internationally adopted children. *Pediatrics*. 2001;108;608-612

Stolley KS. Statistics on adoption in the United States. *Future Child*. 1993;3:36-42

CHAPTER 27

Early Brain Development and Child Care

Edward L. Schor, MD

LEARNING OBJECTIVES

The reader of this chapter will:

- Become familiar with recent research regarding early brain development.
- Understand implications of early brain development for child care.
- Understand implications of early brain development on violence and violence prevention.

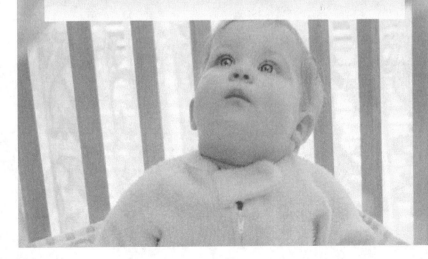

INTRODUCTION

Nearly everyone accepts that early life experiences have profound effects on children's later social and academic success. In the past decade, bridges between cognitive psychology and neuroscience have substantially advanced our understanding of why this is so.[1] Simply, the human brain is relatively undeveloped at birth, its potential waiting to unfold as its structure takes shape, and depends on individual experience to guide its growth. Experiences and sensory inputs (visual, auditory, tactile, olfactory, and taste) organize patterns of communication between neurons. These neural patterns become the determinants of how we think, feel, and behave.

That mental functions are mapped onto brain structures has extremely important implications for parents and child care providers, especially during children's first 3 years of life, when brain development progresses so rapidly. At birth, children's brains are about 25% of their adult weight; by 3 years of age, approximately 90% of adult brain size has been achieved.[2]

At birth, children's brains are about 25% of their adult weight; by 3 years of age, approximately 90% of adult brain size has been achieved.

USE-DEPENDENT BRAIN DEVELOPMENT

Some patterns of neural anatomy and functioning are genetically anticipated, and the developing brain needs only the expected stimuli to firmly establish a capability. For some abilities, physical maturation places time limits and creates "sensitive periods" for normal development. For example, the development of amblyopia in children is evidence that visual pathways, if functional at birth but deprived of adequate stimulation, will wither and vision will be lost if these pathways fail to receive expected sensory input. Similarly, the almost magical acquisition of language is severely impaired if children are not exposed to language before approximately 10 years of age; appropriate syntax is learned best before 6 years of age. From a developmental perspective, the potential to fully use the genetic endowment guiding brain development, as well as the brain's plasticity, diminishes over time. It is important in early childhood that environmental conditions are created that foster optimal brain development.

The more primitive functions of the brain, those residing primarily in the brain stem, postnatal midbrain, and limbic system, are established during intrauterine development and are far less susceptible to subsequent experience than are higher functions of the neocortex. At birth, positron emission tomography scans demonstrate that the areas of highest brain metabolism are in the phylogenetically oldest structures (eg, primary sensorimotor cortex, thalamic nuclei, brainstem, and cerebellar vermis). The brain of a newborn infant has approximately 100 billion neurons, the same number of brain cells it will have for the rest of the child's life.

Brain metabolism seems to coincide with the rate of synapse formation. The rate of synapse proliferation varies greatly according to the region of the brain and the age of the child. This aspect of brain development is not a steady process; rather, it is characterized by periods of exuberant growth. Many more synapses are produced during infancy than will ultimately remain. This overproduction and subsequent elimination or pruning of neuronal processes and their synaptic contacts is largely a postnatal process.

Brain maturation, as assessed by glucose metabolism, progresses in concert with the usual behaviors observed in infants. For example, between 6 and 8 months of age, the frontal cortex begins to show a maturational rise in metabolism. This coincides with the more complex interactions infants of that age have with their surroundings.[2] By 2 years of age, brain metabolic rates reach those of adults and exceed adult levels by 3 years of age. At approximately 4 years of age, a plateau of neural activity is reached that extends until near puberty. During these middle years, children's rate of brain metabolism is approximately 225% that of adults. After this period of intense activity, metabolic rates decrease to adult levels by late adolescence.

For those concerned with influencing the developmental course of children, the single most important concept derived from neuroscientific research is that experience shapes the brain. Nerve cells store information in a fashion that is contingent on previous patterns of activity.[3] The brain organizes in a "use-dependent" way, mirroring the pattern, quality, and quantity of the experiences of the infant. Repeated use during critical periods leads to retention and increased efficiency of synaptic connections; connections used less frequently are more susceptible to elimination. Thus, neuronal circuits are fine tuned by early life experiences, making the neuronal architecture of each individual unique.[2]

STABILITY OF FUNCTIONING

Cognition

The newborn's brain, unlike most other organs, is neither structurally nor functionally mature. Consequently, there is considerable opportunity for cumulative environmental influences, either good or bad, to modify many of the measurable consequences of brain development. Infants' scores on traditional developmental tests of cognitive abilities are only weakly associated with IQ measurements in later childhood. However, some cognitive patterns persist. Infants who rapidly lose interest in familiar stimuli and who rapidly regain interest when presented with new stimuli tend to show higher IQ scores later.[4]

Personal Characteristics

Similar to IQ, measures of temperament are only modestly consistent over time, although continuity in behavioral style increases with age. Temperament is modified by a child's analysis of a situation and by their self-concept and self-efficacy. Because these are altered by experience, it follows that aspects of temperament, the intensity of a child's emotional reactions, activity level, or approach to new situations will also change over time. Important adults in their environment can promote children's healthy psychosocial development by recognizing and adapting to the children's temperaments. Children's self-esteem and self-efficacy are especially important factors in their ability to deal with social risk factors and stressful events. Child-rearing that promotes these aspects of a positive self-image contribute to the development of effective social skills and sustained social success.

Problem Behaviors

Longitudinal research has demonstrated a high stability of problem behaviors among boys from preschool ages to adolescence. Aggressive behavior and conduct disorders, in particular, tend to be quite persistent over time. Persistence is most likely when the problems in early childhood involve a combination of hyperactivity, inattention, impulsivity, and aggression and when this constellation is associated with family stress and discord.[4]

STRESS AND VIOLENCE

All children are exposed to stress. When stress is modulated by the presence of an emotionally responsive, caring adult, children learn to modulate their own physiology and, thus, their emotional response to stress. They also learn that they can rely on others in their environment for assistance. Learning to cope successfully with stress is an essential developmental skill. Overwhelming stress has long-term physiologic and social consequences. Children exposed to chronic violence seem to adapt by adopting a persistently vigilant state.[3] Basal heart rates and blood pressure are elevated. They become chronically hypersensitive to external stimuli. These acquired traits interfere with learning and with the ability to form and maintain relationships. In stressful situations, such children are more likely to respond aggressively.

INTERVENTIONS

There is abundant evidence that children's brain development and associated physical and social health is influenced by the nurturing and stimulation they receive. Environmental effects are variable, but several patterns stand out.[4] Experiences during early infancy are less likely to have substantial long-term effects than are similar experiences from the toddler period forward. Brief, severe stressful experiences may sometimes have long-term consequences, but persistent environmental exposure is more likely to create enduring effects. Experiences in childhood may persist long after the environment has changed.

Touch

Children who are rarely touched develop brains 20% to 30% smaller than normal for their age. On the other hand, research has shown that weight gain by premature infants can be increased nearly twofold merely by applying a regular dose of gentle touching.

Play and Environmental Stimulation

Animal research shows that young animals provided the opportunity for interesting play have brains with 25% more synapses per neuron. Human studies of children of mothers with long-standing depression (who are less likely to respond sensitively or provide their children with optimal cognitive stimulation) are more likely to have difficulty with the expression and regulation of emotions. The period during which children are most susceptible to the risk of the consequences of maternal depression is between 6 and 18 months of age. Children who are rarely spoken or responded to, who are exposed to few toys, and who have little opportunity to explore and experiment with their environment may fail to develop to their full social and intellectual capacity. On the other hand, excessive stimulation or an environment that does not provide age- and developmentally appropriate experiences and expectations can also interfere with children's psychologic development.

Language Stimulation

Infants seem to be conditioned to patterns of speech in the womb. Within the first week of life they show preference for the language spoken by their parents as opposed to a foreign one. By 12 months of age, infants will lose the ability to discriminate sounds that are not significant in their language. When mothers frequently speak to their infants, children learn almost 300 more words by 2 years of age than do their peers who are spoken to less frequently.[5]

Early Intervention

There is ample evidence that environmental influences can have a lasting effect on intelligence. These effects are most evident when interventions begin early in life and persist through childhood and adolescence. High-quality, intensive child care and family support beginning in infancy can significantly increase IQ scores and decrease grade retention and the need for special education in school.[6] Equally important is the finding that a similar intervention introduced after 5 years of age fails to yield similar significant benefits.

ESSENTIAL CHARACTERISTICS OF POSITIVE PARENTING AND CAREGIVING

There is extensive literature on the qualities of parenting that lead to positive outcomes for children. Warm, affectionate, responsive, and flexible parenting is more likely to yield creative, cooperative, happy, achievement-oriented children with high self-esteem and good problem-solving skills.[7] When this type of nurturing is provided in a consistent, predictable way and combined with enriched experiences in a safe setting, optimal brain organization and function is likely to result. What is true for parenting also applies to child care provided by someone other than a child's parents.

IMPLICATIONS FOR EARLY EDUCATION AND CHILD CARE

Children's readiness for kindergarten has little to do with academic skills. Rather, children need to be: 1) physically healthy; 2) able to communicate their needs, wants, and thoughts; 3) enthusiastic and curious in approaching new activities; 4) able to follow directions; 5) not disruptive; 6) sensitive to other children's feelings; and 7) able to take turns and share. Most of these skills are social and reflect the emotional environment and social relationships that the child has had in the 0 to 5 years when the brain is so rapidly developing.

CONCLUSIONS AND RECOMMENDATIONS

High-quality child care is structured in a way that promotes emotional development through social interactions. At its best, child care is individualized education in the context of a relationship with a trusted adult. Parents and child care providers who strive to provide effective child rearing must learn to respond to children's cues in a developmentally appropriate way. High-quality child care, which must be a partnership between parents and other caregivers, can help children become creative, responsible, empathic, and intelligent contributors to society.

REFERENCES

1. West J, Hausken EG, Collins M. *Readiness for Kindergarten: Parent and Teacher Beliefs.* Washington, DC: US Department of Education, National Center for Education Statistics; 1993. Publication No. NCES 93-257

2. Chugani HT. Neuroimaging of developmental nonlinearity and developmental pathologies. In: Thatcher RW, Lyon GR, Rumsey J, Krasnegor N, eds. *Developmental Neuroimaging: Mapping the Development of Brain and Behavior.* San Diego, CA: Academic Press; 1996

3. Rutter M, Rutter M. *Developing Minds: Challenge and Continuity Across the Life Span.* New York, NY: Basic Books; 1993

4. Shore R. *Rethinking the Brain: New Insights into Early Development.* New York, NY: Families and Work Institute; 1997

5. Huttenlocher J, Levine S, Vevea J, et al. Environmental input and cognitive growth: a study using time-period comparisons. *Child Dev.* 1998;69:1012-1029
6. Campbell FA, Ramey CT. Effects of early intervention on intellectual and academic achievement: a follow-up study of children from low-income families. *Child Dev.* 1994;65:684-698
7. Baumrind D. Familial antecedents of adolescent drug use: a developmental perspective. In: Jones CL, Battjes RJ, eds. *Etiology of Drug Abuse: Implications for Prevention.* Rockville, MD: US Department of Health and Human Services; 1987. Publication No. ADM 87-1335

ADDITIONAL RESOURCES

Bowman BT, Donovan MS, Burns MS, eds. *Eager to Learn: Educating Our Preschoolers.* Washington, DC: National Academies Press; 2000

Perry BD. The memories of states: how the brain stores and retrieves traumatic experience. In: Goodwin J, Attias R, eds. *Splintered Reflections: Images of the Body in Trauma.* New York, NY: Basic Books; 1999:9-38

Shonkoff JP, Phillips DA, eds. *From Neurons to Neighborhoods: The Science of Early Childhood Development.* Washington, DC: National Academies Press; 2000

Glossary

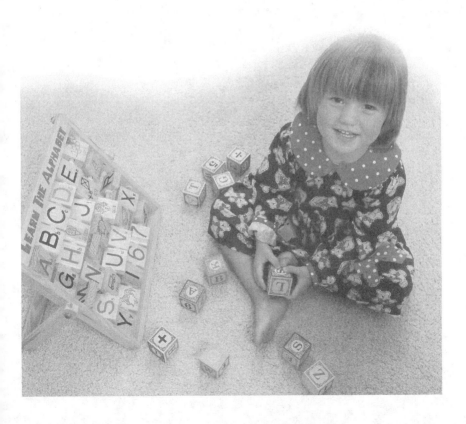

Antisiphon ballcock–An automatic valve in the toilet tank, the opening and closing of which is controlled by a spherical float at the end of a lever. The antisiphon ballcock prevents dirty water from being admixed with clean water.

Asphyxial crib death–Death attributed to an item inside the crib that caused deprivation of oxygen or obstruction to normal breathing of an infant.

Bleach solution–For disinfecting environmental surfaces (one quarter cup of household liquid chlorine bleach [sodium hypochlorite] per gallon of water) prepared fresh daily. See also disinfectant.

Body fluids–Urine, feces, saliva, blood, nasal discharge, eye discharge, and injury or tissue discharge.

Capture velocity–Airflow that will collect the pollutant (such as dust or fumes) that you want removed.

Care coordinator–This term is used by some agencies or caregivers in place of, or in association with, the term case manager. The term care coordinator implies that someone is assigned to work with the child's family or alternative caregiver to assist in coordinating services internally within an agency directly providing services or with other service providers for the child and family. The term care coordinator is usually preferred over the term case manager, because the latter implies management of a case rather than assisting people.

Caregiver/child care provider–Used here to indicate the primary staff who work directly with children (ie, director, teacher, aide, or others in the center and the child care provider in small and large family child care homes).

Case manager–See *care coordinator.*

Center–A facility that provides care and education for any number of children in a nonresidential setting and is open on a regular basis (ie, it is not a drop-in facility).

Child abuse–For the purposes of this manual, its definition is considered to be that contained in the laws of the state in which the standards will be applied. Although these differ somewhat, most of them contain basic elements as follows:

> *Emotional abuse–*Acts that damage a child in psychologic ways but do not fall into other categories of abuse. Most states require for prosecution that psychologic damage be very definite and clearly diagnosed by a psychologist or psychiatrist; this category of abuse is rarely reported and even more rarely a cause of protective action.

Neglect–Neglect is divided into 2 categories: general neglect and severe neglect.

General neglect–Failure to provide the common necessities, including food, shelter, a safe environment, education, and health care but without resultant or likely harm to the child.

Severe neglect–Neglect that results or is likely to result in harm to the child.

Physical abuse–An intentional (nonaccidental) act affecting a child that produces tangible physical harm.

Sexual abuse–Any sexual act performed with a child by an adult or by another child who exerts control over the victim. (Many state laws provide considerable detail about the specific acts that constitute sexual abuse.)

Child-staff ratio–The maximum number of children permitted per child care provider.

Children with special health care needs–Children with developmental disabilities, mental retardation, emotional disturbance, sensory or motor impairment, or significant chronic illness who require special health surveillance or specialized programs, interventions, technologies, or facilities.

Cohorting (toys)–Keeping toys and other items used by a group of children together for use only by that group of children to prevent transmission of communicable disease.

Disinfectant–A solution capable of eliminating virtually all germs from inanimate surfaces through the use of chemicals (eg, products registered with the US Environmental Protection Agency as *disinfectants*) or physical agents (eg, heat). In the child care environment, a 1:64 dilution of domestic bleach made by mixing a solution of a quarter cup household liquid chlorine bleach with 1 gallon of tap water and prepared fresh daily is an effective method to remove germs from environmental surfaces and other inanimate objects that have been contaminated with body fluids (see *body fluids*), provided that the surfaces have first been cleaned of organic material before applying bleach and at least 2 minutes of contact time with the surface occurs. (Because complete elimination of all germs may not be achieved using the 1:64 dilution of domestic bleach solution, technically, the process is called sanitizing, not disinfecting. The term sanitize is used in standards most often, but *disinfect* may appear in other or earlier publications when addressing sanitation in child care.) To achieve maximum germ reduction with bleach, the precleaned surfaces should be left moderately or glistening wet with the bleach solution and allowed to air dry or be dried only after at least 2 minutes of contact time. A slight chlorine odor should emanate from this solution. If there is no chlorine smell, a new solution needs to be made, even if the solution was prepared fresh that day. The 1:64 diluted solution will contain 500 to 800 parts per million chlorine bleach.

Two minutes of contact with a coating of a sprayed 1:64 diluted solution of a quarter cup household liquid chlorine bleach in 1 gallon of tap water prepared fresh daily is an effective method of surface-sanitizing of environmental surfaces and other inanimate objects that have first been thoroughly cleaned of organic soil. By itself, bleach is not a good cleaning agent. Household bleach is sold in the conventional strength of 5.25% hypochlorite and a more recently marketed "ultra" bleach that contains 6% hypochlorite solution. In child care, either may be used in a 1:64 dilution.

Bleach solutions much less concentrated than the recommended dilution have been shown in laboratory tests to kill high numbers of bloodborne viruses, including human immunodeficiency virus and hepatitis B virus. This solution is not toxic if accidentally ingested by a child. However, because this solution is moderately corrosive, caution should be exercised in handling it and when wetting or using it on items containing metals, especially aluminum. DO NOT MIX UNDILUTED BLEACH OR THE DILUTED BLEACH SOLUTION WITH OTHER FLUIDS, ESPECIALLY ACIDS (EG, VINEGAR), AS THIS WILL RESULT IN THE RAPID EVOLUTION OF HIGHLY POISONOUS CHLORINE GAS.

Commercially prepared detergent-sanitizer solutions or detergent cleaning, rinsing and application of a nonbleach sanitizer that is at least as effective as the chlorine bleach solution is acceptable as long as these products are nontoxic for children, are used according to the manufacturer's instructions, and are approved by the state or local health department for use as a disinfectant in place of the bleach solution.

These methods are used for toys, children's table tops, diaper changing tables, food utensils, and any other object or surface that is significantly contaminated with body fluids. Sanitizing food utensils can be accomplished by using a dishwasher or equivalent process, usually involving more dilute chemicals than are required for other surfaces.

Drop-in care–A facility providing care that occurs for fewer than 30 days per year per child on a consecutive or intermittent basis or on a regular basis.

Functional outcomes–Health status measures that go beyond traditional physiologic assessments. By incorporating a multidimensional definition of health that encompasses physical, psychologic, and social aspects, functional outcome measures can capture the broader impact of disease and treatment on life from a child's (or parent's) own perspective. Such tools enable children and parents to offer input on their quality of life and their capacity to function in normal social roles.

Ground-fault circuit interrupter (GFCI)–A piece of equipment in an electrical line that offers protection against electrocution if the line comes into contact with water.

Health consultant–A health care professional (physician, certified pediatric or family nurse practitioner, physician assistant, or registered nurse) who has pediatric or child care experience and is knowledgeable in child care, licensing, and community resources. The health consultant provides guidance and assistance to child care staff on health aspects of the facility.

Health plan–A written document that describes emergency health and safety procedures and policies covering the management of mild illness, injury prevention, and occupational health and safety.

Individual Education Plan (IEP)–A written document derived from Part B of the Individuals With Disabilities Education Act [Pub L No. 94-142]) that is designed to meet a child's individual educational program needs. The main purposes for an IEP are to set reasonable learning goals and to state the services that the school district will provide for a child with special educational needs. Every child who is qualified for special educational services provided by the school is required to have an IEP.

Individual Family Service Plan (IFSP)–A written document derived from Part C of the Individuals With Disabilities Education Act that is formulated in collaboration with the family to meet the needs of a child with a developmental disability or delay to assist the family in its care for a child's special educational, therapeutic, and health needs and to deal with the family's needs to the extent to which the family wishes assistance.

Infant–A child between the time of birth and the age of ambulation (usually between birth and 18 months of age).

Large family child care home–Usually, care and education for 7 to 12 children (including preschool children of the caregiver) in the home of the caregiver, who employs 1 or more qualified adult assistants to meet the child-staff ratio requirements. This type of care is likely to resemble center care in its organization of activities.

Lead agency–This term refers to an individual state's choice for the agency that will receive and allocate the federal and state funding for children with special educational needs. The federal funding is allocated to individual states in accordance with the Individuals With Disabilities Educational Act (IDEA).

Mainstreaming–Describes the philosophy and activities associated with providing services to persons with disabilities in community settings, especially in school programs, in which such children or other persons are integrated with persons without disabilities and are entitled to attend programs and to have access to all services available in the community.

Occupational therapy–Treatment based on the participation in occupational activities of a typical child (such as play, feeding, toileting, and dressing). Child-specific exercises are developed to encourage children with mental or physical disabilities to contribute to their own recovery and development.

Sanitize–To remove filth or soil and small amounts of certain bacteria. For an inanimate surface to be considered sanitary, the surface must be clean and the number of germs must be decreased to such a level that disease transmission by that surface is unlikely. This procedure is less rigorous than is disinfection (see *disinfect*) and is applicable to a wide variety of routine housekeeping procedures involving, for example, bedding, bathrooms, kitchen countertops, floors, and walls. To clean, detergent or abrasive cleaners may be used but an additional sanitizer solution must be applied to sanitize. A number of EPA-registered "detergent-disinfectant" products are also appropriate for sanitizing. Directions on product labels should be followed closely.

Small family child care home–Usually, the care and education of 1 to 6 children (including preschool children of the caregiver) in the home of the caregiver. Caregivers model their programs on a nursery school or on a skilled parenting model.

Small family child care home network–A group of small family child care homes in 1 management system.

Staff–Used here to indicate all personnel employed by the facility, including child care providers and personnel who do not provide direct care to the children (such as cooks, drivers, and housekeeping personnel).

Standard precautions–Precautions that apply to contact with nonintact skin, mucous membranes, blood, all body fluids, and excretions except sweat, whether or not they contain visible blood. The general methods of infection prevention are indicated for all people in the child care setting and are designed to decrease the risk of transmission of microorganisms from recognized and unrecognized sources of infection. Although standard precautions were designed to apply to hospital settings, with the exceptions detailed in this definition, they also apply in child care settings. Standard precautions involve use of barriers (as in universal precautions) as well as cleaning and sanitizing contaminated surfaces.

Child Care Adaptation of Standard Precautions (exceptions from the use in hospital settings):

a) In child care settings, use of nonporous gloves is optional except when blood or blood-containing body fluids may be involved.

b) In child care settings, gowns and masks are not required.

c) In child care settings, appropriate barriers include materials, such as disposable diaper table paper, disposable towels, and surfaces that can be sanitized.

Transmission-based precautions–Precautions, in addition to standard precautions, that are required where airborne, droplet, and contact transmission of infectious organisms may occur. In addition to hand washing, cleaning and sanitation of surfaces, transmission-based precautions include use of a room shared only by those who are infected with the same infectious agent (with negative-pressure ventilation when airborne spread is involved), use of masks for infections spread by the airborne and droplet routes, and use of gowns and gloves for diseases spread by contact. Use of gloves for diaper changing is not mandatory in these circumstances. Transmission-based precautions are applicable to child care where children are receiving care who would otherwise be excluded because they have a communicable disease.

Appendices

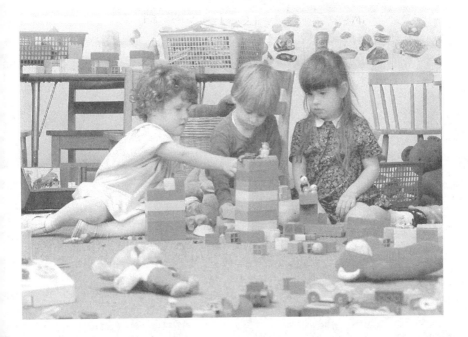

Appendix

Appendix A. Child-Staff Ratio and Group Size

Standard 1.001 Ratios for Small Family Child Care Homes	Age	Standard 1.002 Ratios for Large Family Child Care Homes and Centers		Standard 1.004 Ratios During Transportation	Standard 1.005 Ratios for Wading and Swimming
		Maximum Child-Staff Ratio	Maximum Group Size	Child-Staff Ratio†	Child-Staff Ratio
If there are no children in care younger than 2 years, **then** provider may have 1–6 children older than 2 years	Birth–12 mo	3:1	6	3:1	1:1
	13–30 mo	4:1	8	4:1	1:1
	31–35 mo	5:1	10	5:1	1:1
If there is 1 child younger than 2 years, **then** the provider may have 1–3 children older than 2 years	3 y	7:1	14	7:1	4:1
	4 y	8:1	16	8:1	4:1
If there are 2 children younger than 2 years, **then** the provider may have no children older than 2 years	5 y	8:1	16	8:1	6:1
	6–8 y	10:1	20	10:1	6:1
	9–12 y	12:1	24	12:1	6:1

Adapted from American Academy of Pediatrics, American Public Health Association, and Maternal and Child Health Bureau. *Caring for Our Children. National Health and Safety Performance Standards: Guidelines for Out-of-Home Child Care Programs*, 2nd ed. Elk Grove Village, IL: American Academy of Pediatrics; 2002:3–6.

†The driver is not included in transportation ratios.

APPENDIX B. The Dirty Dozen...

Are they hiding in your child's playground?

The National Playground Safety Institute (NPSI) has identified 12 of the leading causes of injury on playgrounds. By familiarizing yourself with the "Dirty Dozen Checklist," you can inspect your local playground to see how safe it is. As parents and caregivers, we are responsible for providing safe play opportunities for our children. Should you identify any of the following hazards on your child's playground, notify the owner or operator of the play area of the condition so that they may take steps to eliminate the hazard.

The Dirty Dozen Checklist

1. **Improper Protective Surfacing**
   The surface or ground under and around the playground equipment should be soft enough to cushion a fall. Improper surfacing material under playground equipment is the leading cause of playground-related injuries. More than 70% of all injuries on playgrounds are from children falling. Hard surfaces, such as concrete, blacktop, packed earth, or grass, are not acceptable under play equipment. A fall onto one of these hard surfaces could be life threatening.
   There are many surfaces that offer protection from falls. Acceptable surfaces are hardwood fiber or mulch, sand, and pea gravel. These surfaces must be maintained at a depth of 12 inches, be free of standing water and debris, and not be allowed to become compacted. There are also synthetic or rubber tiles and mats that are appropriate for use under play equipment.

2. **Inadequate Fall Zone**
   A fall zone or use zone is the area under and around the playground equipment where a child might fall. A fall zone should be covered with protective surfacing material and extend a minimum of 6 feet in all directions from the edge of stationary play equipment such as climbers and chin-up bars. The fall zone at the bottom or exit area of a slide should extend a minimum of 6 feet from the end of the slide for slides 4 feet or less in height. For slides higher than 4 feet, take the entrance height of the slide and add 4 feet to determine how far the surfacing should extend from the end of the slide. Swings require a much greater area for the fall zone. The fall zone should extend 2 times the height of the pivot or swing hanger in front of and behind the swing's seats. The fall zone should also extend 6 feet to the side of the support structure.

3. **Protrusion and Entanglement Hazards**
   A protrusion hazard is a component or piece of hardware that might be capable of impaling or cutting a child if a child should fall against the hazard. Some protrusions are also capable of catching strings or items of clothing that might be worn around a child's neck. This type of entanglement is especially hazardous because it might result in strangulation. Examples of protrusion and entanglement hazards include bolt ends that extend more than 2 threads beyond the face of the nut, hardware configurations that form a hook or leave a gap or space between components, and open "S" type hooks. Rungs or handholds that protrude outward from a support structure may be capable of penetrating the eye socket. Special attention should be paid to the area at the top of slides and sliding devices. Ropes should be anchored securely at both ends and not capable of forming a loop or a noose.

4. **Entrapment in Openings**
   Enclosed openings on playground equipment must be checked for head entrapment hazards. Children often enter openings feet first and attempt to slide through the opening. If the opening is not large enough, it may allow the body to pass through the opening and entrap the head. Generally, there should be no openings on playground equipment that measure between 3.5 inches and 9 inches. Where the ground forms the lower boundary of the opening is not considered to be hazardous. Pay special attention to openings at the top of a slide, openings between platforms, and openings on climbers where the distance between rungs might be less than 9 inches.

5. Insufficient Equipment Spacing

Improper spacing between pieces of play equipment can cause overcrowding of a play area, which may create several hazards. Fall zones for equipment that is higher than 24 inches above the ground cannot overlap. Therefore, there should be a minimum of 12 feet between 2 play structures. This provides room for children to circulate and prevents the possibility of a child falling off of one structure and striking another structure. Swings and other pieces of moving equipment should be located in an area away from other structures.

6. Trip Hazards

Trip hazards are created by play structure components or items on the playground. Exposed concrete footings, abrupt changes in surface elevations, containment borders, tree roots, tree stumps, and rocks are all common trip hazards that are often found in play environments.

7. Lack of Supervision

The supervision of a playground environment directly relates to the overall safety of the environment. A play area should be designed so that it is easy for a parent or caregiver to observe the children at play. Young children are constantly challenging their own abilities, very often not being able to recognize potential hazards. It is estimated that more than 40% of all playground injuries are directly related to lack of supervision in some way. Parents must supervise their children in some way on the playground!

8. Age-Inappropriate Activities

Children's developmental needs vary greatly from age 2 to age 12. In an effort to provide a challenging and safe play environment for all ages, it is important to make sure that the equipment in the playground setting is appropriate for the age of the intended user. Areas for preschool-aged children should be separate from areas intended for school-aged children.

9. Lack of Maintenance

In order for playgrounds to remain in safe condition, a program of systematic preventive maintenance must be present. There should be no missing, broken, or worn-out components. All hardware should be secure. The wood, metal, or plastic should not show signs of fatigue or deterioration. All parts should be stable with no apparent signs of loosening. The surfacing material must also be maintained. Check for signs of vandalism.

10. Pinch, Crush, Shearing, and Sharp Edge Hazards

Components in the play environment should be inspected to make sure there are no sharp edges or points that could cut skin. Moving components, such as suspension bridges, track rides, merry-go-rounds, seesaws, and some swings, should be checked to make sure there are no moving parts or mechanisms that might crush or pinch a child's finger.

11. Platforms with No Guardrails

Elevated surfaces such as platforms, ramps, and bridgeways should have guardrails that would prevent accidental falls. Preschool-aged children are more at risk from falls, and equipment intended for this age group should have guardrails on elevated surfaces higher than 20 inches. Equipment intended for school-aged children should have guardrails on elevated surfaces higher than 30 inches.

12. Equipment Not Recommended for Public Playgrounds

Accidents associated with the following types of equipment have resulted in the Consumer Product Safety Commission recommending that they not be used on public playgrounds:
- Heavy swings such as animal figure swings and multiple occupancy/glider-type swings
- Free-swinging ropes that may fray or form a loop

APPENDIX B. The Dirty Dozen..., continued

- Swinging exercise rings and trapeze bars are considered athletic equipment and are not recommended for public playgrounds. Overhead hanging rings that have a short amount of chain and are intended for use as a ring trek (generally 4 to 8 rings) are allowed on public playground equipment.

If any of the "Dirty Dozen" playground hazards are present, you should inform the owner or operator of the unsafe condition.

Additional Resource Materials:

- **National Playground Safety Institute (NPSI)**

  The National Playground Safety Institute (NPSI) is sponsored by the National Recreation and Park Association (NRPA). The NPSI's mission is to promote children's rights to play in a safe environment and to nationally promote the importance of play in their development. The NPSI promotes the latest public playground industry standards and guidelines as the most desirable standard of care for public-use playgrounds. For a listing of playground-related publications available through NRPA, contact:

  National Recreation and Park Association
  22377 Belmont Bridge Road
  Ashburn, Virginia 20148
  703/858-2148

- **US Consumer Product Safety Commission (CPSC)**

  For a copy of the Consumer Product Safety Commission's *Handbook for Public Playground Safety,* contact:

  US Consumer Product Safety Commission
  Washington, DC 20207
  800/638-2772

- **American Society for Testing and Materials (ASTM)**

  The American Society for Testing and Materials (ASTM) developed a standard for the manufacturing of public playground equipment titled "Standard Consumer Safety Performance Specifications for Playground Equipment for Public Use." For a copy of this standard, contact the ASTM and ask for the F 1487-95 Standard.

  ASTM
  100 Barr Harbor Drive
  West Conshohocken, PA 19428-2959
  610/832-9500

Adapted with permission from National Recreation and Park Association. *The Dirty Dozen.* Ashburn, VA: National Recreation and Park Association.

APPENDIX C. Child Health Assessment

National Health and Safety Performance Standards

CHILD HEALTH ASSESSMENT

Parents & Child Care Providers fill-in this part.

CHILD'S NAME: (LAST)	(FIRST)	PARENT/GUARDIAN
DATE OF BIRTH:	HOME PHONE:	ADDRESS:
CHILD CARE FACILITY NAME:		
FACILITY PHONE:	COUNTY:	WORK PHONE:

To Parents: Submission of this form to the child care provider implies consent for the child care provider to discuss the child's health with the child's clinician.

PA child care providers must document that enrolled children have received age appropriate health services and immunizations that meet the current schedule of the American Academy of Pediatrics 141 Northwest Point Blvd., Elk Grove Village, IL 60007. The schedule is available at <www.aap.org> or Faxback 847/758-0391 (document #9535 and #9807). Print copies provided by DPW have the schedule on the back of the form.

| Health history and medical information pertinent to routine child care and emergencies (describe, if any): ☐NONE | Date of most recent well-child exam: |
| Allergies to food or medicine (describe, if any): ☐NONE | Do not omit any information. This form may be updated by health professional. (Initial and date new data.) Child care facility needs 2 copies. |

Parents may write immunization dates, health professionals should verify and complete all data.

LENGTH/HEIGHT	WEIGHT	HEAD CIRCUMFERENCE	BLOOD PRESSURE
IN/CM % ILE	LB/KG % ILE	IN/CM % ILE	(BEGINNING AT AGE 3) /

PHYSICAL EXAMINATION	✓ = NORMAL	IF ABNORMAL - COMMENTS
HEAD/EARS/EYES/NOSE/THROAT		
TEETH		
CARDIORESPIRATORY		
ABDOMEN/GI		
GENITALIA/BREASTS		
EXTREMITIES/JOINTS/BACK/CHEST		
SKIN/LYMPH NODES		
NEUROLOGIC & DEVELOPMENTAL		

IMMUNIZATIONS	DATE	DATE	DATE	DATE	DATE	COMMENTS
D TaP/DTP/Td						
POLIO						
HIB						
HEP B						
MMR						
VARICELLA						
PNEUMOCOCCAL						
OTHER						

SCREENING TESTS	DATE TEST DONE	NOTE HERE IF RESULTS ARE PENDING OR ABNORMAL
LEAD		
ANEMIA (HGB/HCT)		
URINALYSIS (UA) (at age 5)		
HEARING (subjective until age 4)		
VISION (subjective until age 3)		
PROFESSIONAL DENTAL EXAM		

HEALTH PROBLEMS OR SPECIAL NEEDS, RECOMMENDED TREATMENT/MEDICATIONS/SPECIAL CARE	(ATTACH ADDITIONAL SHEETS IF NECESSARY)

☐NONE   NEXT APPOINTMENT - MONTH/YEAR:

MEDICAL CARE PROVIDER: SIGNATURE OF PHYSICIAN OR CPNP:	SIGNATURE OF PHYSICIAN OR CPNP:	
ADDRESS:		
	PHONE	LICENSE NUMBER:	DATE FORM SIGNED:

Reprinted with permission from Pennsylvania Department of Public Welfare, 2001

APPENDIX D. Sample Letter to Families About Exposure to Communicable Disease

Name of Child Care Program: _____

Address of Child Care Program: _____

Telephone Number of Child Care Program: _____

Date: _____

Dear Parent or Legal Guardian:

A child in our program has or is suspected of having: _____

Information about this disease:

The disease is spread by: _____

The symptoms are: _____

_____

The disease can be prevented by: _____

_____

_____

What the program is doing: _____

_____

_____

_____

What you can do at home: _____

_____

_____

If your child has any symptoms of this disease, call your doctor to find out what to do. Be sure to tell your doctor about this notice. If you do not have a regular doctor to care for your child, contact your local health department for instructions on how to find a doctor, or ask other parents for names of their children's doctors. If you have any questions, please contact:

_____ at (____)_____
(Caregiver's name)   (Telephone number)

Reprinted from American Academy of Pediatrics, Pennsylvania Chapter. Appendix K. In: *Model Child Care Health Policies.* 4th ed. Rosemont, PA: American Academy of Pediatrics, Pennsylvania Chapter; 2002

APPENDIX E. Immunization for Child Care Staff

Child care providers will be exposed to infectious diseases more frequently than will someone who has less contact with children. Child care providers should know their immunization status and whether they had specific childhood diseases such as varicella and measles. Child care providers can be tested to determine immunity to some of these diseases if immune status is unknown. The Advisory Committee on Immunization Practices of the Centers for Disease Control and Prevention has not developed official recommendations for immunization of child care providers. The table on the next page lists the immunizations that the Centers for Disease Control and Prevention believes are appropriate for child care providers on the basis of the official recommendations for immunization of adults in other occupations and settings.

Tuberculosis Screening

Persons beginning work as child care providers should have a Mantoux intradermal skin test (1-step method) using tuberculin purified protein derivative to assess their tuberculosis status, unless there is documentation of a previous positive skin test or of tuberculosis that has been appropriately treated. Persons older than 60 years or those with immune deficiency of any etiology should be tested by the 2-step method. Using this method, if the first test result is negative, the skin test is repeated after an interval of at least 1 week. Also, in family child care home settings, all persons 12 years and older who are present while the children are in care should also be tested for tuberculosis, even if they are not providing child care. Mantoux skin testing need not be repeated on a regular basis unless required by the state or local health department.

Anyone who has a positive result from the skin test should be evaluated by chest radiography and cleared by a physician and/or the local health department before providing care to children. Individuals with previous positive Mantoux skin test results but no evidence of active disease should be evaluated annually by their health care professional to determine risk of contagion. Anyone who has symptoms of tuberculosis, such as a cough that will not go away, coughing up blood, weight loss, night sweats, or persistent fatigue, should not attend, work, or volunteer at a child care facility until they have been evaluated by a physician. Persons who have active tuberculosis should not return to a child care setting until the local health department has determined that they are no longer contagious.

Recommended Immunization Schedule for Child Care Providers, continued

Immunization	How Often	Why
Influenza	All child care providers, especially those who have chronic health conditions, who will be in their second or third trimester of pregnancy, or who are older than 50 years, should be immunized against influenza. Immunization is given yearly, in October or November (before the flu season).	Influenza causes fever, chills, headache, muscle ache, sore throat, cough, and cold symptoms. Influenza may lead to pneumonia, other severe illness, and hospitalization among infants and children younger than 24 months, pregnant women in their second or third trimester during influenza season, the elderly, and those with chronic illnesses or weak immune systems.
Measles, Mumps, Rubella (MMR)	Child care providers should be immunized or certified by a health care professional to be immune to measles, mumps, and rubella. Providers born before 1957 can be considered immune to measles and mumps. Others can be considered immune if they have a history of physician-diagnosed measles or mumps or laboratory evidence of immunity. Measles, mumps, and rubella vaccines are usually given together as MMR. Susceptible individuals (without evidence of immunity) should receive 2 doses of MMR, at least a month apart.	Measles: 2–3 people out of every 1000 who contract measles die from complications such as pneumonia or encephalitis. Encephalitis is an inflammation of the brain that can lead to convulsions, deafness, or mental retardation. Measles during pregnancy increases the risk of premature labor, spontaneous abortion, and low birth weight. Mumps: 15% of cases are in adolescents and adults. Mumps may cause inflammation of the pancreas or sexual organs and may cause permanent deafness or sterility. Rubella: 15% of young adults are susceptible. Rubella may cause miscarriage, stillbirth, and multiple birth defects (congenital disorders, mental retardation) if contracted during the first trimester of pregnancy.
Tetanus, Diphtheria (Td)	Child care providers should have a record of receiving a series of 3 doses (usually given during childhood) and a booster dose given within the past 10 years.	Tetanus (lockjaw) causes painful muscular contractions. 40%–50% of persons who contract tetanus die. Diphtheria affects throat and nasal passages, interferes with breathing, and produces a toxin that damages the heart, kidneys, and nerves. 10% of cases are fatal.

Recommended Immunization Schedule for Child Care Providers, continued

Immunization	How Often	Why
Poliovirus	Child care providers should have a record of a primary series of 3 doses (usually given during childhood) and a supplementary dose given at least 6 months after the third dose in the primary series.	Poliovirus attacks the nervous system and can cause paralysis.
Hepatitis A	Hepatitis A vaccine is not routinely recommended for child care providers but may be indicated if the local health department determines that the risk of hepatitis A in the community is high. Any person who travels frequently should consider getting hepatitis A vaccine. Any person with chronic liver disease (chronic hepatitis B or C infection, cirrhosis, etc) or individuals living with such persons should also be immunized.	Hepatitis A is a liver infection that causes fever, loss of appetite, nausea, diarrhea, and a generally ill feeling that may persist for weeks. During an outbreak in a child care setting, hepatitis A spreads easily and quickly. However, in the absence of an outbreak, the risk to child care providers does not seem to be increased. Hepatitis A may cause severe, even fatal disease in individuals with liver damage.
Varicella	Child care providers with a history of chickenpox can assume they are immune. All other providers should consider having blood tests to determine whether they are susceptible and in need of immunization. Alternatively, persons who believe they have never had chickenpox or are unsure can be immunized.	Chickenpox can be a severe disease in adults. Child care providers are at high risk of being exposed to chickenpox in the child care setting.
Hepatitis B	Child care providers who may have contact with blood or blood-contaminated body fluids or who work with developmentally disabled or aggressive children should be immunized against hepatitis B with 1 series of 3 doses of vaccine.	Hepatitis B causes serious illness, and 1 in 20 persons will develop chronic hepatitis, which can destroy the liver and increase the risk of liver cancer. Persons who develop chronic hepatitis B are infectious to others.

Provider Exclusion and Readmittance Criteria

A child care provider should be temporarily excluded from providing care to children if he or she has 1 or more of the following conditions.

Condition	Exclude From Child Care Facility
Chickenpox	Until 6 days after the start of rash or when sores have dried or crusted.
Shingles	Only if sores cannot be covered by clothing or a dressing; if not, exclude until sores have crusted and are dry. A person with active shingles should not care for immune-suppressed children.
Rash with fever or joint pain	Until diagnosed not to be measles or rubella.
Measles	Until 4 days after rash starts (if staff is immunocompetent).
Rubella	Until 6 days after rash starts.
Mumps	Until 9 days after glands begin to swell.
Diarrheal illness	If 3 or more episodes of loose stools during previous 24 hours, or if blood in stools, until diarrhea resolves. If *Escherichia coli* O157:H7 or *Shigella* species present, until diarrhea resolves and 2 stool cultures are negative. If *Salmonella typhi* present, 3 negative cultures are required before return.
Vomiting	If 2 or more episodes of vomiting during the previous 24 hours, until vomiting resolves or is determined to be attributable to such noninfectious conditions as pregnancy or a digestive disorder.
Hepatitis A	For 1 week after jaundice appears or as directed by health department.
Pertussis	Until after 5 days of appropriate antibiotic therapy.
Impetigo (a skin infection)	Until 24 hours after antibiotic treatment begins.
Active tuberculosis	Until the local health department approves return to the facility.
Strep throat (or other streptococcal infection)	Until 24 hours after initial antibiotic treatment and fever has ended.
Scabies, head lice	Until after the first treatment has been completed.
Purulent conjunctivitis	Until 24 hours after treatment has begun.
Respiratory illness	If illness limits staff ability to provide child care and compromises the health and safety of children.
Herpes labialis (cold sores)	No exclusion necessary. Staff should cover and not touch the lesion, practice careful hand washing, and not kiss or nuzzle infants or children (particularly children with dermatitis).
Other conditions mandated by state public health law.	As required by law (consult your local health department).

Source: Centers for Disease Control and Prevention; and American Academy of Pediatrics, American Public Health Association, and Maternal and Child Health Bureau. *Caring for Our Children. National Health and Safety Performance Standards: Guidelines for Out-of-Home Child Care Programs.* 2nd ed. Elk Grove Village, IL: American Academy of Pediatrics; 2002:129–130

APPENDIX F. Medication Policy

A. Principle:

This facility will administer medication to children with written approval of the parent and an order from a health provider for a specific child or a specific condition for any child in the facility for whom a plan has been made and approved by _____ (Staff title/name). Because administration of medication poses an extra burden for staff, and having medication in the facility is a safety hazard, medication administration in child care will be limited to situations in which an agreement to give medicine outside child care hours cannot be made. Whenever possible, the first dose of medication should be given at home to see if the child has any type of reaction. Parents or legal guardians may administer medication to their own child during the child care day.

B. Procedure:

_____ (Staff title/name) will administer medication only if the parent or legal guardian has provided written consent, the medication is available in an original labeled prescription or manufacturer's container that meets safety check requirements.* The facility must have on file the written or telephone instructions of a licensed clinician to administer the specific medication. (Sample form in *Model Child Care Health Policies* from the Pennsylvania Chapter, American Academy of Pediatrics).

1) For prescription medications, parents or legal guardians will provide caregivers with the medication in the original, child-resistant container that is labeled by a pharmacist with the child's name, the name and strength of the medication; the date the prescription was filled; the name of the health care provider who wrote the prescription; the medication's expiration date; and administration, storage, and disposal instructions. For over-the-counter medications, parents or legal guardians will provide the medication in a child-resistant container. The medication will be labeled with the child's first and last names; specific, legible instructions for administration and storage supplied by the manufacturer; and the name of the health care provider who recommended the medication for the child.

2) Instructions for the dose, time, method to be used, and duration of administration will be provided to the child care staff in writing (by a signed note or a prescription label) or dictated over the telephone by a physician or other person legally authorized to prescribe medication. This requirement applies both to prescription and over-the-counter medications.

3) A physician may state that a certain medication may be given for a recurring problem, emergency situation, or chronic condition. The instructions should include the child's name; the name of the medication; the dose of the medication; how often the medication may be given; the conditions for use; and any precautions to follow. Example: children may use sunscreen to prevent sunburn; children who wheeze with vigorous exercise may take one dose of asthma medicine before vigorous active (large muscle) play; children who weigh between 25 and 35 pounds may be given 1 teaspoon of acetaminophen 160 mg/5 mL every 4 hours for fever for up to 2 doses. A child with a known serious allergic reaction to a specific substance who develops symptoms after exposure to that substance may receive epinephrine from a staff member who has received training in how to use an auto-injection device prescribed for that child (eg, Epipen). A child may only receive medication with the permission of the child's parent

*Safety check:
1. Child-resistant container
2. Original prescription of manufacturer's label with the name and strength of the medication and physician's directions for use (phone or written)
3. Name of child on container is correct for both first and last names
4. Current date on prescription/expiration label covers period when medication is to be given
5. Name and phone number of licensed health professional who ordered medication on container or on file
6. Instructions are clear for dose, route, and time to give medication

APPENDIX F. Medication Policy, continued

or legal guardian and when the staff person who will give the medication has demonstrated to a licensed health professional the skills required.

4) Medications will be kept at the temperature recommended for that type of medication, in a sturdy, child-resistant, closed container that is inaccessible to children and prevents spillage.

5) Medication will not be used beyond the date of expiration on the container or beyond any expiration of the instructions provided by the physician or other person legally permitted to prescribe medication. Instructions which state that the medication may be used whenever needed will be renewed by the physician at least annually.

6) A medication log will be maintained by the facility staff to record the instructions for giving the medication, consent obtained from the parent or legal guardian, amount, the time of administration, and the person who administered each dose of medication. Spills, reactions, and refusal to take medication will be noted on this log (sample form in *Model Child Care Health Policies* from Pennsylvania Chapter, American Academy of Pediatrics).

7) Medication errors will be controlled by checking the following 5 items each time medication is given:
   a) Right child
   b) Right medicine
   c) Right dose
   d) Right time
   e) Right route of administration

When a medication error occurs, the regional poison control center and the child's parents will be contacted immediately. The incident will be documented in the child's record at the facility.

Adapted from American Academy of Pediatrics, Pennsylvania Chapter. Medication Policy. In: *Model Child Care Health Policies.* 4th ed. Rosemont, PA: American Academy of Pediatrics, Pennsylvania Chapter; 2002:7–8

APPENDIX G. Child Care Staff Health Assessment

National Health and Safety Performance Standards

Child Care Staff Health Assessment

********* **Employer should complete this section.** ********

Name of person to be examined: _____

Employer for whom examination is being done: _____

Employer's Location: _____ Phone number: _____

Purpose of examination: ☐ pre-employment (with conditional offer of employment) ☐ annual re-examination

Type of activity on the job: ☐ lifting, carrying children ☐ close contact with children ☐ food preparation

☐ desk work ☐ driver of vehicles ☐ facility maintenance

**** **Part I and Part II below must be completed and signed by a licensed physician or CRNP.** ****

*Based on a review of the medical record, health history, and examination, does this person
have any of the following conditions or problems that might affect job performance or require accommodation?*

Date of exam: _____

Part I: Health Problems (circle)

Visual acuity less than 20/40 (combined, obtained with lenses if needed)?.. yes .... no

Decreased hearing or difficulty functioning in a noisy environment (less than 20 db at 500, 1000, 2000, 4000 Hz)? .... yes .... no

Respiratory problems (asthma, emphysema, airway allergies, current smoker, other)?... yes .... no

Heart, blood pressure, or other cardiovascular problems? .... yes .... no

Gastrointestinal problems (ulcer, colitis, special dietary requirements, obesity, other)? .... yes .... no

Endocrine problems (diabetes, thyroid, other)?... yes .... no

Emotional disorders or addiction (depression, substance dependency, difficulty handling stress, other)? .... yes .... no

Neurologic problems (epilepsy, Parkinsonism, other)? .... yes .... no

Musculoskeletal problems (low back pain or susceptibility to back injury, neck problems, arthritis, limitations on activity)? ... yes .... no

Skin problems (eczema, rashes, conditions incompatible with frequent handwashing, other)?.............................. yes .... no

Immune system problems (from medication, inherent susceptibility to infection, illness, allergies)?...................... yes .... no

Need for more frequent health visits or sick days than the average person?.. yes .... no

Other special medical problem or chronic disease that requires work restrictions or accommodation? .... yes .... no

Part II: Infectious Disease Status

Immunizations now due/overdue for:

dT (every 10 years) .... yes .... no

MMR (2 doses for persons born after 1989; 1 dose for those born in or after 1957)............................. yes .... no

polio (OPV or IPV in childhood)... yes .... no

hepatitis B (3 dose series).. yes .... no

varicella (2 doses or had the disease) .... yes .... no

influenza .... yes .... no

pneumococcal vaccine .... yes .... no

Female of childbearing age susceptible to CMV or parvovirus?... yes .... no

Evaluation of tuberculosis status shows a risk for communicable TB?....................................... yes .... no

Mantoux test date_____ Result_____

Tuberculosis transmission shall be controlled by requiring regular and substitute staff members and volunteers to have their tuberculosis status assessed with a one-step or two-step Mantoux intradermal skin test prior to beginning employment unless they produce documentation of the following:
a) A positive Mantoux intradermal skin test result in the past, or
b) Tuberculosis disease that has been treated appropriately in the past.
The one-step Mantoux intradermal tuberculin test shall suffice except that for individuals over 60 years of age or those who have a medical condition that reduces their immune response, the use of the two-step method is required. Individuals with a positive Mantoux intradermal skin test or tuberculosis disease in the past shall be evaluated with chest radiographs and shall be cleared for work by their physician or a health department official.

Please attach additional sheets to explain all "yes" answers above. Include the plan for follow up.

MD
DO
CRNP

_____   _____   _____   _____
(Date)   (Signature)   (Printed last name)   (Title)

Phone number of physician or CRNP: _____

I have read and understand the above information.

_____   _____
(Date)   (Patient's Signature)

Reference: Pennsylvania Chapter, American Academy of Pediatrics. *Model Child Care Health Policies.* 3rd ed. Washington D.C: National Association for the Education of Young Children, 1997.
This form was adapted from *Model Child Care Health Policies,* June 1997, by the Early Childhood Education Linkage System (ECELS), a program funded by the Pennsylvania Depts. of Health & Public Welfare and contractually administered by the PA Chapter, American Academy of Pediatrics.

APPENDIX H. Special Care Plan

Facility Name: _____

Facility Address: _____

Child's Name: _____

Date of Birth: _____ Times and Days in Child Care: _____

1. Describe the child's special need during group care:_____

   _____

2. Child's present functional level and skills:_____

   _____

3. What emergency or unusual episode might arise while the child is in care?
   How should the situation be handled? _____

   _____

   (Prepare and maintain information on the "Emergency Form for Children With Special Needs" available from the
   American Academy of Pediatrics at http://aappolicy.aapjournals.org/cgi/content/full/pediatrics;104/4/e53/F1)

4. Accommodation which the facility must provide for this child:_____

   _____

   a) Are there particular instructions for sleeping, toileting, diapering, or feeding? _____

      _____

   b) Will the child require medication while in care? If so, attach the physician's instructions for
      use of the child's medication. _____

      _____

   c) Are special emergency and/or medical procedures required?
      If so, what procedures are required? _____

      _____

   d) What special training, if any, must staff have to provide that care? _____

      _____

   e) Are special materials/equipment needed? _____

      _____

5. Other specialists working with the child (eg, occupational therapist, physical therapist): _____

   _____

Primary Case Manager:_____ Phone: _____
                        (usually the doctor in charge)

APPENDIX H. Special Care Plan, continued

Address:_____

On-site child care facility case manager:_____ Phone: _____

Authorization for Release of Information

I, _____ give permission for
(parent or legal guardian)

_____
(professional/facility)

to release to _____ the following information
(child care program)

_____

The information will be used solely to plan and coordinate the care of my child and will be kept
confidential and may only be shared with _____
(staff title/name)

Name of Child: _____

Address:_____

City: _____ State: _____ Zip Code: _____

Date of Birth: _____

_____
Parent/Legal Guardian Signature   Date

_____
Witness Signature   Date

_____
Staff member to be contacted for additional information

Reprinted from American Academy of Pediatrics, Pennsylvania Chapter. Appendix D. In: *Model Child Care Health Policies.* 4th ed. Rosemont, PA: American Academy of Pediatrics, Pennsylvania Chapter; 2002

Resources

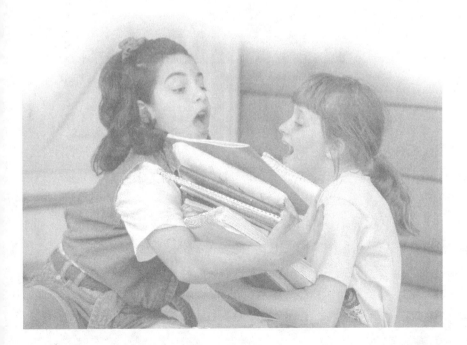

American Academy of Pediatrics (AAP)
141 Northwest Point Boulevard
Elk Grove Village, IL 60007-1098
Phone: 847/434-4000
Fax: 847/434-8000
Web site: http://www.aap.org/

American Dietetic Association (ADA)
120 South Riverside Plaza
Suite 2000
Chicago, IL 60606-6995
Phone: 800/877-1600
Fax: 312/899-1979
Web site: http://www.eatright.org/

American With Disabilities Act Accessibility Guidelines (ADAAG)
US Department of Justice
Civil Rights Division
Disability Rights Section – NYAV
950 Pennsylvania Avenue, NW
Washington, DC 20530
Phone: 800/514-0301
TDD: 800/514-0383
Web site: http://www.usdoj.gov/crt/ada/adahom1.htm

American Public Health Association (APHA)
800 1 Street, NW
Washington, DC 20001-3710
Phone: 202/777-APHA
Fax: 202/777-5234
E-mail: comments@apha.org
Web site: http://www.apha.org

Centers for Disease Control and Prevention (CDC)
1600 Clifton Road NE
Atlanta, GA 30333
Phone: 800/311-3435
Web site: http://www.cdc.gov

Child Care Aware
1319 F Street, NW
Suite 500
Washington, DC 20004
Phone: 800/424-2246
Fax: 202-393-1144
E-mail: info@childcareaware.org
Web site: http://www.childcareaware.org

Child Care Bureau
Administration for Children and Families, US Department of Health
  and Human Services
370 L'Enfant Promenade SW
Washington, DC 20447
Phone: 202/690-6782
Fax: 202/690-5600
E-mail: ccb@acf.dhhs.gov
Web site: http://www.acf.dhhs.gov/programs/ccb

Child Care Law Center
221 Pine Street, Third Floor
San Francisco, CA 94104
Phone: 415/394-7144
Fax: 415/394-7140
E-Mail: info@childcarelaw.org
Web site: http://www.childcarelaw.org

Children's Defense Fund
25 E Street, NW
Washington, DC 20001
Phone: 202/628-8787
E-mail: cdfinfo@childrensdefense.org
Web site: http://www.childrenssdefense.org

Consumer Product Safety Commission (CPSC)
Phone: 800/638-2772
E-mail: info@cpsc.gov
Web site: http://www.cpsc.gov

Cooperative Extension System's National Network for
  Child Care (NNCC)
Web site: http://www.nncc.org

Early Childhood Education Linkage System (ECELS)
Healthy Child Care America
Pennsylvania Chapter, American Academy of Pediatrics
Rosemont Business Campus
Building 2, Suite 307
919 Conestoga Road
Rosemont, PA 19010
Phone: 610/520-3662
Web site: http://www.paaap.org

Food and Nutrition Information Center
Agricultural Research Service, US Department of Agriculture
National Agricultural Library, Room 105
10301 Baltimore Avenue
Beltsville, MD 20705-2351
Phone: 301/504-5755
Fax: 301/504-6927
E-mail: agref@nal.usda.gov
Web site: http://www.nal.usda.gov/fnic

The Healthy Child America Campaign
American Academy of Pediatrics
141 Northwest Point Boulevard
Elk Grove Village, IL 60007-1098
Phone: 888/227-5409
Fax: 847/228-6432
Web site: http://www.healthychildcare.org

The Healthy Child America Back to Sleep Campaign
Web site: http://www.healthychildcare.org/section_SIDS.cfm

National Association of Child Care Resources and Referral Agencies
1319 F Street NW
Suite 500
Washington, DC 20004-1106
Phone: 202/393-5501
Fax: 202/393-1109
E-mail: info@naccrra.org
Web site: http://www.naccrra.org

National Association for the Education of Young Children (NAEYC)
1509 16th Street NW
Washington, DC 20036
Phone: 800/424-2460
E-mail: naeyc@naeyc.org
Web site: http://www.naeyc.org

National Association of Family Child Care (NAFCC)
5202 Pinemont Drive
Salt Lake City, UT 84123
Phone: 801/269-9338
Fax: 801/268-9507
E-mail: nafcc@nafcc.org
Web site: http://www.nafcc.org

National Association of Pediatric Nurse Practitioners (NAPNAP)
20 Brace Road
Suite 200
Cherry Hill, NJ 08034-2633
Phone: 856/857-9700
Fax: 856/857-1600
E-mail: info@napnap.org
Web site: http://www.napnap.org

National Association for Sick Child Daycare (NASCD)
1716 5th Avenue North
Birmingham, AL 35203
Phone: 202/324-8447
Fax: 202/324-8050
E-mail: gwj@nascd.com
Web site: http://www.nascd.com

National Child Care Information Center
243 Church Street, NW, 2nd Floor
Vienna, VA 22180
Phone: 800/616-2242
Fax: 800/716-2242
TTY: 800/516-2242
Web site: http://www.nccic.org

National Child Care Association (NCCA)
1016 Rosser Street
Conyers, GA 30012
Phone: 800/543-7161
Fax: 770/388-7772
Web site: http://www.nccanet.org

National Clearinghouse on Child Abuse and Neglect Information
330 C Street, SW
Washington, DC 20447
Phone: 800/394-3366
Fax: 703/385-3206
Web site: http://www.nccanch.acf.hhs.gov

National Head Start Association
1651 Prince Street
Alexandria, VA 22314
Phone: 703/739-0875
Fax: 703/739-0878
Web site: http://www.nhsa.org/index.htm

NATIONAL HIGHWAY TRAFFIC SAFETY ADMINISTRATION (NHTSA)
Web site: http://www.nhtsa.dot.gov

NHTSA Region I (Connecticut, Maine, Massachusetts, New Hampshire, Rhode Island, Vermont)
55 Broadway
Kendall Square—Code 903
Cambridge, MA 02142
Phone: 617/494-3427
Fax: 617/494-3646
E-mail: region1@nhtsa.dot.gov

NHTSA Region II (New York, New Jersey, Puerto Rico, Virgin Islands)
222 Mamaroneck Avenue, Suite 204
White Plains, NY 10605
Phone: 914/682-6162
Fax: 914/682-6239
E-mail: region2@nhtsa.dot.gov

NHTSA Region III (Delaware, District of Columbia, Maryland, Pennsylvania, Virginia, West Virginia)
10 South Howard Street, Suite 6700
Baltimore, MD 21201
Phone: 410/962-0090
Fax: 410/962-2770
E-mail: region3@nhtsa.dot.gov

NHTSA Region IV (Alabama, Florida, Georgia, Kentucky, Mississippi, North Carolina, South Carolina, Tennessee)
61 Forsyth Street, SW, Suite 17T30
Atlanta, GA 30303
Phone: 404/562-3739
Fax: 404/562-3763
E-mail: region4@nhtsa.dot.gov

NHTSA Region V (Illinois, Indiana, Michigan, Ohio, Wisconsin)
19900 Governors Drive, Suite 201
Olympia Fields, IL 60461
Phone: 708/503-8822
Fax: 708/503-8991
E-mail: region5@nhtsa.dot.gov

NHTSA Region VI (Arkansas, Louisiana, New Mexico, Oklahoma, Texas, Indian Nations)
819 Taylor Street, Room 8A38
Fort Worth, TX 76102-6177
Phone: 817/978-3653
Fax: 817/978-8339
E-mail: region6@nhtsa.dot.gov

NHTSA Region VII (Iowa, Kansas, Missouri, Nebraska)
901 Locust Street, Room 466
Kansas City, MO 64106
Phone: 816/329-3900
Fax: 816/329-3910
E-mail: region7@nhtsa.dot.gov

NHTSA Region VIII (Colorado, Montana, North Dakota, South Dakota, Utah, Wyoming)
555 Zang Street, Room 430
Lakewood, CO 80228
Phone: 303/969-6917
Fax: 303/969-6294
E-mail: region8@nhtsa.dot.gov

NHTSA Region IX (Arizona, California, Hawaii, Nevada, Samoa, Guam, Mariana Island)
201 Mission Street, Suite 2230
San Francisco, CA 94105
Phone: 415/744-3089
Fax: 415/744-2532
E-mail: region9@nhtsa.dot.gov

NHTSA Region X (Alaska, Idaho, Oregon, Washington)
3140 Jackson Federal Building
915 Second Avenue
Seattle, WA 98174
Phone: 206/220-7640
Fax: 206/220-7651
E-mail: region10@nhtsa.dot.gov

National Dissemination Center for Children with Disabilities
PO Box 1492
Washington, DC 20013-1492
Phone: 800/695-0285
Fax: 202/884-8441
E-mail: nichcy@aed.org
Web site: http://www.nichcy.org

National Institute of Child Health and Human Development
PO Box 3006
Rockville, MD 20847
Phone: 800/370-2943
Fax: 301/496-7101
E-mail: NICHDInformationResourceCenter@mail.nih.gov
Web site: http://www.nichd.nih.gov

National Resource Center for Health and Safety in Child Care
UCHSC at Fitzsimons
Campus Mail Stop F541, PO Box 6508
Aurora, CO 80045-0508
Phone: 800/598-5437
Fax: 303/724-0960
Web site: http://nrc.uchsc.edu

National SIDS Resource Center
2070 Chain Bridge Road, Suite 450
Vienna, VA 22182
Phone: 866/866-7437
Fax: 703/821-2098
E-mail: sids@circlesolutions.com
Web site: http://www.sidscenter.org

National Training Institute for Child Care Health Consultants
Department of Maternal and Child Health
University of North Carolina at Chapel Hill
116A S Merritt Mill Road, Box 8126
Chapel Hill, NC 27599-8126
Phone: 919/966-3780
Fax: 919/843-4752
E-mail: nticchc@sph.unc.edu
Web site: http://www.sph.unc.edu/courses/childcare/

Tribal Child Care Technical Assistance Center (TriTAC)
Pawhushka Office:
PO Box 1221
Pawhushka, OK 74056

McLean Office:
6858 Old Dominion Drive, Suite 302
McLean, VA 22101
Phone: 800/388-7670
E-mail: tritac2@aol.com
Web site: http://nccic.org/tribal

Zero to Three
National Center for Infants, Toddlers and Families
2000 M Street NW, Suite 200
Washington, DC 20036
Phone: 202/638-1144
Web site: http://www.zerotothree.org

Index

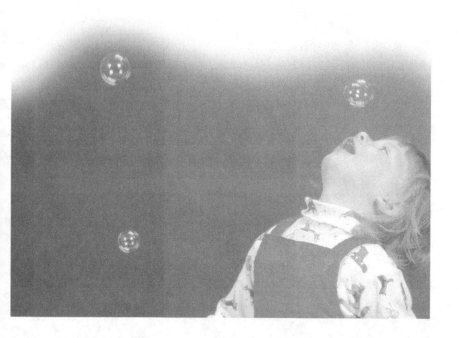

Wood mulch pits, 50
Work and Family Connection, 6
Workers' compensation, 333
Workforce. *See also* Child care staff; Staff
    child care, in child care centers, 315
    mothers in, 3, 84, 164, 177, 237, 238, 247
    two-wage earner families in, 247
Workplace option for sick care, 306

Y
YMCAs/YWCAs, 414

Z
Zero to Three, National Center for Infants,
        Toddlers, and Families, 16,
        448, 450, 509
Zero to Three National Training Institute, 410